Visual Impairment and Blindness - What We Know and What We Have to Know

Edited by Giuseppe Lo Giudice and Angel Catalá

Published in London, United Kingdom

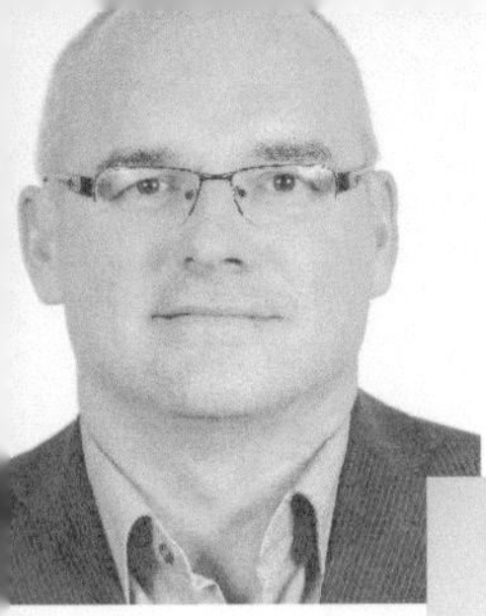
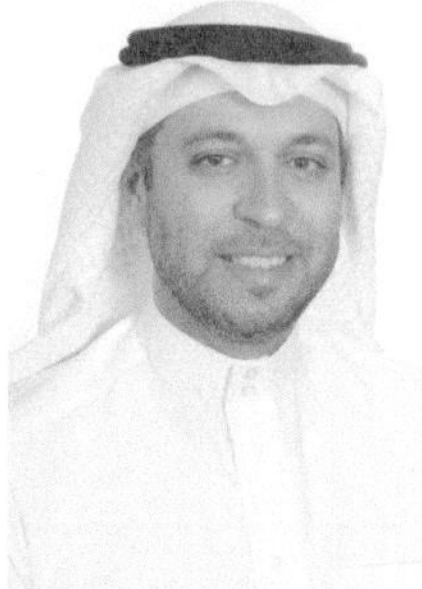
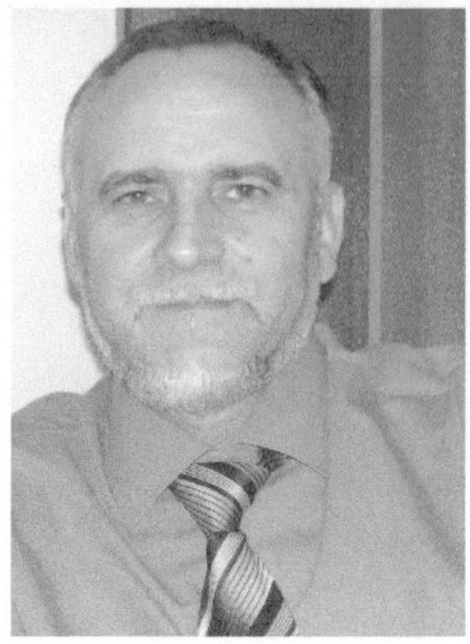
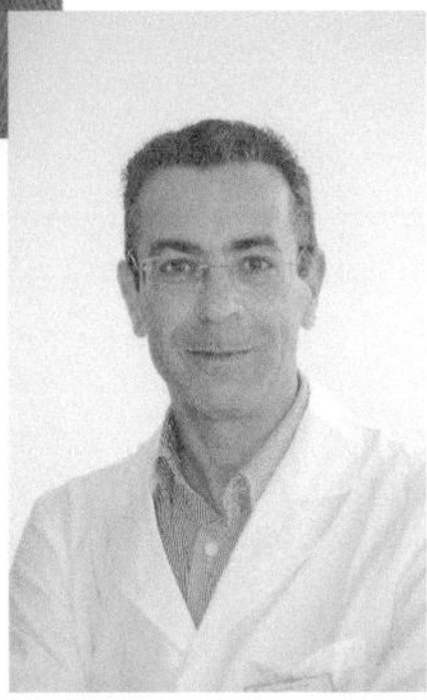
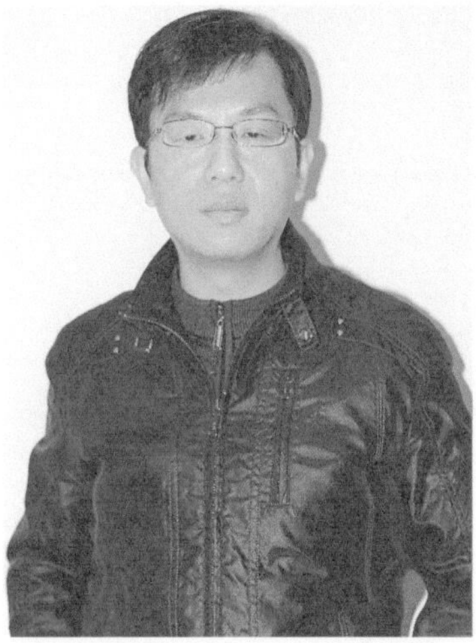
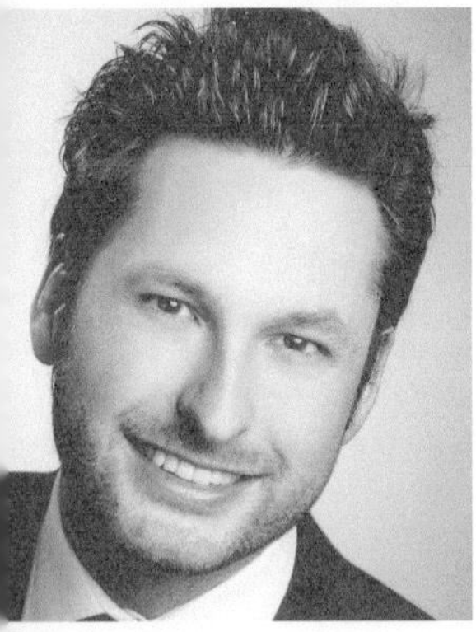
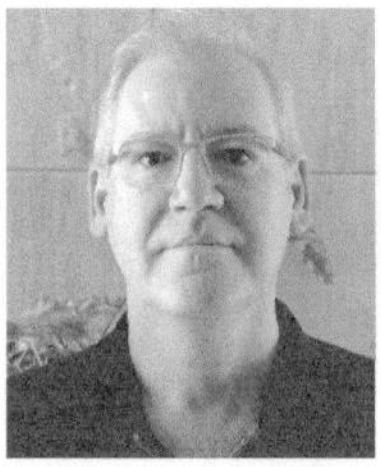

IntechOpen

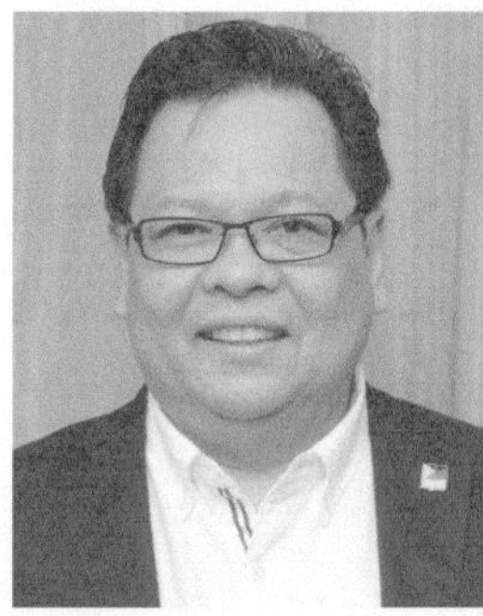
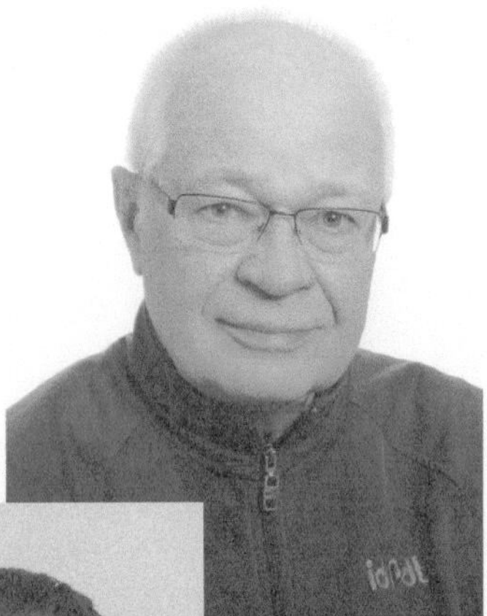
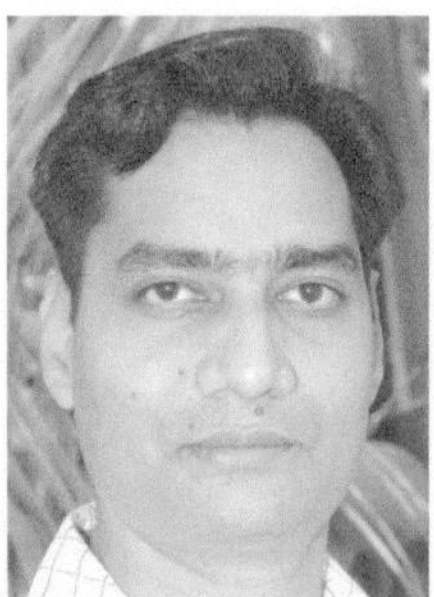
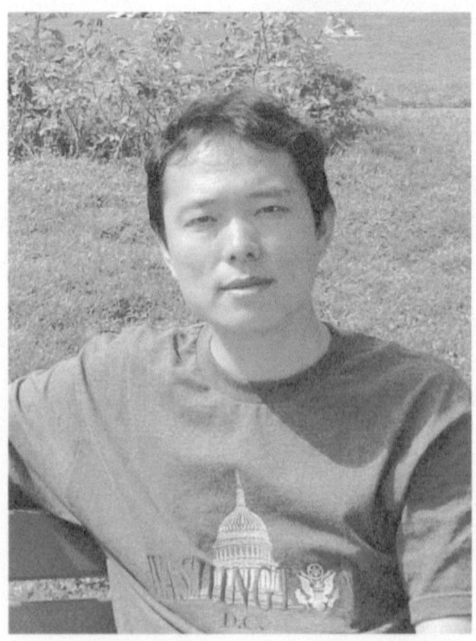
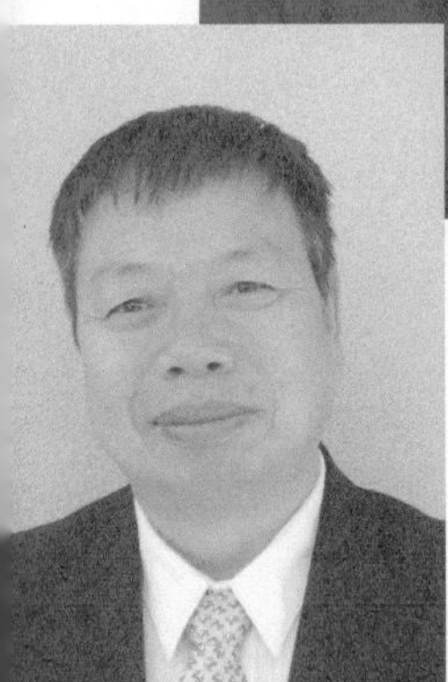
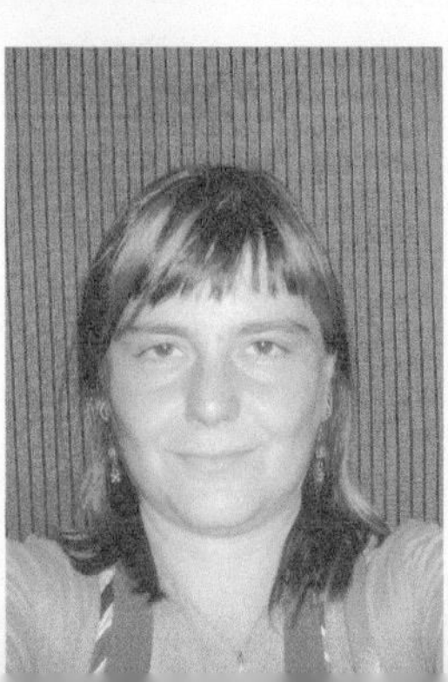

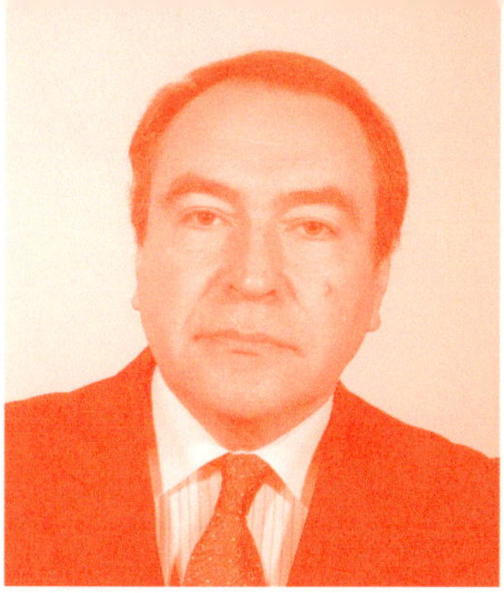
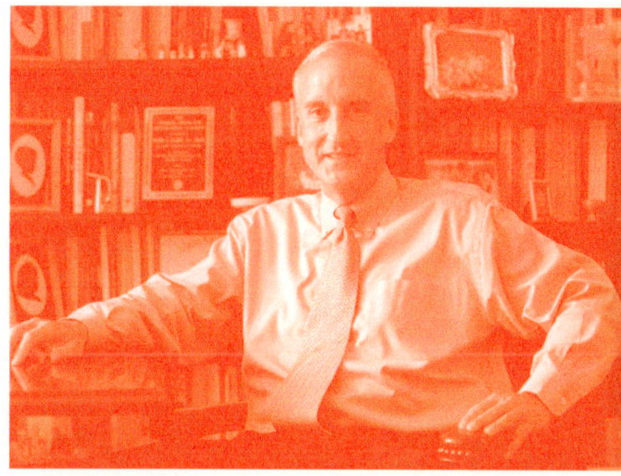
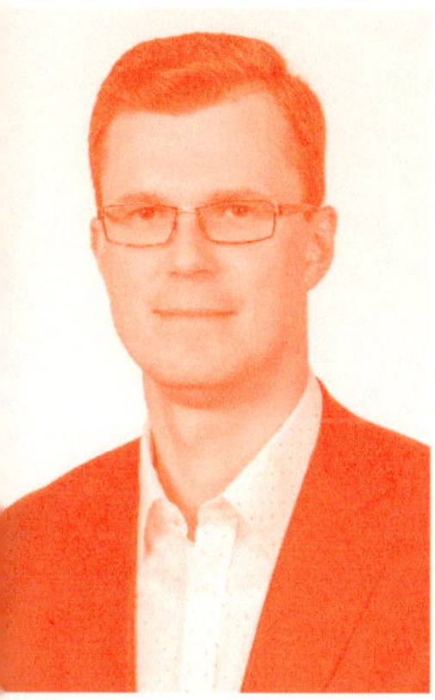
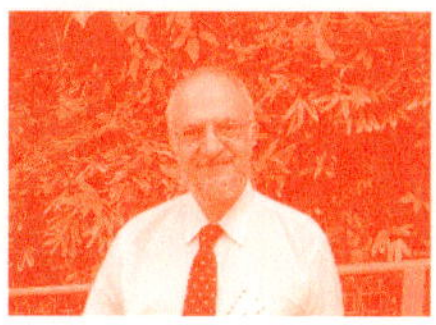
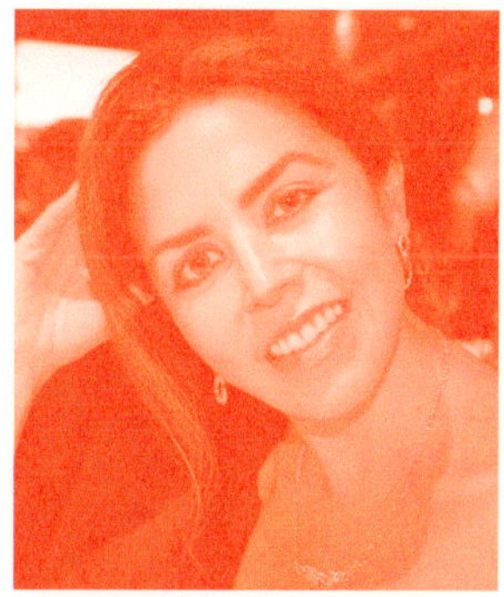

Supporting open minds since 2005

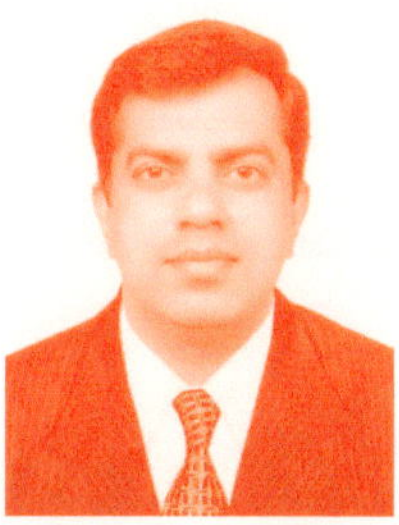
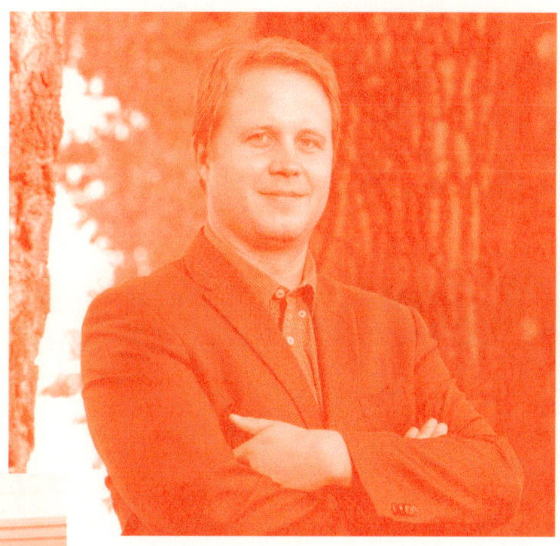
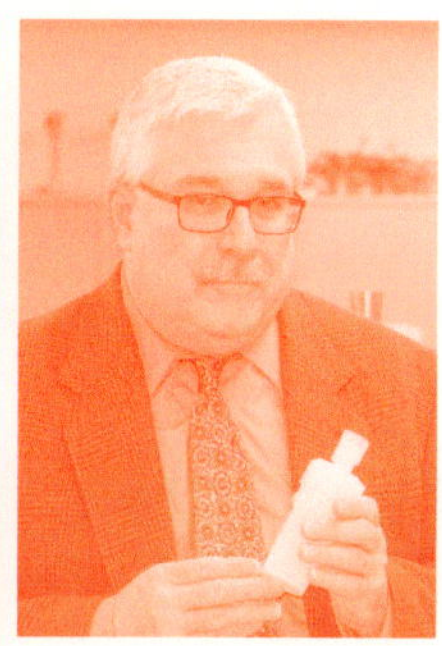
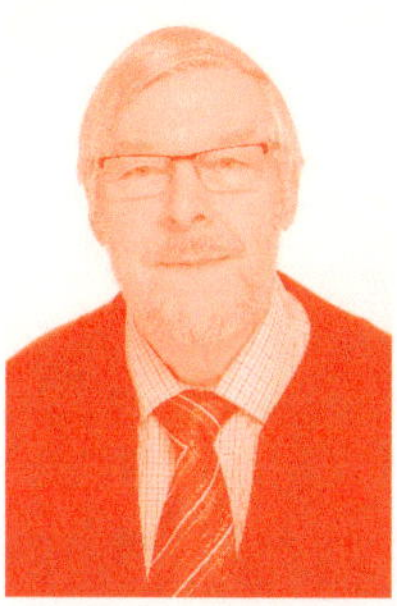
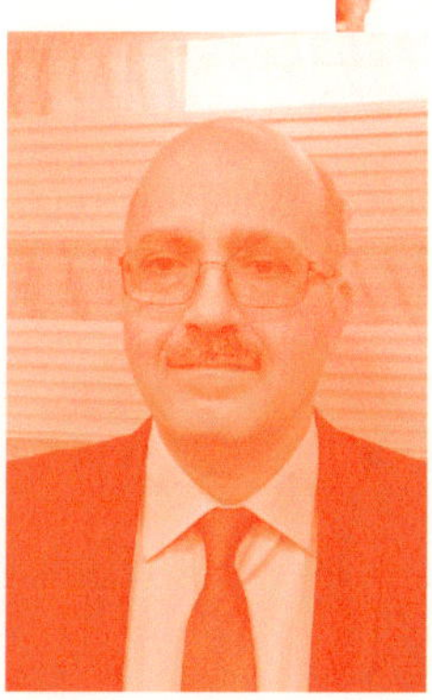
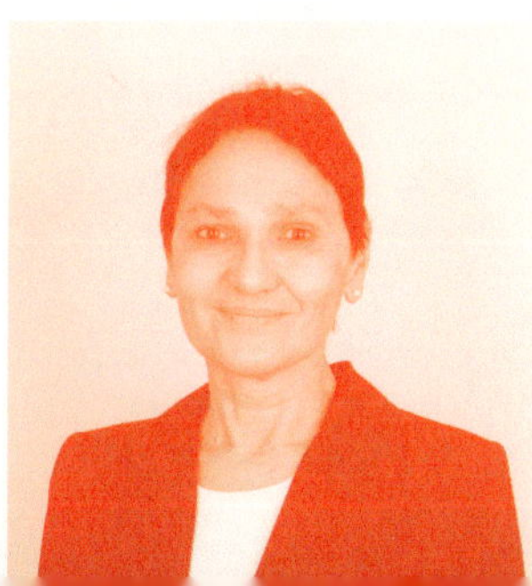
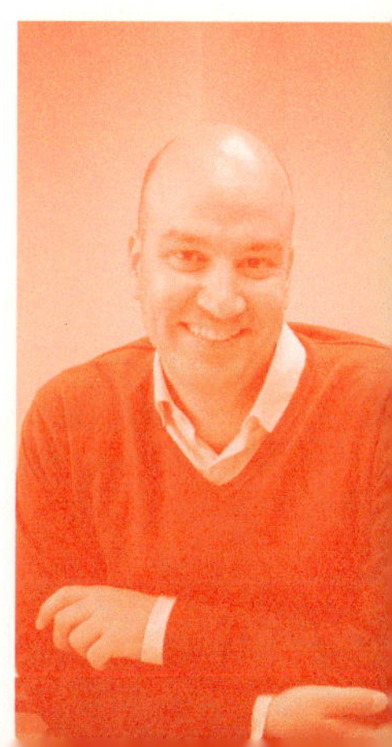

Visual Impairment and Blindness - What We Know and What We Have to Know
http://dx.doi.org/10.5772/intechopen.73976
Edited by Giuseppe Lo Giudice and Angel Catalá

Contributors
Sean Adrean, Siyang Chaili, Andi Arus Victor, Tanya Beelders, Angela Stott, Wan Jin Jahng, Souhail Guennouni, Anass Mansouri, Ali Ahaitouf, Giuseppe Lo Giudice, Poemen Chan, Claire Chow, Maria Iribarne, Maya Pandova, Angel Catala, Monica Gori, Maria Bianca Amadeo, Claudio Campus, Maria Begoña Coco, Juan Oliveros, Luis Leal, Nadiuska Cristine Platero, Joaquín Herrera Medina, Giulia Cappagli, Md Masum Billah, Zulkhairi Mohd Yusof, Kushsairy Kadir, Abdul Malik Mohd Ali, Giovanni Sato, Roberta Rizzo, Vatookarn Roongpoovapatr, Pinnita Prabhasawat, Saichin Isipradit, Mohamed Abou Shousha, Puwat Charukamnoetkanok, Humberto Dória Silva, Eduardo Dória Silva, Cristiana Pereira Dória, Maria Tamires Dória Silva, Cristiane Pereira Dória, Josefina Mejias Smith, Luis Izquierdo, Marta Hadid, Maria Henriquez, Nataraj Vijapur, R. Srinivasa Rao Kunte, Susanne Zimmermann-Janschitz, Diego Montagud-Martínez, Vicente Ferrando, Salvador Garcia-Delpech, Juan A. Monsoriu, Walter Furlan, Weilue He, Srinivas R. Sripathi, Madu Joshua, Ruonan Zhang, Fabunmi Tosin, Patrick Ambrose, Diana R. Gutsaeva, Giulio Sandini

First published in London, United Kingdom, 2020 by IntechOpen
IntechOpen is the global imprint of INTECHOPEN LIMITED, registered in England and Wales, registration number: 11086078, 7th floor, 10 Lower Thames Street, London, EC3R 6AF, United Kingdom
Printed in Croatia

British Library Cataloguing-in-Publication Data
A catalogue record for this book is available from the British Library

Additional hard and PDF copies can be obtained from orders@intechopen.com

Visual Impairment and Blindness - What We Know and What We Have to Know
Edited by Giuseppe Lo Giudice and Angel Catalá
p. cm.
Print ISBN 978-1-83880-257-8
Online ISBN 978-1-83880-258-5
eBook (PDF) ISBN 978-1-83962-953-2

For EU product safety concerns:
IN TECH d.o.o., Prolaz Marije Krucifikse Kozulić 3, 51000 Rijeka, Croatia, info@intechopen.com or visit our website at intechopen.com.

Meet the editors

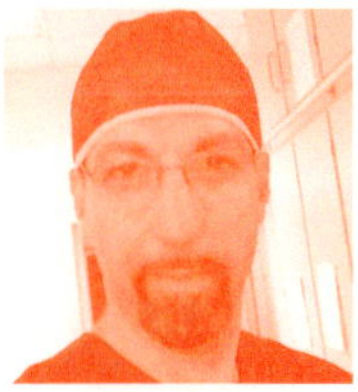

Guiseppe Lo Giudice, MD, is Assistant Professor of Ophthalmology at San Antonio Hospital, Padua. He received his medical degree from the University of Messina, Italy, and completed his residency in ophthalmology at the Department of Ophthalmology, University of Padua, Italy. After completing his residency, Dr. Lo Guidice became an Assistant in Ophthalmology at Conegliano Hospital and then a fellow at the Ophthalmology Department of the Gironcoli Ophthalmic Centre, Conegliano, Treviso, Italy. His major field of interest is developing new treatments for retinal diseases (proliferative retinopathies, AMD, and diabetic retinopathy). He has more than 20 years of clinical research experience in clinical trials and laboratory work. He has performed more than 7000 anterior segment surgeries (cataract surgery, phacotrabeculectomy, trabeculectomy, etc.) in the last 5 years. In the last 3 years, Dr. Lo Guidice has performed more than 700 vitreo-retinal surgeries for retinal pucker, retinal detachment, and vitreoretinal proliferative disease at San Antonio Hospital.

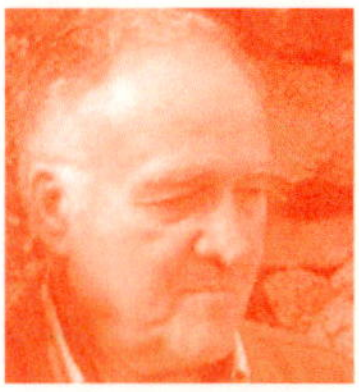

Angel Catalá, PhD, was born in Rodeo, San Juan, Argentina. He received a PhD in Chemistry from the Universidad Nacional de La Plata, Argentina, in 1965. From 1964 to 1974, he worked as Assistant in Biochemistry at the School of Medicine, Universidad Nacional de La Plata. From 1974 to 1976, he was a fellow of the National Institutes of Health (NIH) at the University of Connecticut Health Center, USA. From 1985 to 2004, he served as a full professor of Biochemistry at the Universidad Nacional de La Plata. He is a member of the National Research Council (CONICET), Argentina, and Argentine Society for Biochemistry and Molecular Biology (SAIB). His laboratory has been interested for many years in lipid peroxidation of biological membranes from various tissues and different species. Dr. Catalá has directed twelve doctoral theses, published more than 100 papers in peer-reviewed journals, several book chapters, and twelve edited books. He received awards at the 40th International Conference Biochemistry of Lipids, Dijon, France (1999). He was also winner of the Bimbo Pan-American Nutrition, Food Science and Technology Award, South America, in 2006 and 2012. In 2006, he received an award in pharmacology in recognition of his meritorious works of research. Dr. Catalá belongs to the editorial boards of the *Journal of Lipids*, *International Review of Biophysical Chemistry*, *Frontiers in Membrane Physiology and Biophysics*, *World Journal of Experimental Medicine*, *Biochemistry Research International*, *World Journal of Biological Chemistry*, *Diabetes and the Pancreas*, *International Journal of Chronic Diseases and Therapy*, and *International Journal of Nutrition*. He is also co-editor of *The Open Biology Journal* and associate editor for *Oxidative Medicine and Cellular Longevity*.

Contents

Preface

Blindness defines either the best-corrected distance visual acuity or presenting distance visual acuity in the better eye. Different visual acuity levels are commonly used to better define blindness ranging between < 20/400 and < 20/200 in the better eye. In contrast, visual impairment defines a visual acuity of 20/60 or less in the better eye.

The prevalence of blindness varies considerably among developed countries. Socio-economic factors are linked to available health and eye care services and thus influence prevalence. For example, a 0.25 prevalence of blindness among the general population living in a well-developed country may translate to a 1.25 prevalence in a country with poor socio-economic status and health care. Differences in prevalence are also due to blindness being secondary to several diseases and conditions, such as cataracts, refractive errors, and corneal scarring (trachoma, corneal infections, and vitamin A deficiency). Visual impairment and blindness is an important public health problem that requires affordable, high-quality clinical and diagnostic capacity, good therapeutic approaches, and rehabilitation.

In this book we provide an overview of the effects of blindness and visual impairment in the context of the most common causes of blindness in older adults and children. These causes may include retinal disorders, cataracts, glaucoma, and macular and corneal degeneration.

Giuseppe Lo Giudice, MD
San Paolo Ophthalmic Center,
San Antonio Hospital,
University of Padua, AOPD,
Italy

Angel Catala
National University of La Plata,
Argentina

Section 1

Cornea and Refractive Concepts

Chapter 1

Infectious Keratitis: The Great Enemy

Vatookarn Roongpoovapatr, Pinnita Prabhasawat, Saichin Isipradit, Mohamed Abou Shousha and Puwat Charukamnoetkanok

Abstract

Infectious keratitis tops the list of diseases leading to visual impairment and corneal blindness. Corneal opacities, predominantly caused by infectious keratitis, are the fourth leading cause of blindness globally. In the developed countries, infectious keratitis is usually associated with contact lens wear, but in developing countries, it is commonly caused by trauma during agricultural work. The common causative organisms are bacteria, fungus, Acanthamoeba, and virus. Severe cases can progress rapidly and cause visual impairment or blindness that requires corneal transplantation, evisceration, or enucleation. The precise clinical diagnosis, accurate diagnostic tools, and timely appropriate management are important to reduce the morbidity associated with infectious keratitis. Despite the advancement of diagnostic tools and antimicrobial drugs, outcomes remain poor secondary to corneal melting, scarring, or perforation. Eye care strategies should focus on corneal ulcer prevention. This review addresses the epidemiology, diagnostic approach, clinical manifestations, risk factors, investigations, treatments, and the update of major clinical trials about common pathogens of infectious keratitis.

Keywords: infectious keratitis, corneal ulcer, corneal scar, blindness, visual impairment

1. Introduction

Infectious keratitis tops the list of diseases leading to visual impairment and corneal blindness. Globally, it is approximated that 1.3 billion people live with visual impairment [1]. The major causes of corneal blindness included infectious keratitis, ocular trauma, trachoma, bullous keratopathy, corneal degenerations, and vitamin A deficiency [2]. Corneal opacities, predominantly caused by infectious keratitis, are the fourth leading cause of blindness globally [3]. Recent paper reported that 3.5% of global blindness could be attributed to corneal opacity [4]. According to the goal of the "Vision 2020: The Right to Sight," which was proposed by WHO, the prevention of avoidable corneal blindness should receive more awareness [5, 6].

Interestingly, the majority of visual impairment is avoidable [1]. Infectious keratitis accounts for 10% of avoidable visual impairment in the world's least-developed countries [3]. The number of people with avoidable visual loss has increased considerably because of population growth and aging. This trend will continue beyond

2020 [7] and will inevitably impact the eye care need in the near future. In the developed countries, infectious keratitis is usually associated with contact lens wear, but in developing countries, it is commonly caused by trauma during agricultural work [8–17]. Infectious keratitis is characterized by a corneal epithelial defect with underlying stromal inflammation caused by replicating microorganisms [14]. Acute eye pain and redness are the common presentation [14]. The common causative organisms are bacteria, fungus, Acanthamoeba, and virus [10, 17]. However, corneal infection involving more than one microorganisms such as bacteria and fungus is relatively uncommon [17] Microbial keratitis requires acute ophthalmic care and aggressive treatment to stop the disease progression and limit the extent of corneal scarring, which can cause loss of vision [14]. The precise clinical diagnosis, accurate diagnostic tools, and timely appropriate management are important to reduce the morbidity associated with infectious keratitis. This review addresses the epidemiology, diagnostic approach, clinical manifestations, risk factors, investigations, treatments, and the update of major clinical trials about common pathogens of infectious keratitis. The purpose of this review is to provide a concise and essential knowledge about common etiologic pathogens of infectious keratitis to improve understanding and reduce morbidity and visual loss due to this condition.

2. Global epidemiology, global etiologies, and burden of diseases

2.1 Global epidemiology

The precise prevalence of infectious keratitis is unknown [18]. The actual prevalence may be higher due to the underreporting or reporting under the term of corneal blindness, which also includes traumatic, infectious, inflammatory, and inherited causes [8]. Overall cases may exceed 2 millions cases per year worldwide [8]. The global incidence of infectious keratitis shows wide disparity among regions. The incidence of infectious keratitis was high in south, south-east, and east Asia, but lower in developed world [8]. The estimated general incidence of infectious keratitis per 100,000 population per year varies from 11 to 27.6 in the United States [19, 20], 40.3–52.1 in the United Kingdom [8, 21], 6.3 in Hong Kong [22], 113 in India [23], 339 in Bhutan [24], 710 in Burma [24], and 799 in Nepal [25]. In contact lens wearers, the incidence is about 6 times higher [8, 18, 20]. It has been reported that nearly 90% of the global cases of ocular trauma and infectious keratitis leading to corneal blindness occur in developing countries [2].

2.2 Global etiologies

The principal organisms of infectious keratitis have regional variation [18]. In developed countries such as Europe [21, 26, 27], North America [28, 29], and Australia [14], the highest proportions of infectious keratitis are attributable to bacteria. This incidence correlated with the prevalence of contact lens wear and high gross national income [30]. On the contrary, in developing countries, the proportions of infectious keratitis attributable to bacteria were less [31–33] than or similar to those from fungus [34]. The Asia Cornea Society Infectious Keratitis Study (ACSIKS) group that included data from 13 study centers and 30 subcenters from 6626 eyes of 6563 subjects demonstrated the similar percentage of bacterial and fungal infections. Overall, bacterial keratitis was diagnosed in 2521 eyes (38.0%) and fungal keratitis in 2166 eyes (32.7%) [34]. But in India and China, fungal keratitis was the majority of nonviral microbial keratitis [34]. Similarly, data from the large trial in India by Lalitha et al. that included 17,948 patients demonstrated that 6218 of 10,207 (60.9%) culture-positive patients had a fungal etiology [31]. The recent studies from China by Lin et al. [35] and Xie et al. [33] reported proportions of fungal keratitis to be 44.6% and 77.9%, respectively. Vision 2020: "The Right to Sight" also suggests that we acquire a clearer and more precise understanding of infectious keratitis in each country [6, 33].

The frequency of causative organisms of keratitis among different geography may vary by countries [30]. In North America, Australia, the Netherlands, and Singapore, the highest proportion of infectious keratitis was bacterial in origin. The highest proportion of pseudomonas keratitis was reported in a study from Bangkok, whereas the highest proportion of staphylococcal ulcers was reported in a study from Paraguay. On the other hand, the highest proportions of fungal keratitis were reported in studies from India and Nepal [30]. Interestingly, recent data from the Asia Cornea Society Infectious Keratitis Study (ACSIKS) group demonstrated that the commonest etiology of infectious keratitis was viral keratitis, which accounted for 47.7% [34]. A recent population-based study in China estimated that the prevalence of herpes simplex keratitis was 0.11%, similar to that in the United States and France [5].

For the worldwide frequency of Acanthamoeba keratitis, around 1% of infectious keratitis was reported [30]. Although the number of infections caused by these organisms is low, Acanthamoeba keratitis is an emerging disease mostly due to the increased use of contact lens worldwide [36]. Cariello et al. reported the higher rate of 7.4% of infectious keratitis caused by Acanthamoeba in Brazil [37].

2.3 Burden of diseases

Despite the fact that infectious keratitis is a significant cause of corneal blindness [2, 38, 39], there has been relatively little evidences available about the definite global burden of infectious keratitis. Moreover, the actual burden may be higher due to the underreport [8] and a fact that most of the patients reside in countries with less-developed economics [38].

Collier et al. reported the burden of this disease in the United States. Infectious keratitis causes an estimated 930,000 doctor's office and outpatient clinic visits and 58,000 emergency department visits per year. Nearly 80% of keratitis visits lead to antimicrobial prescriptions. The direct health care costs for keratitis and contact lens disorders were approximately 175 US dollars. Moreover, it consumed over 250,000 hours of clinician time annually [8, 40].

Data from the national surveys in China and India reported that infectious keratitis is responsible for the major burden of corneal blindness [5, 23, 41]. However, in other endemic areas of infectious keratitis such as China and India, the actual costs were not available. It may be underreported or underestimated in poor rural and agricultural farm-based populations [8]. The cost of infectious keratitis is magnified as it usually affects the poorest populations during their most productive years [8, 42]. Moreover, the cost may be derived from poor access to health care, corticosteroid abuse, inadequate empiric antibiotics, and difficulty to obtain diagnostic cultures that leads to delay presentation of or fulminant infection [8, 42].

3. Diagnostic approach

It is helpful for ophthalmologists to be familiar with the typical signs and symptoms of different organisms that are responsible for infectious keratitis. The provisional diagnosis may help to ensure the prompt management prior to the revelation of the definite diagnosis from investigations.

3.1 History

The common symptoms of infectious keratitis include pain, foreign body sensation, redness of conjunctiva and eyelids, tearing, discharge, photophobia, blurry vision, eyelids swelling, and notice of a white mark on the cornea [24, 43, 44]. In Acanthamoeba keratitis, the patients usually have severe pain out of proportion to the corneal lesion because of perineuritis. Bacterial keratitis usually has an acute onset, and gradual onset of symptoms usually suggests nonbacterial causes such as atypical keratitis or fungal keratitis [43]. Careful history taking about risk factors of infectious keratitis will help confirm the diagnosis. The important risk factors such as history of eye trauma, contact lens wear and hygiene, history of ocular surface disease, previous bacterial or HSV keratitis, history of corticosteroid abuse, hot tub exposure, prior ocular surgery, systemic diseases such as diabetes, immunodeficiency, and vitamin A deficiency will aid in the clinical diagnosis [43–45].

3.2 Physical examination

If the ophthalmologist is familiar with the characteristics of different etiologic agents of infectious keratitis, this helps confirm the diagnosis and determine the possible etiologic organisms. A thorough physical examination from general appearance and eye examination will aid in the provisional clinical diagnosis [43–45]. Visual acuity will be invariably affected depending on the location of the lesion and degree of intraocular inflammation [43]. Intraocular pressure should be examined unless corneal perforation is suspected such as deep lesion on slit lamp examination, and visible protrusion of intraocular content unless corneal perforation is suspected [43]. Ocular hypotony will be present in perforation cases. On the other hand, a high intraocular pressure can be suggestive of HSV, which is associated with trabeculitis [43]. External examination for the general appearance, lid closure, blinking, and corneal sensation are vital to determine the predisposing factors. For example, the patient that has a lagophthalmos is usually prone to an infectious keratitis at inferior cornea. A slit lamp examination is also crucial to determine the etiology of a suspected lesion. Eyelids may appear swollen, and conjunctiva may reveal injection and tearing and/or mucopurulent discharge. Ciliary flush is common. Cornea examination should document the characteristics of the lesion such as the size, shape, border, density, location, depth, and color. For instances, Pseudomonas ulcer usually shows the classic clinical feature of "ground glass appearance," which is a diffuse ulceration with stromal infiltrate or edema involving adjacent or whole cornea [24]. The classical clinical picture of the filamentous fungal keratitis is dry, raised infiltrate with feathery edges. A brown or dark pigmentation may be presented in dematiaceous fungal keratitis and can be an important diagnostic clue [24, 46]. The size and border of the lesion should be documented because it can suggest a positive response to a treatment if the size is decreased and/or the border is consolidated [44]. The depth of the lesion should be evaluated. In fungal keratitis, if the lesion is superficial, it may have a better response to the antifungal eye drop treatment than the deeper lesion because of poor ocular penetration and unpredictable bioavailability of antifungal agents [47]. If there is a significant corneal thinning and/or descemetocele, urgent management is required. The patient may have decreased visual acuity if the infiltration is located over the pupil or have a significant intraocular inflammation [24]. Fluorescein staining and cobalt blue light aid in the document of epithelial defect and detect the corneal perforation by Seidel test [24, 44]. The anterior chamber should be documented for a cell, flare, and/or hypopyon. Essential history and physical examination are listed in **Table 1**.

Essential history	Essential physical examination

• Duration of symptoms
• Eye trauma
• Contact lens wear (types and hygiene)
• Swimming, using a hot tub, or showering while wearing contact lenses
• Past ocular diseases
  ○ Previous infection, e.g., bacteria, fungus, herpes simplex virus (HSV)
• Past ocular surgery
• Previous and current eye drops usage
  ○ Current treatment
  ○ Contaminated ocular medication
  ○ Topical nonsteroidal anti-inflammatory drugs (NSAIDs)
  ○ Topical anesthetics
  ○ Topical corticosteroids
  ○ Preservatives
  ○ Glaucoma medications
• Past medical history
  ○ Medical conditions
  ○ Immunosuppression
• Medication allergies
	• Visual acuity
	• Intraocular pressure (contraindicated in corneal perforation)
	• External examination
	  ○ General appearance, lid closure, blinking, corneal sensation
	• Slit lamp examination
	  ○ Eyelid margins
	  ○ Eye lashes abnormality
	  ○ Discharge
	  ○ Conjunctival injection, ciliary flush
	  ○ Characteristics of lesion, size, shape, border, density, location, depth, color
	  ○ Endothelial plaque
	  ○ Seidel test
	  ○ Pupillary examination
	  ○ Anterior chamber reaction
	  ○ Sclera
	  ○ Foreign body
	• Complete eye examinations
	• Contralateral eye for clues to etiology
	• Signs of previous corneal or refractive surgery

References based on references [43, 44].

Table 1.
Essential history and examination in infectious keratitis patient.

3.3 Microbiological investigations

Most of the bacterial keratitis cases resolve with the empiric topical antibiotics before the results of culture are available [26, 44].

The smears and cultures are indicated as follows [44, 48]:

1. A corneal infiltrate is central, large, and/or is associated with significant stromal involvement or melting.

2. The keratitis is chronic or unresponsive to broad-spectrum antibiotic therapy.

3. History of corneal surgeries is found.

4. Atypical clinical features that are suggestive of fungal, amoebic, or mycobacterial keratitis are identified.

5. There are multiple locations of cornea infiltrates.

Corneal culture helps to identify the causative organisms and determine antibiotics sensitivity [44]. Moreover, culture can help in modifying therapy in unresponsive cases and eliminating unnecessary medications to decrease ocular surface toxicity [44]. Corneal scraping should be obtained from the advancing borders of infected cornea. The hypopyon in bacterial keratitis cases is usually sterile, and aqueous and vitreous tapping should not be done unless suspected of microbial endophthalmitis. Cultures should be performed before starting antimicrobial therapy, and if cultures are negative, the ophthalmologist may consider stopping antibiotic treatment for 12 to 24 hours and then re-culturing the infectious keratitis [44]. The stain provides provisional diagnosis of pathogenic organisms of infectious keratitis. However, cultures were the gold standard to identify the definitive pathogens and provided antibiotics susceptibility testing [26, 49]. Data from the large trial that enrolled 3300 eyes with infective keratitis in India demonstrated that the sensitivity of KOH was higher in the detection of fungi than that of Gram-stained smears (99.3%; 95% CI 98.6 to 99.6) and (89.2% (95% CI 87.3 to 90.8), respectively [50]. The Gram stain has diagnostic accuracy of 60–75% for bacteria keratitis detection and 35–90% for fungal keratitis [51]. The KOH alone has 62–99% sensitivity and 73–99% specificity for fungal keratitis detection [51]. Giemsa stain has 40–85% sensitivity and 70–96% specificity in detecting fungal keratitis [51].

All media are examined for growth daily and are incubated for 1–2 weeks before considering negative culture. Bacteria such as atypical mycobacteria, Nocardia spp., and Acanthamoeba grow slowly and require prolonged incubation [52]. Nonnutrient agar plate should be observed for at least 10 days [49]. Fungus grows within 24 hours to maximum of 2 weeks, so prolonged incubation at least for two to 3 weeks before the culture is considered negative [49]. The vital stains and cultures that are used for infectious keratitis are concluded in **Table 2**.

Even among the cornea specialists, they can correctly differentiate bacterial keratitis from fungal keratitis in less than 70% of cases [55]. Classic clinical figures may be obscured in large keratitis due to tissue destruction [53]. Acanthamoeba keratitis may be responsible for many cases of clinically presumed herpes simplex keratitis [54]. Cultures and smears are the gold standard to diagnose bacterial and fungal keratitis, but fungal cultures consume several days to weeks to obtain growth and can be falsely negative for deep infiltrates [56]. In these cases, other investigations such as in vivo confocal microscopy (IVCM) and PCR may have a role.

3.3.1 In vivo confocal microscopy (IVCM)

Bacteria and virus cannot be identified by IVCM but Acanthamoeba and fungal filaments are large enough and can be visualized [56]. Early detection of Acanthamoeba keratitis is associated with favorable outcome. Two most commonly used types of corneal IVCM include slit-scanning (ConfoScan; Nidek Technologies) and laser-scanning (Heidelberg Retina Tomograph with Rostock Corneal Module) [56]. In vivo confocal microscopy provides a rapid, noninvasive diagnostic tool and monitors treatment response, which has 85.7 to 88.3% sensitivity and 81.4 to 91.1% specificity for fungal keratitis detection and 88.2 to 88.3% sensitivity and 91.1 to 98.2% specificity for Acanthamoeba keratitis diagnosis [53–55, 57]. However, the branching angle of Fusarium and Aspergillus spp. was not easily differentiated by IVCM, and culture remains essential to address fungal species [58]. Amoebas are visible as double-walled cysts or as brightly reflective ovoid structures [54, 59]. However, diagnostic performance of IVCM is highly dependent on the operator's experience [60].

Type		Organism visualized
Stains	Gram stain	Most of the pathogenic bacteria, fungi, Acanthamoeba
	Giemsa stain	Chlamydia trachomatis Herpes simplex virus Varicella zoster virus Acanthamoeba
	Potassium hydroxide (KOH)	Fungi, Acanthamoeba
	Calcofluor white	Fungi, Acanthamoeba
	Special stains • Ziehl-Neelsen and/ or Kinyoun stain • Immunoflorescence stain • Periodic acid Schiff (PAS) stain • Gomori methenamine silver (GMS) stain	• Mycobacterium and Nocardia • Chlamydiae and viruses • Fungi • Fungi, Acanthamoeba
Cultures	Blood agar	Aerobic and facultatively anaerobic bacteria, fungi such as *P. aeruginosa*, *S. aureus*, *S. epidermidis*, and *S. pneumoniae*
	Chocolate agar	Aerobic and facultatively anaerobic bacteria including *H. influenzae*, *N. gonorrhea*
	MacConkey agar	Lactose fermenting (e.g., *Escherichia coli*, Enterobacter, Klebsiella) VS Lactose nonfermenting bacteria (Salmonella, Shigella, Proteus spp., Pseudomonas)
	Thioglycolate broth	Aerobic and facultatively anaerobic bacteria
	Sabouraud dextrose agar	Fungi
	Optional culture media • Lowenstein Jensen medium • Nonnutrient agar	• *Mycobacterium* and Nocardia spp. • Acanthamoeba

References based on [18, 24, 43, 48–54].

Table 2.
Common stains and cultures used to identify common pathogens of infectious keratitis.

3.3.2 PCR

Although not yet widely available, the advantages of PCR are rapid specific identification and requiring small clinical sample [51, 61, 62]. PCR is generally a required test for viral diagnosis and detection of organisms that are difficult to culture such as Microsporidia, *Mycobacterium tuberculosis*, fungi, and Acanthamoeba [52, 61, 63, 64]. PCR can be used as adjunct to smear and culture especially in cases where routine diagnostic procedures failure [65]. When compared to standard culture technique, real-time PCR had 100% sensitivity and 96% specificity in the diagnosis of Acanthamoeba keratitis [63].

4. Etiological agents of infectious keratitis

The common causative organisms of infectious keratitis are bacteria, fungus, Acanthamoeba, and virus [5, 14, 18, 34]. This review addresses the epidemiology, clinical manifestations, risk factors, and treatment of each pathogen. The classic clinical features of common causative organisms of infectious keratitis are show in **Figure 1**.

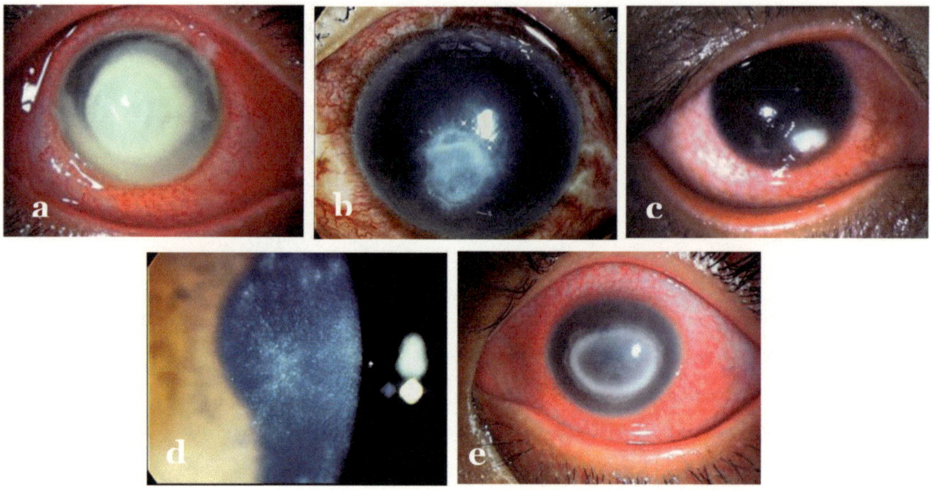

Figure 1.
The classic clinical features of common causative organisms of infectious keratitis: (a) Bacterial keratitis. (b) Fungal keratitis. (c) Herpes necrotizing stromal keratitis. (d) Early Acanthamoeba keratitis. (e) Late Acanthamoeba keratitis.

4.1 Bacterial keratitis

4.1.1 Epidemiology

Bacterial pathogens are responsible for a majority of infectious keratitis cases especially in developed countries and in contact lens wearers [21, 26, 27, 30, 43]. The keratitis can occur after a break in the corneal epithelium that allows bacteria to enter [43, 45]. The important pathogens of bacterial keratitis can be classified as follows: [18].

1. Gram-positive bacteria

    - Gram-positive cocci, e.g., *Staphylococcus aureus*, *Coagulase-negative staphylococcus, Streptococcus pneumoniae*

    - Gram-positive bacilli, e.g., *Nontuberculous mycobacteria (Mycobacterium fortuitum, Mycobacterium chelonae), Nocardia* spp.

2. Gram-negative bacteria

    - Gram-negative bacilli; *e.g., Pseudomonas aeruginosa, Enterobacteriaceae, Moraxella, Haemophilus*

    - Gram-negative cocci; e.g., *Neisseria gonorrhea*

The major bacterial causes are *Staphylococcus aureus*, *Coagulase-negative staphylococcus, Streptococcus pneumoniae Pseudomonas aeruginosa, and Streptococcus* spp. [18, 24, 66, 67].

4.1.2 Manifestations

The patient with bacterial keratitis usually presents with rapid onset of pain, photophobia, blurry vision, and eye redness. Slit lamp examination usually reveals clearly defined infiltrations with stromal edema and inflammation (**Figure 1**) [43, 45]. The classic clinical figures for Gram-positive cocci are "localized round or oval ulceration, grayish-white stromal infiltrates, distinct borders with minimal surrounding stromal haze, or no edema" [18, 24]. *Nontuberculous mycobacteria* usually have a "cracked wind-shield"-type of appearance. *Nocardia* spp. usually has a multiple small white infiltrate that resembles "wreath pattern." Gram negative bacterial infection usually presented as a dense stromal suppuration, hazy surrounding cornea, "immune ring" [18]. Pseudomonas keratitis may develop as ring abscess without epithelial defect [24]. Gram-negative bacterial keratitis can perforate within few days if not properly managed [24]. Keratitis caused by Gram-negative cocci usually present with lid edema and copious purulent discharge, perforate rapidly, and may have bilateral involvement [24]. However, the slit-lamp manifestation alone may not specify the definite pathogens. For instance, satellite lesions, immune ring, and endothelial plaques may be present in both bacterial and fungal keratitis and cannot help to differentiate between bacterial and fungal keratitis [24]. Appropriate microbiological investigation is needed to confirm the specific pathogens. Even among the cornea specialists, they can correctly differentiate culture-proven bacterial keratitis and smear-positive fungal keratitis in photographs in less than 70% of cases [55]. In the case that the keratitis is unresponsive to the initial treatment or has an atypical course, the mixed-organism infection such as bacterial combined with fungal keratitis should be suspected [17].

4.1.3 Risk factors

The keratitis usually occurs after a break in the corneal epithelium [45, 68]. The major risk factors are contact lens wear, corneal abrasions, and ocular trauma [43, 45]. Other important risk factors include prior ocular surgery, chronic ocular disease, use of corticosteroids, contaminated ocular medications, and diabetes [66]. Contact lens wear and lagophthalmos were identified as the major risk factors for the development of Gram-negative infection [18, 66]. Preexisting ocular disease and previous HSV keratitis were associated with Gram-positive infectious keratitis [18, 68].

4.1.4 Treatment

Topical antibiotic eye drops can achieve high tissue concentration and are the preferred method of treatment in most cases [69]. Topical fluoroquinolones usually prescribed as first-line empiric initial treatment of suspected bacterial keratitis are at least as effective as combined fortified antibiotics [69]. Even though the susceptibility of Gram-negative bacteria to fluoroquinolone monotherapy was high, the susceptibility of Gram-positive bacteria was less and more variable [11, 68]. Because of shift in antibiotics resistance patterns, in some regions, fluoroquinolone monotherapy is not recommended for severe infectious keratitis, but combined fortified antibiotics should be prescribed instead [11]. Fortified topical antibiotics should be considered for large and/or visually significant keratitis, unresponsive to initial treatment, especially if a hypopyon is present [11, 44]. In contact lens wearers, the disease pattern and etiologic organisms may be altered to increase incidence of *Pseudomonas aeruginosa* [70]. Fluoroquinolones and aminoglycosides are good empirical antibiotics for infectious keratitis treatment [70]. In noncontact lens wearers, it tends to be caused by other organisms such as *coagulase-negative Staphylococci, Staphylococcus aureus, and Streptococcus pneumoniae*, which are largely sensitive to fluoroquinolones [70]. In terms of patients' tolerance to medications, fluoroquinolones are more favorable than combined fortified antibiotics [69]. The initial empirical therapy should be prescribed until definite microbial identity and sensitivity are disclosed [11]. For central or severe keratitis, a loading dose every 5–15 minutes followed by frequent applications such as every hour is recommended [24, 44]. Subconjunctival antibiotics may be useful in impending scleral spreading and questionable adherence to topical treatment. In cases of scleral or intraocular extension of infection, perforation, or systemic infection, systemic therapy may be helpful [24, 44]. Oral tetracycline class antibiotics (including doxycycline) could be used to inhibit corneal stromal thinning by matrix metalloproteinases [71].

Reevaluation depends on the extent and severity of disease. The initial treatment should be modified when the eye shows a lack of improvement or stabilization within 48 hours [44]. Coexisting conditions and/or complications, such as glaucoma, corneal perforation, endophthalmitis, and eye lid abnormalities, should be treated promptly. The progressive corneal stromal thinning should be managed by application of tissue adhesive, penetrating keratoplasty, or lamellar keratoplasty [44]. Therapeutic keratoplasty may be indicated in cases of large corneal perforation or uncontrolled infection [24, 44]. Corneal transplantation in active infection has high failure rate [34]. However, the result is usually better than fungal keratitis, and 40–50% of these patients recover useful vision [24].

4.2 Fungal keratitis

4.2.1 Epidemiology

Fungal keratitis, potentially blinding condition, is an important cause of infectious keratitis [72]. Fungal keratitis is very common, accounts for 30–62% of infectious keratitis, in tropical region, but is uncommon in temperate climates [72]. The important pathogens of fungal keratitis can be classified as follows [18, 24, 45, 61, 72]:

Filamentous fungi such as *Aspergillus* spp., *Fusarium* spp., *Curvularia* spp., and *Scedosporium* spp. are frequent causes.

Yeasts such as *Candida albicans*, *Candida* spp., and *Cryptococcus* spp., are less common [18]. The fungi invade the ocular surface only when it is compromised or has a defect in the epithelial barrier and access into the corneal stroma [72]. However, the keratitis may present as chronic infiltration or even with an intact epithelium [56].

4.2.2 Manifestations

Symptoms of fungal keratitis typically are not as acute as other microbial keratitis [72]. The pain, redness, and lid edema are similar with bacterial keratitis. Early fungal keratitis may appear like a dendritic ulcer of herpes simplex virus. The feathery edge is a pathognomonic clinical feature [24]. Satellite lesions, immune ring, and unlevelled hypopyon may support the diagnosis but not specific clinical figures [24]. The surface is raised with grayish-white creamy infiltrates, which may or may not appear dry [24]. The keratitis due to pigmented fungi such as Curvularia spp., Bipolaris, and Exserohilum spp. will appear as brown or dark, raised, dry, rough, leathery plaque on the corneal surface [24, 46]. A recent report from the Mycotic Ulcer Treatment Trial II (MUTT II) stated that the presence of hypopyon at baseline indicated 2.28 times the odds of the patient developing corneal perforation and/or needing therapeutic keratoplasty [73].

4.2.3 Risk factors

Fungal keratitis must be suspected if the patient is in agricultural work [24]. For filamentous fungi, trauma with subsequent exposure to plant or vegetable material is usually the only predisposing factor, although previous use of corticosteroids, native medicine, and contact lens wear are increasing in importance as risk factors [24, 45, 61]. For yeast, there is usually some systemic or ocular surface compromise [61].

4.2.4 Treatment

The currently available antifungal drugs have multiple drawbacks such as poor ocular penetration, unpredictable bioavailability, and adverse effects associated with systemic medications [47]. Filamentous fungal keratitis is difficult to treat despite the use of topical and systemic antifungal agents and adjuvant surgery, such as corneal transplantation [61]. About one-third of fungal keratitis patients have pharmacological failure that required surgical interventions to get rid of infection [72]. Thus, early diagnosis of fungal keratitis is the most important determinant of their prognosis [56]. Topical corticosteroids are contraindicated in the treatment of fungal keratitis and also in the early postoperative therapeutic keratoplasty [72]. For filamentous fungi, the first-line drug is 5% natamycin, and the second-line drugs are 1% itraconazole and 2% Econazole [18]. There is evidence that natamycin is more effective than voriconazole in the treatment of filamentous fungal keratitis especially in Fusarium keratitis [74, 75]. *Candida keratitis* is usually initially treated with 0.15% amphotericin B followed by fluconazole eye drop if the first-line drug is not responsive [18]. The systemic antifungal agents, including oral ketoconazole, itraconazole, voriconazole, and posaconazole, are needed for severe keratitis or cases with extension beyond the anterior chamber [18, 43]. Seventy percent of Fusarium keratitis with deep lesion does not respond to sole medical treatment, and surgical intervention may be required [61]. More than 80% of Aspergillus keratitis responds to medical therapy alone; however, in deep keratitis, surgical intervention is needed [61]. For Candida keratitis, medical therapy generally has a favorable response, and the presence of deep lesions is not a major issue [61]. Severe fungal keratitis patients that are still smear-positive despite being pretreated with appropriate antifungal agents may benefit from aggressive multimodality therapy [76]. Various drugs and route of antifungal agents for fungal keratitis are available as listed below [9, 18, 47, 60, 61, 75, 77–79].

1. Topical: natamycin (5%), amphotericin B (0.15–0.3%), Econazole (1%), Flucytosine (1%), clotrimazole (1%), miconazole (1%), ketoconazole (1–2%), itraconazole (1%), fluconazole (1%), voriconazole (1–2%), and caspofungin (0.5%)

2. Subconjunctiva: fluconazole (0.5–1.0 mL of a 2% solution), miconazole (10 mg in 0.5 mL), and voriconazole (10 mg)

3. Intravenous: amphotericin B and miconazole (600–1200 mg/day), and voriconazole (6 mg/kg)

4. Oral: ketoconazole (200–600 mg/day), itraconazole (100–200 mg/day), fluconazole (50–200 mg/day), and voriconazole (400 mg/day)

5. Intrastromal injection: voriconazole (50 μg per 0.1 mL) and amphotericin B (5–10 μg per 0.1 mL)

6. Intracameral: voriconazole (50 μg /0.1 mL) and amphotericin B (5–10 μg/0.1 mL)

Surgical debridement of the epithelium and base of the fungal keratitis is crucial in the management because it debulks the organisms and enhances drug penetration into cornea [79]. Surgery for fungal keratitis, ranging from lamellar or penetrating keratoplasty to evisceration or enucleation, plays a role as an adjunct to medical therapy for initial management and when medical therapy fails or impending corneal perforation [51, 61, 79]. The prognosis of fungal keratitis is worse than bacterial keratitis [80]. The course is favorable with medical treatment in 50—70% of cases. A surgery is required in 30 to 54% of cases [80]. These infections may lead to loss of the globe in 10 to 25% of cases [80]. High risk of developing corneal perforation and the need to undergo therapeutic penetrating keratoplasty (TPK) are due to infiltrate size of more than 6.6 mm, an infiltrate involving the posterior one-third of the stroma, and the presence of a hypopyon [73]. Unfortunately, recurrence keratitis can occur approximately 6–7% after therapeutic keratoplasty [81]. Hypopyon, corneal perforation, and corneal infection expanding to limbus and lens infection are predominant risk factors for the recurrence of fungal keratitis after corneal transplantation [81]. After therapeutic keratoplasty, systemic and topical antifungal treatments should be used for 2 weeks routinely and possibly for 6 to 8 weeks in high-risk cases [81]. Generally, if no typical signs of recurrence were present 2 weeks after surgery, low-concentration topical steroids may be administered with caution [81].

4.3 Viral keratitis

4.3.1 Epidemiology

Herpes simplex virus (HSV) is a common cause of viral keratitis and the most common cause of unilateral infectious corneal blindness in the world [5, 9]. Varicella-zoster and cytomegalovirus can also cause viral keratitis but are much less common [9]. The prevalence of viral keratitis was 0.11% in a recent population-based study [5]. The majority of corneal HSV-1 infection is not the outcome of primary ocular infection, but in response to reactivation of latent virus from the trigeminal ganglion [82]. However, recurrent corneal epithelial infection with HSV-1 can have stromal involvement known as herpes stromal keratitis (HSK), which can be necrotizing, nonnecrotizing, or a mix of both [82, 83]. One study with HSV stromal keratitis reported that disease was of the necrotizing type in 7%, nonnecrotizing in 88%, and a mix of the two in 5% [84]. In this review, we address only the herpes necrotizing stromal keratitis that may mimic infectious keratitis from other organisms.

4.3.2 Manifestations

Viral keratitis differs from bacterial and fungal keratitis in that it can become recurrent and chronic [9]. In necrotizing HSV stromal keratitis, necrosis, ulceration, and dense leukocytic infiltration of the stroma are present and often associated with an overlying epithelial defect and neovascularization [18, 83, 85]. The viral keratitis diagnosis is usually based on clinical findings [43] and diagnosis by exclusion. However, in atypical cases, the investigations such as tissue culture, ELISA, and PCR may aid in the diagnostic confirmation [43].

4.3.3 Risk factors

The risk of HSV reactivation can occur after excimer laser refractive surgery such as LASIK or PRK. The exposure to ultraviolet light during corneal collagen cross-linking

(CXL) can reactivate latent HSV infection [86]. Previous stromal keratitis increased the risk of stromal keratitis, and the risk was strongly related to the number of previous episodes [86, 87].

4.3.4 Treatment

Both immune and active viral replications are responsible for the disease pathogenesis [83]. In contrast to nonnecrotizing stromal keratitis where topical corticosteroid is the mainstay treatment, oral acyclovir is used to control the viral invasion and replication in cornea, while low-dose topical corticosteroids are given to control inflammation in necrotizing stromal keratitis [18]. Topical CsA administration can resolve stromal inflammation and neovascularization in 50 and 64% of cases, respectively [83]. Without timely and effective treatment, necrotizing HSV stromal keratitis can rapidly lead to corneal perforation [83]. Amniotic membrane transplantation onto the ocular surface promotes corneal epithelial healing and reduces stromal inflammation, angiogenesis, and scarring [83]. Various oral antiviral agents to treat active viral replication and prevent recurrences are available as mentioned below [86]:

1. Acyclovir: 800 mg, 3–5 times/day, 7–10 days

2. Valacyclovir: 1 g, 3 times per day, 7–10 days

3. Famciclovir: 500 mg, 2 times/day, 7–10 days

Data from the Herpetic Eye Disease (HEDS) study concluded that the HSV stromal keratitis patients who received 400 mg oral acyclovir twice per day for 12 months had reduced rate of recurrent HSV stromal keratitis by about 50%. The research about HSV vaccination is underway, and no vaccine is currently available [83, 86, 88].

4.4 Acanthamoeba keratitis

4.4.1 Epidemiology

Acanthamoeba is a free-living protozoan found in soil and in freshwater that can cause keratitis primarily in contact lens (CLs) wearers [45]. The epidemiological features of Acanthamoeba keratitis may vary among different geographic regions, climate, and living environments [36].

Acanthamoeba is responsible for less than 5% of infectious keratitis [24].

4.4.2 Manifestations

The classic presentation of patients with Acanthamoeba keratitis is pain out of proportion to ophthalmological finding, photophobia, and slow progressive course [36, 43, 45]. The keratitis usually presents in one eye, but in CL users, it can present with bilateral involvement [36]. The examination may reveal various findings depending on the stage of ocular involvement. Within the first month, the disease can manifest as diffuse punctate epithelial lesions, dendritic-like lesions (mimic herpes simplex epithelial keratitis), epithelial or subepithelial infiltrates, or perineural infiltrates, and ring-shaped stromal infiltrates may be presented [45, 89]. After a month, the disease is characterized by ring-shaped stromal infiltrates, anterior uveitis, endothelial plaque, and disciform keratitis

[36]. Limbitis is a common feature in both early and advance disease [36]. If not managed properly, the disease can progress and late stage findings can develop such as scleritis, iris atrophy, anterior synechiae, secondary glaucoma, mature cataract, chorioretinitis, and retinal vasculitis [89].

4.4.3 Risk factors

The majority of cases are found in contact lens wearers [43]. Infections related to contact lens are often associated with improper wear such as poor cleaning, overuse, and sleeping or swimming with them [36]. Other risk factors for Acanthamoeba keratitis are cornea trauma or exposure to contaminated fresh water, soil, or vegetation and after corneal laser refractive surgery [36, 43, 90].

4.4.4 Treatment

There are two principal issues that lead to severe visual outcomes that are misdiagnosis or late diagnosis, and lack of a fully effective therapy for highly resistant cyst stage of Acanthamoeba [36]. The current diagnostic techniques are insensitive and poor turn around time. Moreover, the better yields and rapid test such as PCR or IVCM are not widely available [62]. This keratitis should be treated as soon as possible to prevent loss of visual acuity or even blindness [36]. Thus, ophthalmologists should be familiar with varied clinical pictures of Acanthamoeba keratitis. Currently, there are n0 FDA-approved medications for Acanthamoeba keratitis [62]. Treatment for Acanthamoeba keratitis includes the following medications [62]:

1. Diamidines (propamidine and hexamidine)

2. Biguanides (polyhexamethylene biguanide and chlorhexidine)

3. Aminoglycosides (neomycin and paromomycin)

4. Imidazole/triazoles (voriconazole, miconazole, clotrimazole, ketoconazole, and itraconazole)

Unfortunately, only the biguanides have been proven to be effective against both the cysts and trophozoite forms of Acanthamoeba [43]. The combination therapy may be of benefit [89]. The earlier the diagnosis, the better the chances of having a good visual prognosis [43]. In the early stage, epithelial debridement and 3 to 4 months of anti-amoebic therapy are enough [45]. Confocal microscopy is the most suitable tool to monitor the keratitis during the course of treatment [62]. However, after a prolonged and maximal medical treatment, recurrence can occur. Topical corticosteroids may mask clinical signs of Acanthamoeba keratitis, encystment, and an increase in number of trophozoites [89]. However, a patient with Acanthamoeba keratitis and severe inflammation may also benefit from this drug [89]. Optical keratoplasty may be considered after 3 to 6 months disease-free interval to avoid the late recurrence [62].

5. Complications of infectious keratitis

Despite timely and appropriate topical antibiotic treatment, surgical interventions such as tectonic or therapeutic keratoplasty may be required to preserve the eye and vision [91]. However, performing keratoplasty in a "hot eye" is associated with an increased risk of recurrence of the disease and graft rejection/failure [91]. The visual outcomes of infectious keratitis may be poor from various complications such as corneal scarring or perforation, irregular astigmatism, development of glaucoma, cataracts, endophthalmitis, and vision loss [92]. Moreover, the advanced infectious keratitis that required therapeutic keratoplasty had decreased quality of life. The characteristics associated with corneal perforation in infectious keratitis were the lack of corneal vascularization, delay in starting initial treatment, and failure to start fortified antibiotics [42, 93]. Inappropriate use of traditional medicines or topical steroids abuse and delay in referral to an ophthalmologist for diagnosis and treatment are all responsible for unnecessary visual loss [24]. The primary care provider should be aware about complication of infectious keratitis. The standardized referral and treatment guideline for patients with infectious keratitis on their first contact at primary care level is needed [93].

6. Prevention of infectious keratitis

Due to the magnitude of the problem, limited access to treatment, inadequate well-trained medical personnel, costs of treatments, and the often poor visual outcomes, prevention may be one of the feasible public health strategies available [5, 34]. Avoiding or correcting predisposing factors may reduce the risk of keratitis [44]. Patients with risk factors for keratitis should be educated about their risk, made familiar with the signs and symptoms of keratitis, and informed that they have to consult an ophthalmologist promptly if they encounter such warning signs or symptoms to minimize permanent visual loss [44, 94]. In the developed countries, infectious keratitis is usually associated with contact lens wear, but in developing countries, it is commonly caused by trauma during agricultural work [8–10, 13]. Interestingly, data from the recent trial reported that "Up to 50% of contact lens wearer are not compliant with hand washing procedures" [95]. Poor hand hygiene is a risk factor of developing infectious keratitis in contact lens wearers [95]. Developing effective prevention strategy that is circulated to contact lens users is crucial to reduce the incidence of infectious keratitis [40]. Although the use of protective eyewear in industrial and agricultural work can prevent ocular injury, the actual utilization of such protective eyewear has been found to be consistently low, even in industrialized countries with robust workplace safety regulations [34]. The protective eyewear during these works should be compelled. The outcome of corneal injury with secondary infection can be improved by early diagnosis and prompt treatment with appropriate antibiotics at the primary level of eye care [24]. Because most cases of infectious keratitis are the result of corneal trauma, the use of 0.5–1% chloramphenicol eye ointment three times per day for 3 successive days for superficial corneal trauma in primary care is recommended by WHO to prevent the development of infectious keratitis [24].

7. Update of major clinical trials about common pathogens

7.1 Steroids for Corneal Ulcers Trial (SCUT)

The large, randomized, placebo-controlled, double-masked multicenter clinical trial that compared 12 months clinical outcomes in patients receiving adjunctive topical 1.0% prednisolone sodium phosphate or topical placebo in the treatment of bacterial keratitis found that adjunctive topical corticosteroid therapy may improve best spectacle-corrected visual acuity (BSCVA) in bacterial corneal keratitis not caused by Nocardia species. But no significant difference was identified by treatment for scar size for non-Nocardia ulcers. However, scar size was larger in Nocardia keratitis [96, 97].

7.2 Mycotic Ulcer Treatment Trial (MUTT) I

The double-masked, multicenter trial that compare topical 5% natamycin vs. 1% voriconazole in the treatment of filamentous fungal keratitis showed a benefit of topical natamycin over topical voriconazole for filamentous fungal keratitis, particularly among those caused by Fusarium. Natamycin-treated cases had significantly better 3-month BSCVA, less likely to have perforation or require therapeutic penetrating keratoplasty than voriconazole-treated cases [74].

7.3 Mycotic Ulcer Treatment Trial (MUTT) II

The randomized, placebo-controlled, double-masked multicenter clinical trial showed that adding oral voriconazole to topical antifungal agents in the treatment of severe filamentous fungal keratitis did not improve the rate of corneal perforation, the need for therapeutic penetrating keratoplasty (TPK), microbiologic cure at 6 days, rate of re-epithelialization, BSCVA, and infiltrate and/or scar size. However, oral voriconazole did increase in nonserious adverse events and cost [98].

7.4 The Herpetic Eye Disease Study (HEDS) I

The Herpetic Eye Disease Study (HEDS) was a series of randomized, double-masked, placebo-controlled clinical trials that studied ocular HSV and is still the gold standard for ocular HSV management [86]. HEDS showed a significant benefit of topical corticosteroids and oral acyclovir for HSV stromal keratitis [84, 99].

7.5 The Herpetic Eye Disease Study (HEDS) II

HEDS II showed that oral acyclovir decreased the recurrence rate of any type of HSV keratitis by 50% approximately [88, 100].

8. Recent treatments of infectious keratitis

The mainstay treatment of infectious keratitis is antimicrobial drugs, which is fraught with drug resistance [11]. However, despite appropriate diagnosis and urgent treatment, medical treatment failure may occur and lead to corneal perforation [101] and/or therapeutic keratoplasty. Novel treatment is emerging to expand the armamentarium of tools to manage infectious keratitis and improve treatment outcomes [101]. The interesting managements in recent years are Photo-Activated Chromophore for Keratitis–Corneal Cross-Linking (PACK-CXL) and photodynamic antimicrobial therapy (PDAT) [91, 101–103].

8.1 PACK-CXL

The mechanism of action of PACK-CXL is antimicrobial activity of UV light, which can directly damage the DNA and RNA of various etiologic organisms [91]. Moreover, synergistic effect is derived from reactive oxygen species released from photoactivated riboflavin, which can directly damage DNA and cell membranes of microorganisms [91]. These effects can increase corneal resistance to enzymatic degradation and increase corneal rigidity. So, it may decrease corneal melting and avoid emergency therapeutic keratoplasty [102, 104]. As microbial resistance to microbicidal therapy increases, CXL might be effective in treating advanced infectious keratitis as an adjuvant and also for treating early-stage bacterial infiltrates as first-line treatment [102, 104]. However, CXL is not routinely used for infectious keratitis because of the uncertainty of its safety and efficacy. A recent systematic review and meta-analysis from Ting et al. demonstrated that adjuvant PACK-CXL could expedite the resolution of bacterial keratitis and potentially fungal keratitis, in terms of size of infiltrates [105, 106]. However, adjuvant PACK-CXL did not shorten the time to corneal healing [107]. Unfortunately, in Acanthamoeba, viral, fungal, and mixed keratitis, treatment outcome was insufficient [91, 103]. However, when rose Bengal was used instead of riboflavin, PACK-CXL was effective against Acanthamoeba [108]. UV radiation in PACK-CXL may exacerbate viral keratitis [109].

8.2 Photodynamic antimicrobial therapy (PDAT)

Since CXL was found to be ineffective against fungal keratitis, potential blinding disease, PDT was proposed as an alternative measure [103]. Photodynamic therapy (PDT) involves the activation of a photosensitizing agent that reacts with oxygen to create reactive oxygen species (ROS). The light using in PDT ranges from ultraviolet-A (UV-A) to near-infrared wavelengths. These ROS react with intracellular components and produce cell inactivation and death [110]. In vitro study demonstrated that Rose Bengal-mediated PDT successfully inhibited the growth of *Fusarium solani, Aspergillus fumigatus*, and *Candida albicans* [103]. Moreover, the Rose Bengal- and riboflavin-mediated PDT demonstrated in vitro inhibition of methicillin-resistant *Staphylococcus aureus* (MRSA) [111]. Riboflavin PDAT strengthens the corneal collagen fibers, delays keratolysis, and prevents a corneal perforation in humans [112]. This can be used as an adjunct treatment in bacterial and fungal keratitis with good long-term outcome [112].

9. Conclusion

Infectious keratitis tops the list of the diseases leading to visual impairment and corneal blindness. The precise clinical diagnosis, accurate diagnostic tools, and timely appropriate management are important to reduce the morbidity associated with infectious keratitis. Although most patients improve after medical and surgical management, their vision may be considerably decreased [15]. A few emerging treatments used to manage infectious keratitis show good preliminary outcomes for selected cases of infectious keratitis, although additional research is required before it is accepted as mainstream treatment for this potentially blinding condition. Therefore, the importance of eye protection [18], hygiene education, and contact lens care and hygiene must be strongly emphasized.

Conflict of interest

The authors declare no conflict of interest.

Author details

Vatookarn Roongpoovapatr[1,2,3]*, Pinnita Prabhasawat[2], Saichin Isipradit[1], Mohamed Abou Shousha[3] and Puwat Charukamnoetkanok[1]

1 Department of Ophthalmology, Mettapracharak (Wat Rai Khing) Hospital, Nakorn-Pathom, Thailand

2 Department of Ophthalmology, Faculty of Medicine, Siriraj Hospital, Mahidol University, Bangkok, Thailand

3 Miller School of Medicine, Bascom Palmer Eye Institute, University of Miami, FL, USA

*Address all correspondence to: drvatookarn@gmail.com

References

[1] WHO. Blindness and vision impairment. 2018; Available from: https://www.who.int/news-room/fact-sheets/detail/blindness-and-visual-impairment

[2] Whitcher JP, Srinivasan M, Upadhyay MP. Corneal blindness: A global perspective. Bulletin of the World Health Organization. 2001;**79**(3):214-221

[3] Pascolini D, Mariotti SP. Global estimates of visual impairment: 2010. The British Journal of Ophthalmology. 2012;**96**(5):614-618

[4] Flaxman SR, Bourne RRA, Resnikoff S, Ackland P, Braithwaite T, Cicinelli MV, et al. Global causes of blindness and distance vision impairment 1990-2020: A systematic review and meta-analysis. The Lancet Global Health. 2017;**5**(12):e1221-e1234

[5] Song X, Xie L, Tan X, Wang Z, Yang Y, Yuan Y, et al. A multi-center, cross-sectional study on the burden of infectious keratitis in China. PLoS One. 2014;**9**(12):e113843

[6] WHO. What is VISION 2020?. Available from: https://www.who.int/blindness/partnerships/vision2020/en/

[7] Sabanayagam C, Cheng C-Y. Global causes of vision loss in 2015: Are we on track to achieve the vision 2020 target? The Lancet Global Health. 2017;**5**(12):e1164-e1165

[8] Ung L, Bispo PJM, Shanbhag SS, Gilmore MS, Chodosh J. The persistent dilemma of microbial keratitis: Global burden, diagnosis, and antimicrobial resistance. Survey of Ophthalmology. 2019;**64**(3):255-271

[9] Austin A, Lietman T, Rose-Nussbaumer J. Update on the Management of Infectious Keratitis. Ophthalmology. 2017;**124**(11):1678-1689

[10] Tananuvat N, Punyakhum O, Ausayakhun S, Chaidaroon W. Etiology and clinical outcomes of microbial keratitis at a tertiary eye-care center in northern Thailand. Journal of the Medical Association of Thailand. 2012;**95**(Suppl 4):S8-S17

[11] Jin H, Parker WT, Law NW, Clarke CL, Gisseman JD, Pflugfelder SC, et al. Evolving risk factors and antibiotic sensitivity patterns for microbial keratitis at a large county hospital. The British Journal of Ophthalmology. 2017;**101**(11):1483-1487

[12] Otri AM, Fares U, Al-Aqaba MA, Miri A, Faraj LA, Said DG, et al. Profile of sight-threatening infectious keratitis: A prospective study. Acta Ophthalmologica. 2013;**91**(7):643-651

[13] Green M, Apel A, Stapleton F. Risk factors and causative organisms in microbial keratitis. Cornea. 2008;**27**(1):22-27

[14] Keay L, Edwards K, Naduvilath T, Taylor HR, Snibson GR, Forde K, et al. Microbial keratitis predisposing factors and morbidity. Ophthalmology. 2006;**113**(1):109-116

[15] Lin SH, Lin CP, Wang HZ, Tsai RK, Ho CK. Fungal corneal ulcers of onion harvesters in southern Taiwan. Occupational and Environmental Medicine. 1999;**56**(6):423-425

[16] Pan X-J, Jiang T, Zhu H, Liu P-P, Zhou Z-Y, Mao AJ. Corneal infection in Shandong peninsula of China: A 10-year retrospective study on 578 cases. International Journal of Ophthalmology. 2016;**9**(1):53-57

[17] Ahn M, Yoon K-C, Ryu SK, Cho NC, You IC. Clinical aspects and prognosis of

mixed microbial (bacterial and fungal) keratitis. Cornea. 2011;**30**(4):409-413

[18] Thomas PA, Geraldine P. Infectious keratitis. Current Opinion in Infectious Diseases. 2007;**20**(2):129-141

[19] Erie JC, Nevitt MP, Hodge DO, Ballard DJ. Incidence of ulcerative keratitis in a defined population from 1950 through 1988. Archives of Ophthalmology. 1993;**111**(12):1665-1671

[20] Jeng BH, Gritz DC, Kumar AB, Holsclaw DS, Porco TC, Smith SD, et al. Epidemiology of ulcerative keratitis in northern California. Archives of Ophthalmology. 2010;**128**(8):1022-1028

[21] Ibrahim YW, Boase DL, Cree IA. Epidemiological characteristics, predisposing factors and microbiological profiles of infectious corneal ulcers: The Portsmouth corneal ulcer study. The British Journal of Ophthalmology. 2009;**93**(10):1319-1324

[22] Lam DSC, Houang E, Fan DSP, Lyon D, Seal D, Wong E, et al. Incidence and risk factors for microbial keratitis in Hong Kong: Comparison with Europe and North America. Eye (London, England). 2002;**16**(5):608-618

[23] Gonzales CA, Srinivasan M, Whitcher JP, Smolin G. Incidence of corneal ulceration in Madurai District, South India. Ophthalmic Epidemiology. 1996;**3**(3):159-166

[24] World Health Organization, Regional Office for South-East Asia. Guidelines for the Management of Corneal Ulcer at Primary, Secondary and Tertiary Care Health Facilities in the South-East Asia Region. Geneva: WHO Regional Office for South-East Asia; 2004. Available from: https://apps.who.int/iris/handle/10665/205174

[25] Upadhyay MP, Karmacharya PC, Koirala S, Shah DN, Shakya S, Shrestha JK, et al. The Bhaktapur eye study: Ocular trauma and antibiotic prophylaxis for the prevention of corneal ulceration in Nepal. The British Journal of Ophthalmology. 2001;**85**(4):388-392

[26] Shalchi Z, Gurbaxani A, Baker M, Nash J. Antibiotic resistance in microbial keratitis: Ten-year experience of corneal scrapes in the United Kingdom. Ophthalmology. 2011;**118**(11): 2161-2165

[27] Ting DSJ, Settle C, Morgan SJ, Baylis O, Ghosh S. A 10-year analysis of microbiological profiles of microbial keratitis: The north east England study. Eye (London, England). 2018;**32**(8):1416-1417

[28] Alexandrakis G, Alfonso EC, Miller D. Shifting trends in bacterial keratitis in South Florida and emerging resistance to fluoroquinolones. Ophthalmology. 2000;**107**(8):1497-1502

[29] Lichtinger A, Yeung SN, Kim P, Amiran MD, Iovieno A, Elbaz U, et al. Shifting trends in bacterial keratitis in Toronto: An 11-year review. Ophthalmology. 2012;**119**(9):1785-1790

[30] Shah A, Sachdev A, Coggon D, Hossain P. Geographic variations in microbial keratitis: An analysis of the peer-reviewed literature. The British Journal of Ophthalmology. 2011;**95**(6):762-767

[31] Lalitha P, Manoharan G, Karpagam R, Prajna NV, Srinivasan M, Mascarenhas J, et al. Trends in antibiotic resistance in bacterial keratitis isolates from South India. The British Journal of Ophthalmology. 2017;**101**(2):108-113

[32] Leck AK, Thomas PA, Hagan M, Kaliamurthy J, Ackuaku E, John M, et al. Aetiology of suppurative corneal ulcers in Ghana and South India, and epidemiology of fungal keratitis. The British Journal of Ophthalmology. 2002;**86**(11):1211-1215

[33] Xie L, Zhong W, Shi W, Sun S. Spectrum of fungal keratitis in North China. Ophthalmology. 2006;**113**(11):1943-1948

[34] Khor W-B, Prajna VN, Garg P, Mehta JS, Xie L, Liu Z, et al. The Asia cornea society infectious keratitis study: A prospective multicenter study of infectious keratitis in Asia. American Journal of Ophthalmology. 2018;**195**:161-170

[35] Lin L, Lan W, Lou B, Ke H, Yang Y, Lin X, et al. Genus distribution of bacteria and fungi associated with keratitis in a large eye center located in southern China. Ophthalmic Epidemiology. 2017;**24**(2):90-96

[36] Juárez MM, Tártara LI, Cid AG, Real JP, Bermúdez JM, Rajal VB, et al. Acanthamoeba in the eye, can the parasite hide even more? Latest developments on the disease. Contact Lens & Anterior Eye. 2018;**41**(3):245-251

[37] Cariello AJ, Passos RM, Yu MCZ, Hofling-Lima AL. Microbial keratitis at a referral center in Brazil. International Ophthalmology. 2011;**31**(3):197

[38] Gupta N, Tandon R, Gupta SK, Sreenivas V, Vashist P. Burden of corneal blindness in India. Indian Journal of Community Medicine. 2013;**38**(4):198-206

[39] Prabhasawat P, Trethipwanit K, Prakairungthong N, Narenpitak S, Jaruroteskulchai S, Anantachai J. Causes of corneal blindness: A multi-center retrospective review. Journal of the Medical Association of Thailand. 2007;**90**(12):2651-2657

[40] Collier SA, Gronostaj MP, MacGurn AK, Cope JR, Awsumb KL, Yoder JS, et al. Estimated burden of keratitis–United States, 2010. Morbidity and Mortality Weekly Report (MMWR). 2014;**63**(45):1027-1030

[41] Gupta N, Vashist P, Tandon R, Gupta SK, Dwivedi S, Mani K. Prevalence of corneal diseases in the rural Indian population: The corneal opacity rural epidemiological (CORE) study. The British Journal of Ophthalmology. 2015;**99**(2):147-152

[42] Burton MJ, Pithuwa J, Okello E, Afwamba I, Onyango JJ, Oates F, et al. Microbial keratitis in east Africa: Why are the outcomes so poor? Ophthalmic Epidemiology. 2011;**18**(4):158-163

[43] Farahani M, Patel R, Dwarakanathan S. Infectious corneal ulcers. Disease-a-Month. 2017;**63**(2):33-37

[44] Lin A, Rhee MK, Akpek EK, Amescua G, Farid M, Garcia-Ferrer FJ, et al. Bacterial Keratitis Preferred Practice Pattern®. Ophthalmology. Jan 2019;**126**(1):1-55

[45] Byrd LB, Martin N, Ulcer C. StatPearls. Treasure Island, FL: StatPearls Publishing; 2019. Available from: http://www.ncbi.nlm.nih.gov/books/NBK539689/

[46] Garg P, Gopinathan U, Choudhary K, Rao GN. Keratomycosis: Clinical and microbiologic experience with dematiaceous fungi. Ophthalmology. 2000;**107**(3):574-580

[47] Sahay P, Singhal D, Nagpal R, Maharana PK, Farid M, Gelman R, et al. Pharmacologic therapy of mycotic keratitis. Survey of Ophthalmology. 2019;**64**(3):380-400

[48] Park J, Lee KM, Zhou H, Rabin M, Jwo K, Burton WB, et al. Community practice patterns for bacterial corneal ulcer evaluation and treatment. Eye & Contact Lens. 2015;**41**(1):12-18

[49] Madhavan HN, Therese KL. Microbiological Procedures for Diagnosis of Ocular Infections. L&T

Microbiology Research Centre Vision Research Foundation l8, College Road, Chennai-600006; Available from: http://www.ijmm.org/documents/ocular.pdf

[50] Bharathi MJ, Ramakrishnan R, Meenakshi R, Mittal S, Shivakumar C, Srinivasan M. Microbiological diagnosis of infective keratitis: Comparative evaluation of direct microscopy and culture results. The British Journal of Ophthalmology. 2006;**90**(10):1271-1276

[51] Chang H-YP, Chodosh J. Diagnostic and therapeutic considerations in fungal keratitis. International Ophthalmology Clinics. 2011;**51**(4):33-42

[52] Sharma S. Diagnosis of infectious diseases of the eye. Eye (London, England). 2012;**26**(2):177-184

[53] Tu EY, Joslin CE. Recent outbreaks of atypical contact lens-related keratitis: What have we learned? American Journal of Ophthalmology. 2010;**150**(5):602-608.e2

[54] Mathers WD, Sutphin JE, Folberg R, Meier PA, Wenzel RP, Elgin RG. Outbreak of keratitis presumed to be caused by Acanthamoeba. American Journal of Ophthalmology. 1996;**121**(2):129-142

[55] Dalmon C, Porco TC, Lietman TM, Prajna NV, Prajna L, Das MR, et al. The clinical differentiation of bacterial and fungal keratitis: A photographic survey. Investigative Ophthalmology & Visual Science. 2012;**53**(4):1787-1791

[56] Erie JC, McLaren JW, Patel SV. Confocal microscopy in ophthalmology. American Journal of Ophthalmology. 2009;**148**(5):639-646

[57] Wikipedia. MacConkey agar. Available from: https://en.wikipedia.org/wiki/MacConkey_agar

[58] Chidambaram JD, Prajna NV, Larke N, Macleod D, Srikanthi P, Lanjewar S, et al. In vivo confocal microscopy appearance of Fusarium and Aspergillus species in fungal keratitis. The British Journal of Ophthalmology. 2017;**101**(8):1119-1123

[59] Parmar DN, Awwad ST, Petroll WM, Bowman RW, McCulley JP, Cavanagh HD. Tandem scanning confocal corneal microscopy in the diagnosis of suspected acanthamoeba keratitis. Ophthalmology. 2006;**113**(4):538-547

[60] Sabour S, Ghassemi F. Sensitivity and specificity of laser-scanning in vivo confocal microscopy for filamentous fungal keratitis: Role of observer experience. American Journal of Ophthalmology. 2017;**182**:201-202

[61] Thomas PA, Kaliamurthy J. Mycotic keratitis: Epidemiology, diagnosis and management. Clinical Microbiology and Infection. 2013;**19**(3):210-220

[62] Boggild AK, Martin DS, Lee TY, Yu B, Low DE. Laboratory diagnosis of amoebic keratitis: Comparison of four diagnostic methods for different types of clinical specimens. Journal of Clinical Microbiology. 2009;**47**(5):1314-1318

[63] Karsenti N, Lau R, Purssell A, Chong-Kit A, Cunanan M, Gasgas J, et al. Development and validation of a real-time PCR assay for the detection of clinical acanthamoebae. BMC Research Notes. 2017;**10**(1):355

[64] Prabhasawat P, Leelaporn A, Tesavibul N, Uiprasertkul M, ChirapapaisanC.Molecularidentification by 16S rDNA sequencing using excised corneal tissues: A useful diagnostic tool for refractory keratitis. Japanese Journal of Ophthalmology. 2010;**54**(1):97-100

[65] Tananuvat N, Salakthuantee K, Vanittanakom N, Pongpom M, Ausayakhun S. Prospective comparison between conventional microbial work-up vs PCR in the diagnosis of

fungal keratitis. Eye (London, England). 2012;**26**(10):1337-1343

[66] Gilani CJ, Yang A, Yonkers M, Boysen-Osborn M. Differentiating urgent and emergent causes of acute red eye for the emergency physician. The Western Journal of Emergency Medicine. 2017;**18**(3):509-517

[67] Teweldemedhin M, Gebreyesus H, Atsbaha AH, Asgedom SW, Saravanan M. Bacterial profile of ocular infections: A systematic review. BMC Ophthalmology. 2017;**17**:212

[68] Termote K, Joe AW, Butler AL, McCarthy M, Blondeau JM, Iovieno A, et al. Epidemiology of bacterial corneal ulcers at tertiary centres in Vancouver, B.C. Canadian Journal of Ophthalmology. 2018;**53**(4):330-336

[69] Hanet M-S, Jamart J, Chaves AP. Fluoroquinolones or fortified antibiotics for treating bacterial keratitis: Systematic review and meta-analysis of comparative studies. Canadian Journal of Ophthalmology. 2012;**47**(6):493-499

[70] Tong W, Chen D, Chai C, Tan AM, Manotosh R. Disease patterns of microbial keratitis in Singapore: A retrospective case series. Contact Lens & Anterior Eye. 2019;**42**(4):455-461

[71] Ralph RA. Tetracyclines and the treatment of corneal stromal ulceration: A review. Cornea. 2000;**19**(3):274-277

[72] Rymgayłło-Jankowska B, Rakowska E, Haszcz D, Kudasiewicz-Kardaszewska A, Suchodoła-Ratajewicz E, Bielińska A, et al. Fungal infections of the cornea–Diagnostics and management. Klinika Oczna. 2007;**109**(10-12):475-478

[73] Prajna NV, Krishnan T, Rajaraman R, Patel S, Shah R, Srinivasan M, et al. Predictors of corneal perforation or need for therapeutic Keratoplasty in severe fungal keratitis: A secondary analysis of the mycotic ulcer treatment trial II. JAMA Ophthalmology. 2017;**135**(9):987-991

[74] Prajna NV, Krishnan T, Mascarenhas J, Rajaraman R, Prajna L, Srinivasan M, et al. The mycotic ulcer treatment trial: A randomized trial comparing natamycin vs voriconazole. JAMA Ophthalmology. 2013;**131**(4):422-429

[75] FlorCruz NV, Evans JR. Medical interventions for fungal keratitis. Cochrane Database of Systematic Reviews. 2015;**4**:CD004241

[76] Sun CQ, Prajna NV, Krishnan T, Rajaraman R, Srinivasan M, Raghavan A, et al. Effect of pretreatment with antifungal agents on clinical outcomes in fungal keratitis. Clinical & Experimental Ophthalmology. 2016;**44**(9):763-767

[77] Heralgi MM, Badami A, Vokuda H, Venkatachalam K. An update on voriconazole in ophthalmology. The official scientific journal of Delhi ophthalmological. Society. 2016;**27**(1):9-15

[78] Müller GG, Kara-José N, Castro RS. Antifúngicos em infecções oculares: drogas e vias de administração. Revista Brasileira de Oftalmologia. 2013;**72**(2):132-141

[79] Cheryl Guttman. Diagnostic and therapeutic advances emerging for fungal keratitis. cornea update [Internet]. Available from: https://pdfs.semanticscholar.org/a078/5015aa09b4f26d17311979cbacd84e22a592.pdf

[80] Bourcier T, Sauer A, Dory A, Denis J, Sabou M. Fungal keratitis. Journal Français d'Ophtalmologie. 2017;**40**(9):e307-e313

[81] Shi W, Wang T, Xie L, Li S, Gao H, Liu J, et al. Risk factors, clinical features, and outcomes of recurrent fungal keratitis after corneal transplantation. Ophthalmology. 2010;**117**(5):890-896

[82] Hazlett L, Suvas S, McClellan S, Ekanayaka S. Challenges of corneal infections. Expert Review of Ophthalmology. 2016;**11**(4):285-297

[83] Knickelbein JE, Hendricks RL, Charukamnoetkanok P. Management of herpes simplex virus stromal keratitis: An evidence-based review. Survey of Ophthalmology. 2009;**54**(2):226-234

[84] Barron BA, Gee L, Hauck WW, Kurinij N, Dawson CR, Jones DB, et al. Herpetic eye disease study. A controlled trial of oral acyclovir for herpes simplex stromal keratitis. Ophthalmology. 1994;**101**(12):1871-1882

[85] Heiligenhaus A, Bauer D, Meller D, Steuhl KP, Tseng SC. Improvement of HSV-1 necrotizing keratitis with amniotic membrane transplantation. Investigative Ophthalmology & Visual Science. 2001;**42**(9):1969-1974

[86] Kalezic T, Mazen M, Kuklinski E, Asbell P. Herpetic eye disease study: Lessons learned. Current Opinion in Ophthalmology. 2018;**29**(4):340-346

[87] Beck RW, Kip KE, Wilhelmus KR. Predictors of Recurrent Herpes Simplex Virus Keratitis: Cornea. Mar 2001;**20**(2): 123-128

[88] Wilhelmus KR, Beck RW, Moke PS, Dawson CR, Barron BA, Jones DB, et al. Acyclovir for the Prevention of Recurrent Herpes Simplex Virus Eye Disease. The New England Journal of Medicine. 30 Jul 1998;**339**(5):300-306

[89] Szentmáry N, Daas L, Shi L, Laurik KL, Lepper S, Milioti G, et al. Acanthamoeba keratitis-Clinical signs, differential diagnosis and treatment. Journal of Current Ophthalmology. 2019;**31**(1):16-23

[90] Sharma DP, Sharma S, Wilkins MR. Microbial keratitis after corneal laser refractive surgery [Internet]. 2011. Available from: https://www.futuremedicine.com/doi/abs/10.2217/fmb.11.61

[91] Ting DSJ, Henein C, Said DG, Dua HS. Photoactivated chromophore for infectious keratitis–Corneal cross-linking (PACK-CXL): A systematic review and meta-analysis. The Ocular Surface. 2019;**8**

[92] Rose-Nussbaumer J, Prajna NV, Krishnan T, Mascarenhas J, Rajaraman R, Srinivasan M, et al. Risk factors for low vision related functioning in the mycotic ulcer treatment trial: A randomised trial comparing natamycin with voriconazole. The British Journal of Ophthalmology. 2016;**100**(7):929-932

[93] Titiyal JS, Negi S, Anand A, Tandon R, Sharma N, Vajpayee RB. Risk factors for perforation in microbial corneal ulcers in North India. The British Journal of Ophthalmology. 2006;**90**(6):686-689

[94] Mascarenhas J, Srinivasan M, Chen M, Rajaraman R, Ravindran M, Lalitha P, et al. Differentiation of etiologic agents of bacterial keratitis from presentation characteristics. International Ophthalmology. 2012;**32**(6):531-538

[95] Fonn D, Jones L. Hand hygiene is linked to microbial keratitis and corneal inflammatory events. Contact Lens & Anterior Eye. 2019;**42**(2):132-135

[96] Srinivasan M, Mascarenhas J, Rajaraman R, Ravindran M, Lalitha P, Glidden DV, et al. Corticosteroids for bacterial keratitis: The steroids for corneal ulcers trial (SCUT). Archives of Ophthalmology. 2012;**130**(2):143-150

[97] Srinivasan M, Mascarenhas J, Rajaraman R, Ravindran M, Lalitha P,

O'Brien KS, et al. The steroids for corneal ulcers trial (SCUT): Secondary 12-month clinical outcomes of a randomized controlled trial. American Journal of Ophthalmology. 2014;**157**(2):327-333.e3

[98] Prajna NV, Krishnan T, Rajaraman R, Patel S, Srinivasan M, Das M, et al. Effect of oral voriconazole on fungal keratitis in the mycotic ulcer treatment trial II (MUTT II): A randomized clinical trial. JAMA Ophthalmology. 2016;**134**(12):1365-1372

[99] Wilhelmus KR, Gee L, Hauck WW, Kurinij N, Dawson CR, Jones DB, et al. Herpetic eye disease study. A controlled trial of topical corticosteroids for herpes simplex stromal keratitis. Ophthalmology. 1994;**101**(12):1883-1895

[100] Beck RW, Asbell PA, Cohen EJ, Dawson CR, Hyndiuk RA, Jones DB, et al. Oral Acyclovir for Herpes Simplex Virus Eye DiseaseEffect on Prevention of Epithelial Keratitis and Stromal Keratitis. Archives of Ophthalmology. 1 Aug 2000;**118**(8):1030

[101] Robaei D, Carnt N, Watson S. Established and emerging ancillary techniques in management of microbial keratitis: A review. The British Journal of Ophthalmology. 2016;**100**(9):1163-1170

[102] Tabibian D, Richoz O, Hafezi F. PACK-CXL: Corneal cross-linking for treatment of infectious keratitis. Journal of Ophthalmic & Vision Research. 2015;**10**(1):77-80

[103] Arboleda A, Miller D, Cabot F, Taneja M, Aguilar MC, Alawa K, et al. Assessment of rose bengal versus riboflavin photodynamic therapy for inhibition of fungal keratitis isolates. American Journal of Ophthalmology. 2014;**158**(1):64-70.e2

[104] Zloto O, Barequet IS, Weissman A, Ezra Nimni O, Berger Y, Avni-Zauberman N. Does PACK-CXL change the prognosis of resistant infectious keratitis? Journal of Refractive Surgery. 2018;**34**(8):559-563

[105] Kasetsuwan N, Reinprayoon U, Satitpitakul V. Photoactivated chromophore for moderate to severe infectious keratitis as an adjunct therapy: A randomized controlled trial. American Journal of Ophthalmology. 2016;**165**:94-99

[106] Bamdad S, Malekhosseini H, Khosravi A. Ultraviolet A/riboflavin collagen cross-linking for treatment of moderate bacterial corneal ulcers. Cornea. 2015;**34**(4):402-406

[107] Said DG, Elalfy MS, Gatzioufas Z, El-Zakzouk ES, Hassan MA, Saif MY, et al. Collagen cross-linking with photoactivated riboflavin (PACK-CXL) for the treatment of advanced infectious keratitis with corneal melting. Ophthalmology. 2014;**121**(7):1377-1382

[108] Atalay HT, Dogruman-Al F, Sarzhanov F, Özmen MC, Tefon AB, Arıbaş YK, et al. Effect of riboflavin/rose Bengal-mediated PACK-CXL on acanthamoeba trophozoites and cysts in vitro. Current Eye Research. 2018;**43**(11):1322-1325

[109] Herpetic keratitis with iritis after corneal crosslinking with riboflavin and ultraviolet A for keratoconus. [cited 23 August 2019]. Available from: https://www-ncbi-nlm-nih-gov.ejournal.mahidol.ac.th/pubmed/?term=Herpetic+keratitis+with+iritis+after+corneal+crosslinking+with+riboflavin+and+ultraviolet+A+for+keratoconus

[110] Dai T, Fuchs BB, Coleman JJ, Prates RA, Astrakas C, St Denis TG, et al. Concepts and principles of photodynamic therapy as an alternative antifungal discovery platform. Frontiers in Microbiology. 2012;**3**:120

[111] Halili F, Arboleda A, Durkee H, Taneja M, Miller D, Alawa KA, et al. Rose Bengal- and riboflavin-mediated photodynamic therapy to inhibit methicillin-resistant *Staphylococcus aureus* keratitis isolates. American Journal of Ophthalmology. 2016;**166**:194-202

[112] Martinez JD, Arboleda A, Naranjo A, Aguilar MC, Durkee H, Monsalve P, et al. Long-term outcomes of riboflavin photodynamic antimicrobial therapy as a treatment for infectious keratitis. American Journal of Ophthalmology Case Reports. 2019;**15**:100481

Chapter 2

How to Improve Visual Acuity in Keratoconic Cornea?

Josefina A. Mejías S, Marta G. Hadid, Luis Izquierdo and Maria Henriquez

Abstract

Keratoconus is one of the most important corneal diseases that causes preventable blindness, so we decided to review the main techniques for improving visual acuity in patients with progressive and nonprogressive keratoconus, in order to expand knowledge in relation to the range of therapeutic possibilities that exist today and the benefits and risks of each of these alternatives.

Keywords: keratoconus, visual acuity, corneal blindness, intrastromal corneal rings, scleral lenses, phakic toric lenses, ICL, artisan, Artiflex, corneal transplant, DALK, penetrating keratoplasty

1. Introduction

Keratoconus is an asymmetric bilateral corneal disease, defined as noninflammatory in which the cornea changes its usual morphology and begins to cause a corneal thinning with protrusion of the thinnest area. It usually begins between the first and second decade of life, without predilection for sex, and progresses gradually until the third decade with deterioration of visual acuity in the form of irregular myopic astigmatism that does not improve with the usual existing correction measures (frame lenses or soft contact lenses) [1, 2].

Histopathological changes include disruption of Bowman's layer, stromal and epithelial thinning, folding or rupture of Descemet's membrane in severe cases, and a variable amount of scarring, especially in the anterior stroma, always with normal endothelium [2].

Some of the risk factors described are eye rubbing, asthma, a history of allergic rhinitis, or allergic conjunctivitis, as well as a family history of keratoconus, although there is no inheritance or genetic pattern involved so far [3, 4].

In relation to the clinic, it is presented as a decrease in progressive visual acuity without improvement with correctors.

About the treatment, there are different approaches according to the objective planned. For correction of visual acuity in mild cases, it can be achieved for rigid gas-permeable lenses; in moderate to severe degrees, contact lenses are also used, but surgical techniques are added such as intrastromal rings, toric intraocular lenses, refractive phakic toric lens surgery, and lamellar and penetrating corneal transplants.

About progressive keratoconus there are two lines of treatment, as a first line to stop the progression of the disease and in the second instance to improve the visual acuity and quality of life of the patient. Currently the only FDA-approved treatment to stop the progression of the disease since April 18, 2016 is corneal collagen cross-linking (CXL) [4].

2. Visual acuity improvement techniques in patients with keratoconus

Intrastromal corneal rings
Toric intraocular lenses of anterior and posterior chamber
Corneoscleral contact lens
Lamellar and penetrating corneal transplant

2.1 Corneoscleral contact lens (CScL)

Keratoconus patients tend to be complicated to treat because they are forced to leave their glasses frequently due to oscillations in their refraction because their measurements are unstable and must continually adapt to new glasses or other types of devices to achieve an optimal visual acuity [5]. The visual correction of the keratoconus will depend on the stage in which it is found; in the early stages astigmatism can be corrected with glasses; however, when it is moderate to severe, contact lenses become the most appropriate option before placement of intrastromal rings or corneal transplantation [6].

Contact lenses for the treatment of keratoconus were induced by Adolf Fick in 1888 [6]. The corneoscleral contact lens (CScL) are rigid oxygen-permeable gas lenses and are composed of fluorosilicone acrylate; these rest partially on the cornea and conjunctival tissue and are used to improve vision in patients with high or irregular astigmatism either secondary to keratoconus, marginal pellucid degeneration, keratoglobus, or posttransplant astigmatism, as well as other pathologies such as Steven-Johnson syndrome, scar pemphigoid, or graft versus host disease may require its use, and also for patients who do not tolerate conventional gas-permeable rigid lenses [7, 8].

There are several types of contact lenses that can be used for the correction of visual acuity, astigmatism, and high-order aberrations in patients with keratoconus such as the corneoscleral contact lenses mentioned above, the mini-scleral contact lens (MSCL), the piggyback contact lens, and the rigid gas-permeable contact lens (RGPCL), being the hybrid contact lens (HCLs), soft toric lenses (STCLs), and corneoscleral contact lens (CScL) the most used for the correction of refractive error reporting excellent comfort and better vision with the corneoscleral contact lenses since the latter tends to be more accessible to use than conventional [5, 6, 9].

There are two types of scleral lenses: those ventilated by air or fenestrated or those ventilated by fluid or not fenestrated; according to Rathi et al. [7], fenestrated lenses tend to compromise visual acuity because air bubbles can enter the visual axis altering vision, while this does not happen with non-fenestrated ones. There is a difference between mini-scleral lenses that have less corneal clearance but are likely to get stuck in the cornea due to the suction vacuum and its smaller diameter [7].

Corneoscleral contact lenses have factors that can affect your refractive performance such as the scleral or haptic portion that rests on the sclera and should be between 12.60 and 13.5 mm, the vault that is involved in the corneal and limbal clearance, the base curvature which should vary between 5.8 and 9.2 mm, the peripheral or scleral curves ranging from 5 to 6 to 11.4 mm, and the central optical portion that should be 0.20–0.27 mm more than the horizontal diameter of the iris, and its powers range from +20.00 to −25.00 D so that when making the calculation of the lens and its adjustment, these three factors must be taken into account [7, 8].

The advantages of these lenses are that they are less mobile, focus better on the cornea, and have no contact with it so it does not cause irritation discomfort since they settle on the conjunctiva and the sclera; the ideal measures are between 15 and 17 mm of diameter or more. One of the advantages of this type of contact lenses is that they create a new ocular surface to compensate for the optical system so they must be filled with liquid before being placed and can be used for a longer time than conventional ones as long as the height of the vault is larger, so it is usually comfortable for some patients given the extended hours of use without complications [5–7, 10].

The disadvantage of soft, silicone hydrogel and permeable gas lenses concerning scleral lenses is that they cannot neutralize irregular astigmatism, so they do not provide visual acuity as suitable as corneoscleral contact lenses [5, 6].

Soft toric lenses (STCLs) are limited for the correction of astigmatism in an irregular cornea but are comfortable and are only indicated in patients with early keratoconus [6]. The corneoscleral contact lenses correct astigmatism through the fluid reservoir, and the haptic should be aligned with the sclera to position it properly and avoid high-order aberrations and correct them [8, 10].

On the other hand, RGPCL improves corneal irregularities through the tear layer between the lens and the anterior corneal surface and decreases higher-order aberrations because they provide a regular refractive surface but tend to be intolerable and are indicated in mild to moderate keratoconus. HCLs have a rigid central part and a soft peripheral part to reduce discomfort and improve visual acuity but still develop many complications. MSCL and CScL improve visual acuity, are comfortable, and delay the need for keratoplasty in the eyes with advanced keratoconus; these lenses rest in the sclera without touching the cornea or limbus but should be used with appropriate ophthalmic solutions to reduce turbidity [6, 8, 10].

In the study of Saraç et al. [6], it was determined that the uncorrected visual acuity (UCVA) of users with MSCL, CScL, and RGPCL was greater than the users of STCL; topographic astigmatism in MSCL and CScL was greater than those of the STCL, but the cones that were in the center had a spectacle-corrected visual acuity (SCVA) lower. In conclusion, MSCL and CScL are good alternatives to RGPCL and HCL for the correction of visual acuity since it achieves more efficient levels of visual acuity than other types. The study it was also determined that patients undergoing corneal collagen crosslinking (CXL) had a better visual acuity than those who had not undergone this treatment, so that a condition to achieve adequate visual acuity can also be submitted to patients to this type of treatment and then adjust the contact lenses.

According to Montalt et al. [10], residual high-order aberrations remained high compared to normal eyes after the use of CScL; this study highlights that although spherical and high-order aberrations were improved after the use of CScL for 1 year, it is not clinically significant since they are only corrected at the time of use without anatomically modifying the cornea after use.

The CScL has decreased the incidence of performing corneal transplants either PK or DALK; these contact lenses are used in mild to moderate keratoconus and constitute a conservative route for treatment, and their advantage is that they are reversible; however, its high cost and perhaps its difficulty in placement may limit its use in some patients. Patients should be informed about the total reversibility of CScL unless adequate visual acuity is not achieved, and the patient must be informed of the complications of transplantation, such as glaucoma, high post-keratoplasty astigmatism, ametropia, or anisometropia, that tend to be difficult to correct to provide a more appropriate visual correction [11].

There are patients who, although they have implanted intracorneal lens segment (ICRS), will require a certain degree of visual correction, and in some cases corneoscleral contact lens, conventional or customized soft lenses, and rigid gas permeable, hybrid or piggyback contact lens can be complemented [8].

It should be noted that after the insertion of the ICRS, the anterior and posterior cornea may undergo certain variations in its surface so that the visual quality, the increase in corneal aberrations, and the alteration of the contrast sensitivity can be affected by the irregularity that this ICRS tends to produce; one option is to place corneoscleral contact lens since acceptable visual acuities and decreased high-order aberrations or vertical coma have been achieved; therefore, despite the fact that the placement of ICRS can contribute to the treatment of keratoconus, they induce aberrations that the ICRS cannot control and can be complemented with CScL [8].

The use of CScL showed no adverse effects such as corneal edema, compromised areas of the cornea, or corneal physiological deterioration. The visual quality was maintained; the number of hours of use of the lens and the comfort was adequate so it is a good option for additional correction in patients who require it [8].

2.2 Intrastromal corneal rings

The intrastromal rings correspond to small circular segments of biocompatible material (polymethylmethacrylate (PMMA)), which are inserted into the corneal thickness, specifically in the stromal layer in order to regularize the surface and improve the main refractive defect. Several studies show successful results in relation to corneal remodeling, but the evidence is scarce to show effect on its progression [1].

It is thought that the insertion of corneal implants results in a flattening of the corneal center with the consequent reduction of myopia and astigmatism that patients with keratoconus usually suffer, also generating a biomechanical support of the thin ectatic cornea. A tunnel is performed in the corneal stroma manually or assisted by femtosecond, and the intrastromal implant is inserted. This implant can be removed at any time, but usually they are removed only in case of complications or displacements of their original position [2].

Changes in the corneal structure can be explained by Barraquer's law, in which when a material is added to the corneal periphery or the same amount of material is removed from the area of the central cornea, a flattening effect is achieved. On the other hand, when a material is added to the center or removed from the corneal periphery, the curvature of the surface protrudes. It is postulated that the corrective results vary according to the thickness and diameter of the segment [12].

Each segment has a double effect: one of flattening, through the virtual line that connects the two terms of the segments, and another of protrusion perpendicular to the line reached by the action of the ring established by the difference between the plane of the segment and the plane of the cornea in the insertion area. With this, each segment flattens the axis parallel to the line and protrudes the perpendicular axis, which is why the segments are implanted in the most protruding axis [12]. In addition, it has been seen that the most flattening action is greater when the arc is longer and, on the contrary, the protrusion action is greater when the arc is smaller. The general flattening is greater with thicker segments [13].

Most publications suggest that the indications for intrastromal segments are patients with moderate keratoconus with a clear optic zone and those who are intolerant of contact lenses. The upper limit of K max should not be greater than 60 D, the patient should not have any scar on the visual axis, and the cornea should be at least 350 mm thick by ultrasonic pachymetry in the optical zone or over the area in which the segments will be installed and the refractive error less than −6 D [14].

The corneal segments can be implanted using manual techniques or assisted by femtosecond laser. It is believed that the creation of the mechanical tunnel is more complex and dependent on the skill of the surgeon; however, the technique with the femtosecond laser is faster and more precise, and with this a better reproducibility is achieved [15].

There are few studies that describe visual and refractive results in relation to implant depth to date, which have delivered results without significant differences [16].

On the other hand, several studies have evaluated with very good results the combination of cross-linking treatments and implants of intrastromal rings, because it is postulated that the first is the only effective treatment to stop the progression of the disease and the second for visual and refractive improvement without having a great implication in its progression [17–21]. ICRs combined with CXL showed that UDVA improved 0.12 logMAR at 12 months of follow-up, CDVA worsened 0.03 logMAR at 12 months of follow-up, but the mean sphere and cylinder component improved 3.03 ± 1.99 and 1.99 ± 0.96 D, respectively, at 12 months of follow-up. Keratometry improved 4.31 ± 2.62 D at 12 months of follow-up. Thus, UDVA, refraction, and keratometry improved to a greater degree than if only the ICR procedure was used [22].

Regarding the complications of the implant of rings, the systematic review by Izquierdo et al. [22] carried out in 1325 eyes showed that complications are rare but do occur. Intraoperative complications are mainly linked to the construction of the tunnel in manual techniques. Decentration of the segments, inadequate depth of the tunnel, and asymmetry of the segments are the most frequent. Postoperative complications include ring segment extrusion, corneal neovascularization, corneal haze, segment migration, corneal melting, and infectious keratitis, among others. Related to the combined procedure, the primary complications in the ICR group were white deposits (57 [5.75%]), epithelial defects (56 [5.65%]), extrusion (21 [2.11%]), decentration (14 [1.41%]), segment migration (6 [0.6%]), and halos and glare (6 [0.6%]). In the ICR and CXL group, the main complications were edema (17 [5.08%]), extrusion (2 [0.59%]), perforation (2 [0.59%]), and corneal melting (1 [0.29%]) [22].

2.3 Phakic anterior IOLS for keratoconus

Several surgical options have been reported for patients undergoing corneal transplants secondary to keratoconus with refractive errors that are difficult to correct or patients with keratoconus and virgin corneas that do not tolerate contact lenses or who want the independence of the glasses. The variety of treatment is wide, such as photorefractive keratectomy, corneal wavefront-guided customized ablation, corneal relaxing incisions, small incision lenticule extraction, or intrastromal corneal rings. However, the previous chamber iris-fixated phakic intraocular lens (ACIF-PIOL) has taken advantage of other correction techniques that can be provided to the patient for their safety and effectiveness [23].

The toric Artisan (Ophtec BV) is a one-piece polymethylmethacrylate intraocular lens with a 5 mm optical zone, and a concave-convex shape is fixed to the iris and corrects a sphere from −23.00 D to +14.00 D and a cylinder of −1.00 D to −7.50 D. While the Artiflex toric intraocular lens (Ophtec BV) has a 6 mm optical zone and a concave-convex shape, it has a flexible polysiloxane optics and two rigid polymethyl methacrylate haptics and corrects spheres from −1.00 D to −13.50 D and cylinders −1.00 D to −5.00 D [24, 25].

This technique has the advantage to preserve the integrity of the post-transplant graft, prevent tissue ablation, having no risk of postoperative turbidity, and correcting high degrees of spherical and astigmatic refraction, and they are stable, safe, and effective and can correct elevated refractive errors [24–27].

It should be noted that the treatment with anterior chamber phakic intraocular lens must be complemented with the corneal collagen cross-linking before implantation to maintain the keratometry and a stable refraction; these phakic lenses are indicated in patients with mild to moderate progressive keratoconus with regular myopic astigmatism. The implementation of pIOL 6 months after the corneal collagen cross-linking is recommended to consider changes in refractive errors and keratometry values that could alter the lens calculation [23–25, 28].

Before placing the ACIF-PIOL, all sutures should be removed in the case of posttransplant patients, and the candidate patients must have a stable keratoconus; these are not recommended in patients with newly diagnosed keratoconus or young patients with progressive keratoconus [24, 25, 27]. The implementation of anterior chamber phakic intraocular lens can improve a UDVA from 20/40 to 20/20 according to the Snellen scale with a nonsignificant loss of endothelial cells; in the same way, an annual request is recommended for studies such as specular microscopy and anterior segment optical coherence tomography to monitor corneal changes [24, 28].

Some complications that may result from the implantation of this type of lens are endothelial cell damage, cataract formation, glare, haptic disintegration, pigmentary dispersion that can cause pigmentary glaucoma, and the corneal incision that can modify residual astigmatism, but they are very rare [26, 27].

In general, visual rehabilitation in patients, after the insertion of the anterior chamber phakic intraocular lens, is quite rapid, with maximization of vision and an optimal focus within the eye, without serious complications, and can be considered as an alternative treatment before transplantation because it is less invasive [25–27].

2.4 Implantable collamer toric lenses

The implantable collamer lens (ICL; Visian; STAAR Surgical, Nidau, Switzerland), which is used as a posterior chamber pIOL, is made from collamer, a biocompatible hydrophilic copolymer of collagen and hydroxyethyl methacrylate with an ultraviolet light. The lens is implanted in phakic patients in the posterior chamber, between the iris and the anterior lens capsule, without making contact with it so as not to cause cataracts or any other complication. There are toric devices, and with spherical correction, the toric models (Visian TICL) were developed in 1998, but only in 2006 it gets approved by the FDA and marketed for use.

A toric ICL is typically indicated for the correction of myopia in adults aged 21–40y with myopia up to −18.0 diopters (D) with up to 6.0 D of astigmatism. Toric ICL cannot correct irregular corneal astigmatism; therefore, it is an alternative method to correct myopia and myopic astigmatism in the eyes with stable KC for partial visual rehabilitation.

Toric models are identical in material, chromophore, haptic design, size, and thickness to spherical models. It has a central convex-concave optical zone with a cylindrical component intended to correct astigmatism. Usually with the identification by extended alignment marks that orient the surgeon with respect to the degrees and direction of rotation that he has to do in relation to the horizontal axis to achieve a correct alignment.

Regarding the calculation of the power of the ICL, it is performed with nomograms provided by the manufacturer according to the patient's refraction, axial length, curvature and corneal thickness, distance to the vertex, depth of the anterior chamber, and the dimensions of white to white and of sulcus to sulcus, so as to determine the most appropriate ICL size for each patient.

A toric ICL corrects only spherical and cylindrical errors of refraction; it cannot correct HOAs caused by an irregular corneal shape. Patients who have a good spectacle-corrected visual acuity would benefit from toric ICL implantation. A toric

ICL does not induce HOAs. The aberrations associated with an irregular cornea in KC that are uncorrected by the pIOL have an effect on the final visual quality. A phakic toric ICL can correct a high degree of myopic astigmatism without inducing new HOA. High corneal irregularity limits the potential visual acuity and may need another surgery to make the cornea more regular [29, 30].

2.5 Penetrating keratoplasty

As we know, the cornea is a transparent dome-shaped surface that, from a microscopic point of view, is composed of six layers that from the outside inward correspond to the stratified epithelium that helps keep the ocular surface smooth and provides a barrier against the external injury; the Bowman layer, an acellular structure that does not regenerate after damage; the stroma, which has anatomical and biochemical properties that maintain the physical stability of the corneal shape and transparency; the Dua layer, which would measure only 15 μm thick and would be located between the stroma and Descemet's membrane; the Descemet's membrane, which is 10 μm thick and can be easily separated from the stroma regenerating rapidly after trauma; and finally the endothelium, a thin layer of cells that maintain the hydration of the corneal stroma in a gradual manner and contribute to maintaining corneal transparency [31].

Due to the layered or lamellar characteristic of the cornea and the partial or complete commitment of the disease or condition that leads to the decision to perform a corneal transplant, two types of management can be distinguished: those that involve all the corneal thickness and which are lamellar, depending on the layer of the cornea affected.

Penetrating corneal transplantation is a surgical procedure in which the entire corneal is replaced by healthy donated tissue [32]. In DALK, the epithelium, the Bowman membrane, and a small part of the stroma are replaced, leaving the Descemet's membrane and the endothelium undamaged.

Penetrating keratoplasty (QPP) has been the technique traditionally used during the twentieth century, independent of the cause of the transplant requirement. The first technically successful cornea transplant with human graft was performed by Power et al. [33]; however, a loss of corneal transparency was recorded at approximately 20 days [34].

Penetrating technique has been associated with multiple surgical complications such as the risk of tissue rejection, infections, and high astigmatism related to the need to ensure a tight seal for the donor graft [35–37].

The aforementioned complications, mainly graft rejection, have led to the development of new surgical techniques in which only the damaged cornea layer is replaced [32]. Lamellar techniques have been gaining popularity in recent decades and have involved preserving the healthy tissue of the recipient cornea by replacing only the compromised portion [38].

If we consider that the visual loss that affects the person with visual disability and that requires a corneal transplant has repercussions in the psychological, social, and labor, severely affecting their quality of life, there is no doubt that vision is one of the most important aspects of the functional activity of people. Our society attaches great importance to visual communication, to the point that those people who cannot make full use of this sense begin to be marginalized from the world around them, directly or indirectly.

2.6 Deep anterior lamellar keratoplasty (DALK)

The objective of the corneal transplant is to achieve an acceptable visual acuity with a minimum of retraction error and with a long duration. DALK was introduced by Eduardo Archila in 1984 [39]; it is a very innovative technique indicated for patients who have no compromise of the corneal endothelium or Descemet's membrane and for mild cases of keratoconus [40–45].

This type of transplant consists of removing the diseased stroma from the cornea and separating it from the Descemet's membrane and the Dua layer and replacing it with donor tissue [39, 43, 45, 46]. In the United States, according to the Eye Bank Association of America, DALK is the main indication of lamellar transplantation, accounting for 43.4% of cases, and in countries such as the United Kingdom, Singapore, and Australia, this technique has taken up the last 10 years [43].

There have been several techniques that have been developed, such as manual dissection/delamination of the corneal stroma or separation of the DM from the stroma using intrastromal injection of fluid, viscoelastic, hydro-delamination, or a big-bubble [40, 43]. Hydro-dissection is better than the others because it allows an easier dissection of the deep stroma and is more controlled than the rest [41], while Romano et al. [43] concluded that there was no significant difference between manual dissection and the big-bubble technique. In the same way, it has been decided that the best technique is with which each surgeon has more experience [41].

Few of the advantages of this technique over penetrating keratoplasty (PKP) are the preservation of the host's endothelium; a low rate of graft rejection; minimal loss of endothelial cells; lower postsurgical risk; a short term of steroid use during the postoperative period, reducing complications such as cataract, glaucoma, and late wound healing; and lower risk of intraocular infections; adding to this, Romano et al. [45] refer that it produces a stronger cornea, being less prone to spontaneous or posttraumatic wounds, as well as a longer graft survival than PKP [39, 43, 44, 47].

However, a fairly long learning curve is required, since the technique can be complicated for some surgeons, and the surgery time is longer than PKP; it also has unpredictable visual results compared to PKP since it takes between 6 and 12 months to reach an acceptable visual acuity and generate high degrees of spherical and astigmatic refractive errors, and this depends on the thickness of the stromal bed or the presence of folds in the Descemet's membrane; there may also be graft tears that require conversion to PKP [42–46].

The stromal bed is one of the factors that determine a good visual acuity after performing a DALK; several studies suggest that for better visual results, you should have a stromal bed less than 20 mm and not more than 65 mm, and these results are comparable to PKP [39, 45–47].

Moreover to the stromal bed and the folds in the Descemet's membrane, other factors that can influence the variation of visual acuity and refractive errors have been determined, such as vitreous length, suture tension, the time at which sutures are removed, previous keratometric values, donor graft size, and donor-recipient disparity, which can modify the radius of corneal curvature [39–45, 48].

Corneal sutures are one of the most common morbidities in terms of poor visual acuity due to myopia and residual astigmatism that remain secondary to their withdrawal; in some studies it is said that residual myopia may become greater than in PK [40]. Therefore, it is recommended that suture removal be initiated in the 1st month of operation and maximum between 18 and 24 months postoperatively [42–44]. This will depend on postoperative topographic astigmatism, which generally varies from >4 D to 6 D, as well as the loosening of sutures or their degradation or vascularization, taking into account that in PKP, the sutures remain longer than in DALK [44, 45]; in any case, each patient should be assessed as graft dehiscence may occur that requires an early adjustment if they are not removed at the appropriate time [40, 42, 43].

Refractive errors are the first causes of patient dissatisfaction. The most common refractive error is myopia due to lengthening of the posterior segment of the eye [40, 44] and can vary from −3.00 to −13.00 D [46]. Javadi et al. [42] determined that the spherical refraction remained stable after 6 months of suture extraction and refer that the refractive instability of DALK may be secondary to the avascular vertical wound between the donor and the recipient causing changes in the wound architecture during healing and in some cases due to the recurrence of keratoconus.

As for the spherical equivalent, Javadi et al. [42] indicate that the changes in it continued until 6 months after suture removal and remained stable afterward, in an average of 5 years, without changes in refractive astigmatism, and in some cases they recommend refractive surgery 6 months after the spherical equivalent is stabilized in patients who require it. Henein C et al. [48] conclude that the spherical equivalent did not vary between PK and DALK.

A preoperative UCVA of 20/100 and a preoperative BCVA of 20/40 are recommended for DALK since this could result in a postoperative UCVA of 20/50 and a BCVA of 20/25 to 20/20 preoperative in a period of 36 months [43]. Javadi et al. [42] said that the patients evaluated obtained a postoperative visual acuity from 20/30 to 20/40 at the end of the 60-month follow-up. And according to Huang et al. [44], there is no difference in refractive errors between DALK and PK and that a graft diameter size of 8.75–10.0 mm can achieve BCVA between 20/40 and 20/25 and less apparent astigmatism than grafts of 8 mm and less spherical aberrations [39]. According to Romano et al. [43], the DALK is comparable with PK in terms of BCVA and refractive results as is Henein et al. [48].

According to a systematic review by Henein et al. [48], it was shown that BCVA and UCVA at 12 months of follow-up favored PK more than DALK, while better postoperative refractive astigmatism, lower episodes of graft rejection, and greater graft survival supported DALK more than PKP. However, the spherical equivalent and the density of endothelial cells did not vary between these two transplant techniques. They also report that the potential factors for postoperative keratometric and refractive astigmatism are the disparity of the donor graft, the bed of the host, and the degree of preoperative ametropia as some authors conclude [42–44, 46, 48].

It has been determined that factors such as central and peripheral corneal thickness, recipient trepanation size, surgical technique, duration of steroid administration and elevated intraocular pressure do not contribute to postoperative refractive outcomes [40, 42, 45].

In a comparative study about visual results between DALK and PKP, it was determined that there were no significant differences in the best-corrected visual acuity between DALK and PKP at 12 and 24 months; however, patients who underwent DALK were more recorded nearsighted without changes in the cylinder, with greater spherical equivalent than PKP [43, 47].

Some complications that can result from DALK are perforations of the recipient bed, double anterior chamber, corneal opacities, stromal rejection, high astigmatism, vascularization and/or loosening of the sutures, and elevation of intraocular pressure, which are usually controlled, have a very low incidence, and tend to be less frequent than the PKP [45–47].

In conclusion, according to several studies, DALK has many advantages over PKP for the treatment of mild or moderate keratoconus, with visual results that tend to be unpredictable but similar to PKP, with a lower incidence of graft rejections and postoperative complications.

3. Conclusions

Up to date, there are several treatments that improve visual acuity in patients with keratoconus. The best method should be selected according to the characteristics of each patient.

Conflict of interest

The authors declare no conflict of interest.

Author details

Josefina A. Mejías S*, Marta G. Hadid, Luis Izquierdo and Maria Henriquez
Research Department, Instituto de Ojos Oftalmosalud, Lima, Peru

*Address all correspondence to: josefina.mejias.smith@gmail.com

References

[1] Mandathara PS, Stapleton FJ, Willcox MDP. Outcome of keratoconus management: Review of the past 20 years' contemporary treatment modalities. Eye Contact Lens. 2017;**43**(3):141-154

[2] Parker JS, van Dijk K, Melles GRJ. Treatment options for advanced keratoconus: A review. Survey of Ophthalmology. 2015;**60**(5):459-480

[3] Henriquez MA, Cerrate M, Hadid MG, Cañola-Ramirez LA, Hafezi F, Izquierdo L. Comparison of eye-rubbing effect in keratoconic eyes and healthy eyes using Scheimpflug analysis and a dynamic bidirectional applanation device. Journal of Cataract and Refractive Surgery. 2019;**45**(8):1156-1162

[4] Gomes JAP, Tan D, Rapuano CJ, Belin MW, Ambrósio R, Guell JL, et al. Global consensus on keratoconus and ectatic diseases. Cornea. 2015;**34**(4):359-369

[5] Bergmanson JPG, Walker MK, Johnson LA. Assessing scleral contact lens satisfaction in a keratoconus population. Optometry and Vision Science Journal, the Official Journal of the American Academy of Optometry. 2016;**93**(8):855-860

[6] Saraç Ö, Kars ME, Temel B, Çağıl N. Clinical evaluation of different types of contact lenses in keratoconus management. Contact Lens & Anterior Eye: The Journal of the British Contact Lens Association. 2019;**42**(5):482-486

[7] Rathi VM, Mandathara PS, Taneja M, Dumpati S, Sangwan VS. Scleral lens for keratoconus: Technology update. Clinical Ophthalmology (Auckland, N.Z.). 2015;**9**:2013-2018

[8] Montalt JC, Porcar E, España-Gregori E, Peris-Martínez C. Visual quality with corneo-scleral contact lenses after intracorneal ring segment (ICRS) implantation for keratoconus management. Contact Lens & Anterior Eye: The Journal of the British Contact Lens Association. 2019;**42**(1):111-116

[9] Downie LE, Lindsay RG. Contact lens management of keratoconus. Clinical & Experimental Optometry. 2015;**98**(4):299-311

[10] Montalt JC, Porcar E, España-Gregori E, Peris-Martínez C. Visual quality with corneo-scleral contact lenses for keratoconus management. Contact Lens & Anterior Eye: The Journal of the British Contact Lens Association. 2018

[11] Koppen C, Kreps EO, Anthonissen L, Van Hoey M, Dhubhghaill SN, Vermeulen L. Scleral lenses reduce the need for corneal transplants in severe keratoconus. American Journal of Ophthalmology. 2018;**185**:43-47

[12] Piñero DP, Alio JL, Barraquer RI, Michael R. Corneal biomechanical changes after intracorneal ring segment implantation in keratoconus. Cornea. 2012;**31**(5):491-499

[13] Sinjab MM. Quick Guide to the Management of Keratoconus—A Systematic. Springer [Internet]; 2016 Available from: http://www.springer.com/la/book/9783642218392

[14] Rabinowitz YS. INTACS for keratoconus. International Ophthalmology Clinics. 2010;**50**(3):63-76

[15] Kubaloglu A, Sari ES, Cinar Y, Cingu K, Koytak A, Coşkun E, et al. Comparison of mechanical and femtosecond laser tunnel creation for intrastromal corneal ring segment implantation in keratoconus: Prospective randomized clinical trial. Journal of Cataract and Refractive Surgery. 2010;**36**(9):1556-1561

[16] Jabbarvand M, Hashemi H, Mohammadpour M, Khojasteh H, Khodaparast M, Hashemian H. Implantation of a complete intrastromal corneal ring at 2 different stromal depths in keratoconus. Cornea. 2014;**33**(2):141-144

[17] Coskunseven E, Jankov MR, Hafezi F, Atun S, Arslan E, Kymionis GD. Effect of treatment sequence in combined intrastromal corneal rings and corneal collagen crosslinking for keratoconus. Journal of Cataract and Refractive Surgery. 2009;**35**(12):2084-2091

[18] Renesto AC, Melo LAS, Sartori MF, Campos M. Sequential topical riboflavin with or without ultraviolet a radiation with delayed intracorneal ring segment insertion for keratoconus. American Journal of Ophthalmology. 2012;**153**(5):982-993.e3

[19] Elbaz U, Shen C, Lichtinger A, Zauberman NA, Goldich Y, Ziai S, et al. Accelerated versus standard corneal collagen crosslinking combined with same day phototherapeutic keratectomy and single intrastromal ring segment implantation for keratoconus. British Journal of Ophthalmology. 2015;**99**(2):155-159

[20] Liu X-L, Li P-H, Fournie P, Malecaze F. Investigation of the efficiency of intrastromal ring segments with cross-linking using different sequence and timing for keratoconus. International Journal of Ophthalmology. 2015;**8**(4):703-708

[21] Henriquez MA, Izquierdo L, Bernilla C, McCarthy M. Corneal collagen cross-linking before Ferrara intrastromal corneal ring implantation for the treatment of progressive keratoconus. Cornea. 2012;**31**(7):740-745

[22] Izquierdo L, Mannis MJ, Mejías Smith JA, Henriquez MA. Effectiveness of intrastromal corneal ring implantation in the treatment of adult patients with keratoconus: A systematic review. Journal of Refractive Surgery (Thorofare, N.J.: 1995). 2019;**35**(3):191-200

[23] Hashmani S, Hashmani N, Memon RS. Corneal collagen cross-linking combined with an artiflex iris-fixated anterior chamber phakic intraocular lens implantation in a patient with progressive keratoconus. Case Reports in Ophthalmology. 2017;**8**(3):482-488

[24] Tiveron MC, Alió Del Barrio JL, Kara-Junior N, Plaza-Puche AB, Abu-Mustafa SK, Zein G, et al. Outcomes of toric iris-claw phakic intraocular lens implantation after deep anterior lamellar keratoplasty for keratoconus. Journal of Refractive Surgery (Thorofare, N.J.: 1995). 2017;**33**(8):538-544

[25] Budo C, Bartels MC, van Rij G. Implantation of Artisan toric phakic intraocular lenses for the correction of astigmatism and spherical errors in patients with keratoconus. Journal of Refractive Surgery (Thorofare, N.J.: 1995). 2005;**21**(3):218-222

[26] Venter J. Artisan phakic intraocular lens in patients with keratoconus. Journal of Refractive Surgery (Thorofare, N.J.: 1995). 2009;**25**(9):759-764

[27] Ormonde S. Refractive surgery for keratoconus. Clinical & Experimental Optometry. 2013;**96**(2):173-182

[28] Izquierdo L, Henriquez MA, McCarthy M. Artiflex phakic intraocular lens implantation after corneal collagen cross-linking in keratoconic eyes. Journal of Refractive Surgery (Thorofare, N.J.: 1995). 2011;**27**(7):482-487

[29] Abdelmassih Y, El-Khoury S, Dirani A, Antonios R, Fadlallah A,

Cherfan CG, et al. Safety and efficacy of sequential intracorneal ring segment implantation and crosslinking in pediatric keratoconus. American Journal of Ophthalmology. 2017

[30] Emerah SH, Sabry MM, Saad HA, Ghobashy WA. Visual and refractive outcomes of posterior chamber phakic IOL in stable keratoconus. International Journal of Ophthalmology. 2019;**12**(5):840-843

[31] Dua HS, Faraj LA, Said DG, Gray T, Lowe J. Human corneal anatomy redefined. Ophthalmology. 2013;**120**(9):1778-1785

[32] Hjortdal J. Corneal Transplantation. Springer [Internet]; 2019. Available from: https://www.springer.com/la/book/9783319240503

[33] Brightbill FS. Corneal Surgery: Theory, Technique and Tissue. Elsevier Health Sciences; 2009. 970 p

[34] Crawford AZ, Patel DV, McGhee CN. A brief history of corneal transplantation: From ancient to modern. Oman Journal of Ophthalmology. 2013;**6**(Suppl 1):S12-S17

[35] Han DCY, Mehta JS, Por YM, Htoon HM, Tan DTH. Comparison of outcomes of lamellar keratoplasty and penetrating keratoplasty in keratoconus. American Journal of Ophthalmology. 2009;**148**(5):744-751.e1

[36] Vedana G, Villarreal G, Jun AS. Fuchs endothelial corneal dystrophy: Current perspectives. Clinical Ophthalmology (Auckland, N.Z.). 2016;**10**:321-330

[37] Nanavaty MA, Shortt AJ. Endothelial keratoplasty versus penetrating keratoplasty for Fuchs endothelial dystrophy. Cochrane Database of Systematic Reviews. 2011;(7):CD008420

[38] Gain P, Jullienne R, He Z, Aldossary M, Acquart S, Cognasse F, et al. Global survey of corneal transplantation and eye banking. JAMA Ophthalmology. 2016;**134**(2):167-173

[39] Ardjomand N, Hau S, McAlister JC, Bunce C, Galaretta D, Tuft SJ, et al. Quality of vision and graft thickness in deep anterior lamellar and penetrating corneal allografts. American Journal of Ophthalmology. 2007;**143**(2):228-235

[40] Feizi S, Javadi MA. Factors predicting refractive outcomes after deep anterior lamellar keratoplasty in keratoconus. American Journal of Ophthalmology. 2015;**160**(4):648-653.e2

[41] Amayem AF, Hamdi IM, Hamdi MM. Refractive and visual outcomes of penetrating keratoplasty versus deep anterior lamellar keratoplasty with hydrodissection for treatment of keratoconus. Cornea. 2013;**32**(4):e2-e5

[42] Javadi MA, Feizi S, Rahmani S, Khajuee-Kermani P. Refractive stability after deep anterior lamellar keratoplasty for keratoconus. Cornea. 2018;**37**(12):1506-1510

[43] Romano V, Iovieno A, Parente G, Soldani AM, Fontana L. Long-term clinical outcomes of deep anterior lamellar keratoplasty in patients with keratoconus. American Journal of Ophthalmology. 2015;**159**(3):505-511

[44] Huang T, Hu Y, Gui M, Zhang H, Wang Y, Hou C. Large-diameter deep anterior lamellar keratoplasty for keratoconus: Visual and refractive outcomes. British Journal of Ophthalmology. 2015;**99**(9):1196-1200

[45] Pedrotti E, Passilongo M, Fasolo A, Ficial S, Ferrari S, Marchini G. Refractive outcomes of penetrating keratoplasty and deep anterior lamellar keratoplasty in fellow eyes for keratoconus. International Ophthalmology. 2017;**37**(4):911-919

[46] Maharana PK, Agarwal K, Jhanji V, Vajpayee RB. Deep anterior lamellar keratoplasty for keratoconus: A review. Eye Contact Lens. 2014;**40**(6):382-389

[47] Bhatt UK, Fares U, Rahman I, Said DG, Maharajan SV, Dua HS. Outcomes of deep anterior lamellar keratoplasty following successful and failed «big bubble». British Journal of Ophthalmology. 2012;**96**(4):564-569

[48] Henein C, Nanavaty MA. Systematic review comparing penetrating keratoplasty and deep anterior lamellar keratoplasty for management of keratoconus. Contact Lens & Anterior Eye: The Journal of the British Contact Lens Association. 2017;**40**(1):3-14

Chapter 3

Diffractive Corneal Inlays: A New Concept for Correction of Presbyopia

Diego Montagud-Martínez, Vicente Ferrando, Salvador Garcia-Delpech, Juan A. Monsoriu and Walter D. Furlan

Abstract

A new class of corneal inlays for treatment of presbyopia is described, which uses diffraction as the working principle. The inlay consists of an opaque disk with a small central aperture surrounded by an array of micro-holes that are distributed following the order of a given Fresnel zone plate having N zones. In this way, the central hole of the disk produces an extension of the depth of focus of the eye for distance vision and contributes to the zero order of diffraction, and the light diffracted by the micro-holes in the periphery produces a real focus for near vision. In our general design, the number of zones and the diameter of the central hole are free parameters that can be used to design customized devices with different addition power and near-focus intensity. Two different designs are analyzed to show this property. In the analysis, we employed a ray tracing software to study the performance of the new inlays in the two different model eyes. The results are compared with those obtained with a model of the small-aperture inlay that is currently in the market. The different merit functions used in the comparison and the image simulations performed with the inlays in the model eyes show the excellent performance of our proposal.

Keywords: presbyopia, corneal inlay, diffractive optics, refractive surgery, cornea

1. Introduction

Affecting approximately 2 billion people worldwide, presbyopia is the most common refractive defect in the population, disturbing the quality of life of people over 45 years. It is expected that this situation will grow to reach 2100 million in 2020 [1]. In fact, presbyopia is a natural condition of the human being due to aging, and it is caused by the loss of ability of the crystalline lens to accommodate.

The treatment of presbyopia has historically been addressed from multiple perspectives: spectacles (reading glasses, bifocals, and progressive), multifocal contact lenses, and refractive surgery. Within this area, the most recent surgical approach is in the use of corneal inlays (CIs) [1, 2]. These implants consist of lenticels of a biocompatible synthetic material that, as the name implies, are placed into the corneal stroma. The main advantage of CI over other surgical therapies, like intraocular lenses, is that it is a minimally invasive and reversible surgery [3]; in addition, CIs are stable and do not require maintenance.

Currently, all CIs are implanted monocularly in the nondominant eye producing a modified variant of the monovision system, which consists in using the dominant eye for distance vision and the nondominant one for intermediate-near vision. Commercial examples of CIs are the Flexivue Microlens® (Presbia Cooperatief, UA, Irvine, CA, USA) [1, 4, 5], the Raindrop® (ReVision Optics, Lake Forest, CA, USA) [1, 5, 6], and the small-aperture corneal inlay (SACI) whose trade name is KAMRA® inlay (Acufocus, Inc., Irvine, CA, USA) [1, 5, 7–10]. The principle of operation of each model is different. The Flexivue inlay is a bifocal device of the center-far type, since it has a central hole for the passage of nutrients that allows the vision of far and a peripheral area for the near vision that contains the power of addition. The Raindrop inlay uses a different refractive principle, which consists of introducing a lenticel of permeable material in the center of the corneal stroma to create a hyperprolate cornea. Therefore, the cornea becomes itself a center-near bifocal lens. Finally, the SACI uses the pinhole effect to extend the depth of focus of the eye in far vision. Indeed, it consists of an opaque ring of 1.6 mm internal diameter and 3.6 mm external diameter, constructed with carbon-doped polyvinylidene fluoride. It has about 8400 micro-holes with diameters between 5 and 10 μm, distributed randomly to allow the passage of nutrients through the stroma, which gives it around 5% transmittance [10]. Surgically, it is introduced at a depth of 200 μm. The SACI is the most successful commercial CI and has been widely studied both clinically and theoretically [1, 5, 7–10]. However, it has certain drawbacks. As it is an opaque ring, the amount of light that reaches the retina of each eye is different, causing a degradation of binocular distance visual acuity [11] and a potential detrimental effect on the binocular summation ratio [12]. Moreover, the SACI produces marked interocular differences in visual latency and a Pulfrich effect [13]. Other visual function that is compromised by the SACI is a deterioration in stereoacuity with respect to natural conditions, especially for near and intermediate distances [14].

In this chapter we describe a new concept of CI developed by our research group that is based on the concept of diffraction. It consists of a variation of an amplitude Fresnel zone plate [15] in which micro-holes conform the clear zones of the zone plate in a similar way as was proposed to construct the so-called photon sieves [16]. Photon sieves were conceived for its use in X-ray microscopy but were also found to have numerous applications in various scientific and technological areas [17–19]. Inspired by this concept, we conceived the first diffractive corneal inlay (DCI) in which the distribution of holes in an opaque ring has been ordered to achieve a bifocal intrastromal lens. In this way, the light diffracted by the inlay (an unwanted effect in the SACI commercial design) generates a focus, which would allow presbyopic patients to see close objects clearly. To demonstrate its properties, in the following sections theoretical and numerical results are compared with the SACI, using two different theoretical eye models implemented in the ZEMAX™ OpticStudio software (EE version 18.7, ZEMAX Development Corporation, Bellevue, Washington, USA). To evaluate the optical quality of ICs, the modulation transfer function (MTF), which defines the visibility of a given optical system for all spatial frequencies [20]; the area under the MTF curve (AMTF), computed for different object vergences; and the point spread function (PSF) [20] that describes the response of an optical system to a point source have been used. In addition, the numerically calculated PSFs have been used to obtain simulated images of an optotype test chart.

2. Diffractive corneal inlay (DCI)

The starting point of the DCI design is an amplitude Fresnel zone plate, which has been devised with the optical power necessary to generate the addition. In it, instead of fully transparent zones, micro-holes are made to allow the passage of

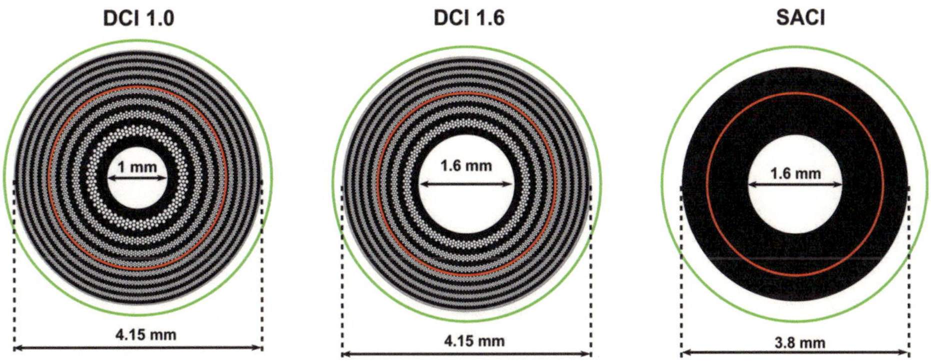

Figure 1.
Design of the analyzed DCIs and the SACI.

light and the nutrients, forming a single structure without any substrate. The DCI [21], in addition to presenting the aforementioned micro-hole structure, has a central hole that acts as a pinhole of variable diameter; thus the DCI presents different diffractive orders. The zero order focuses the light for distant vision, while the +1 order forms the near focus. By varying the number of rings, the number and size of the micro-holes, as well as the internal diameter of the central hole, the diffraction efficiency of the far, and near foci can be modified.

Here we evaluated two DCI models in comparison with a SACI with the dimensions of the KAMRA® (see **Figure 1**). Both DCIs were designed to provide a near focus corresponding to an addition of +2.50 D, and both have an external diameter of 4.15 mm. DCI 1.0 has a central hole of 1.00 mm diameter surrounded by 8 rings with a total of 6394 holes. DCI 1.6 was designed with a central hole of 1.6 mm diameter surrounded by 7 rings conformed by a total of 5989 holes. A complete opaque with the dimensions of the SACI, as shown in **Figure 1**, was evaluated in parallel for comparison.

3. Focusing properties: axial irradiance

To evaluate the focusing properties of the DCIs, we first computed the axial irradiances provided by them in air under monochromatic illumination for a wavelength of 555 nm using the Fresnel approximation [9]. **Figure 2** shows the

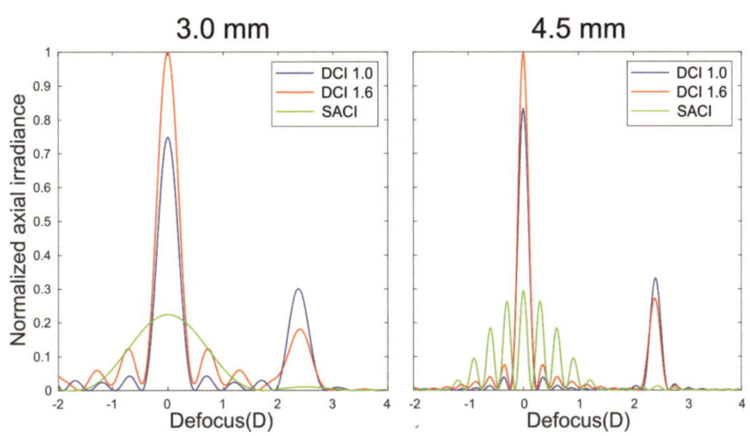

Figure 2.
Normalized axial irradiances of the three CIs for pupil diameters of 3.0 mm (left) and 4.5 mm (right).

results, computed for CIs with external pupils of 3.0 and 4.5 mm diameter (see the red and green circles in **Figure 1**). As can be seen, the profile of the DCIs is clearly bifocal, while that of the SACI is, as expected, of a typical extended focus one. Note also that both DCIs have a more intense focus than the SACI in distant vision (zero defocus).

4. MTFs and AMTFs

The MTFs and AMTFs of the inlays have been calculated using the ZEMAX™ OpticStudio software, in which two theoretical eye models have been implemented: the Liou-Brennan Model Eye (LBME) [22] and the ZEMAX Model Eye (ZME) [23].

The ZME is an eye model included in the software package. **Table 1** shows the data sheet used for the simulations with the ZME.

The LBME is one of the most popular theoretical models because it has the most realistic biometrical data obtained from 45-year-old people (young presbyopes). It takes into account the alpha angle [22] (the angle between the visual axis and the optical axis), the 0.5-mm nasal displacement of the pupil, and the gradient refractive index of the crystalline lens. Its optical parameters are shown in **Table 2**. The major difference between both models relies in the corneal asphericities (Q) that induce different values for the spherical aberration (SA) in each eye.

Surface	Radius (mm)	Asphericity (Q)	Thickness (mm)	Refractive index
Anterior cornea	7.80	−0.50	0.200	1.377
Anterior CI	7.80	−0.50	0.005	1.377
Posterior CI	7.80	−0.50	0.315	1.377
Posterior cornea	6.70	−0.30	3.100	1.337
Iris	—	—	0.100	1.337
Anterior lens	10.00	0.00	3700	1420
Posterior lens	−6.00	−3.25	16.580	1.336

Table 1.
Parameters of ZME.

Surface	Radius (mm)	Asphericity (Q)	Thickness (mm)	Refractive index
Anterior cornea	7.77	−0.18	0.200	1.376
Anterior CI	7.77	−0.18	0.005	1.376
Posterior CI	7.77	−0.18	0.295	1.376
Posterior cornea	6.40	−0.60	3.16	1.336
Iris	—	—	0.00	—
Anterior lens	12.4	−0.94	1.59	$1.368 + 0.049057z - 0.015427 z^2 - 0.001978 r^2$
Lens	Infinity	—	2.43	$1.407 - 0.006605z^2 - 0.001978 r^2$
Posterior lens	−8.10	0.96	16.26	1.336

Table 2.
Parameters of LBME, the pupil is decentered 0.5 mm nasally, and the incidental beams have an angle of entry of 5°.

In these model eyes, both DCIs and the SACI have been inserted virtually at a distance of 200 μm from the anterior surface of the cornea, simulating the surgical procedure of the SACI [5]. In the simulation in ZEMAX, the inlays have been introduced as *.uda* (user-defined aperture) files. To simulate a thickness of 5 μm for the CIs, two CI surfaces were introduced into each eye model, as can be seen in **Tables 1** and **2**. The CIs were centered on the visual axis of each model eye.

The MTFs have been calculated for far and near foci and also for different vergences between +0.50 D and − 3.50 D in steps of 0.10 D, in order to calculate the AMTF. The AMTFs have been obtained integrating the MTF values for a frequency range from 9.49 to 59.86 cycles per degree (cpd), corresponding to visual acuities (VA) between 0.5 logMAR and −0.2 logMAR, respectively.

Figure 3 shows the MTFs at the far and near foci for 3.0-mm pupils. As can be seen, both model eyes predict a similar behavior for the three ICs in both far and near foci. It should be mentioned that for the LBME, the represented MTFs in **Figure 3** are computed as the mean values between the sagittal and the tangential MTF curves. In addition, as explained in previous sections, the higher internal diameter of the DCI 1.6 causes a higher amount of light that focuses on the far distance image with respect

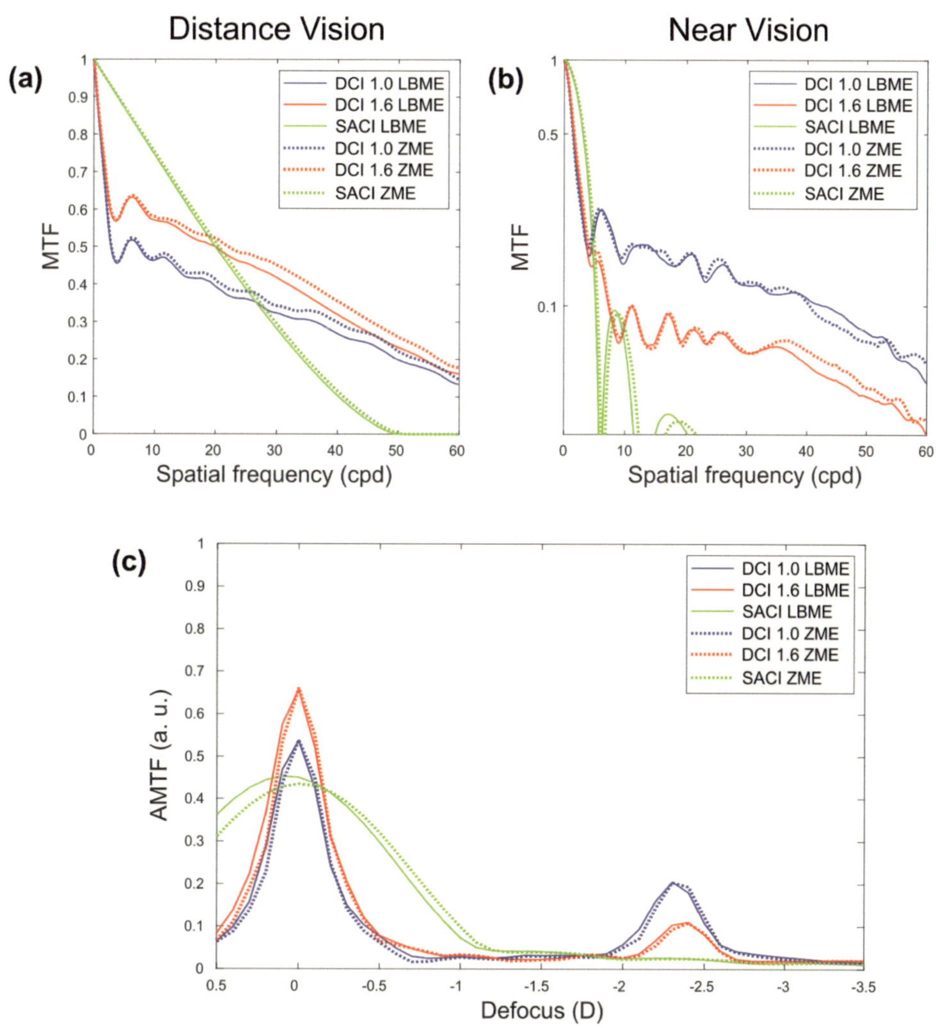

Figure 3.
A 3.0-mm pupil: (a) MTF distance vision, (b) MTF near vision, and (c) AMTF for different defocus conditions of the three CIs: DCI 1.0 (blue), DCI 1.6 (red), and SACI (green) for LBME (continuous lines) and ZME (dashed lines).

to the DCI 1.0. For this reason, the MTF at the far focus of the DCI 1.6 is the better one. The opposite is true for the near focus, while SACI theoretically presents an extended focus, as can be seen in the AMTF; it does not have a defined focus for near vision. In contrast, the diffractive profile of the DCIs generates the near focus that can be seen in **Figure 3c**. The MTF for the near-vision focus of DCI 1.0 is better than for DCI 1.6 because the total area of the inlay is higher. On the other hand, differences between both eye models are hardly observed, because for a 3.0-mm pupil, the influence of the LBME asymmetry and the SA is both minimal.

Figure 4 shows the same merit functions as in **Figure 3** but is calculated for 4.5-mm pupils. The influence of the SA on the eye models can be seen in **Figure 4c**. While the AMTFs of the three CIs in the ZME maintain their focus of vision at distance (zero defocus), in the LBME, the AMTF peaks of the far focus are shifted 0.1 D due to the influence of the SA; however, in the near focus, this effect is not so obvious. It is important to note the effect of the pupil size on the depth of focus of the inlays. As can be seen in the comparison between **Figure 3c** and **4c**, the AMTF

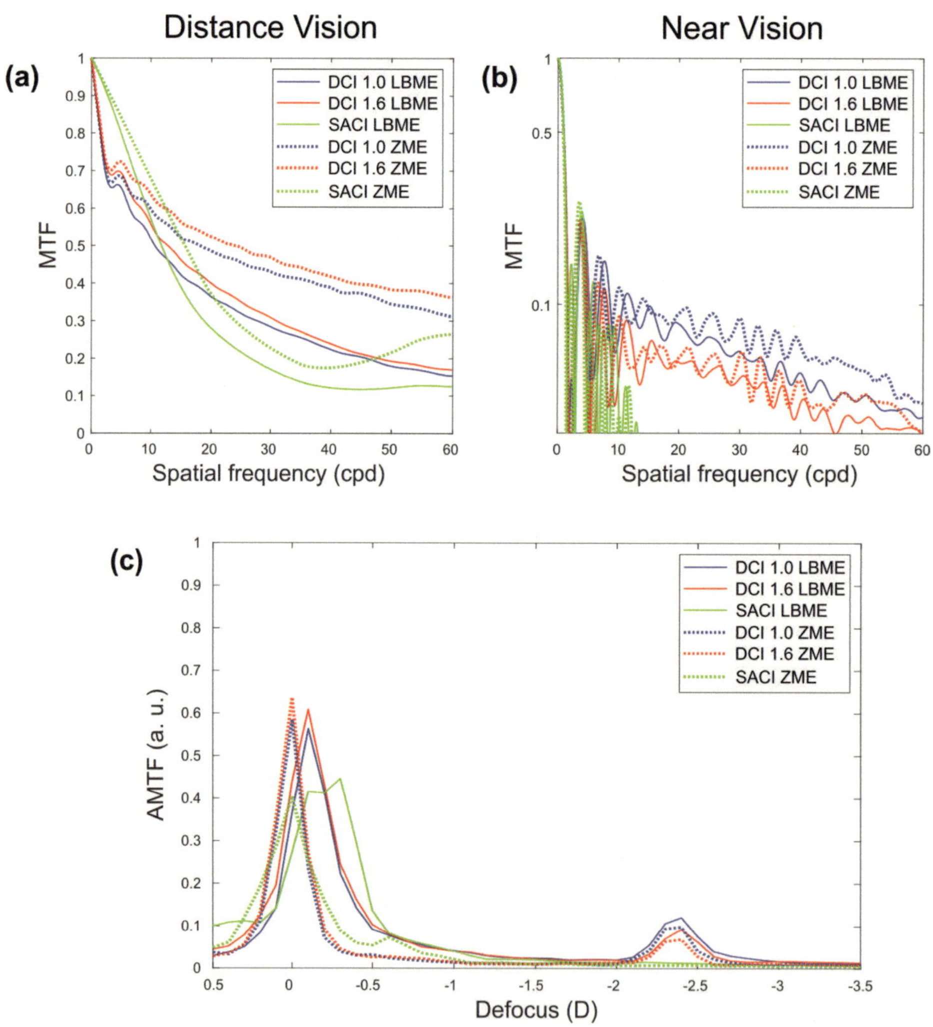

Figure 4.
A 4.5-mm pupil: (a) MTF distance vision, (b) MTF near vision, and (c) AMTF for different defocus conditions of the three CIs: DCI 1.0 (blue), DCI 1.6 (red), and SACI (green) for LBME (continuous lines) and ZME (dashed lines).

of both ICDs is less affected than the AMTF of the SACI, since for the latter the depth of focus is severely reduced.

5. PSF and image simulation

As stated above, the PSF describes the ability of an optical system (in our case an eye model with a CI) to form a good image of a point source. An ideal PSF corresponds to a diffraction-limited system and is known as the airy disk, with a high-intensity central peak, which is more or less concentrated depending on the pupil size. For real systems the PSF spreads out; as more extended is the PSF, the system is worse.

Figures 5 and **6** show the PSFs obtained for the 3.0 and 4.5-mm pupils, respectively, of the three ICs in both eye models. PSFs calculated with ZEMAX were weighted according to the axial irradiances calculated in Section 3 for each CI. Considering that the foci in distance and in near vision have different range intensities, different normalizations were performed in order to compare them. In this way, the PSFs at the far and near foci are normalized to the maximum value of the DCI 1.6 PSF in the ZME, and the PSFs of the near-vision focus are normalized to the maximum of the PSF of the near-focus DCI 1.6 of the ZME in each focus, respectively. This means that in **Figures 5** and **6**, the eye models of the three CIs in each focus can be only compared, but far and near PSFs have different normalizations.

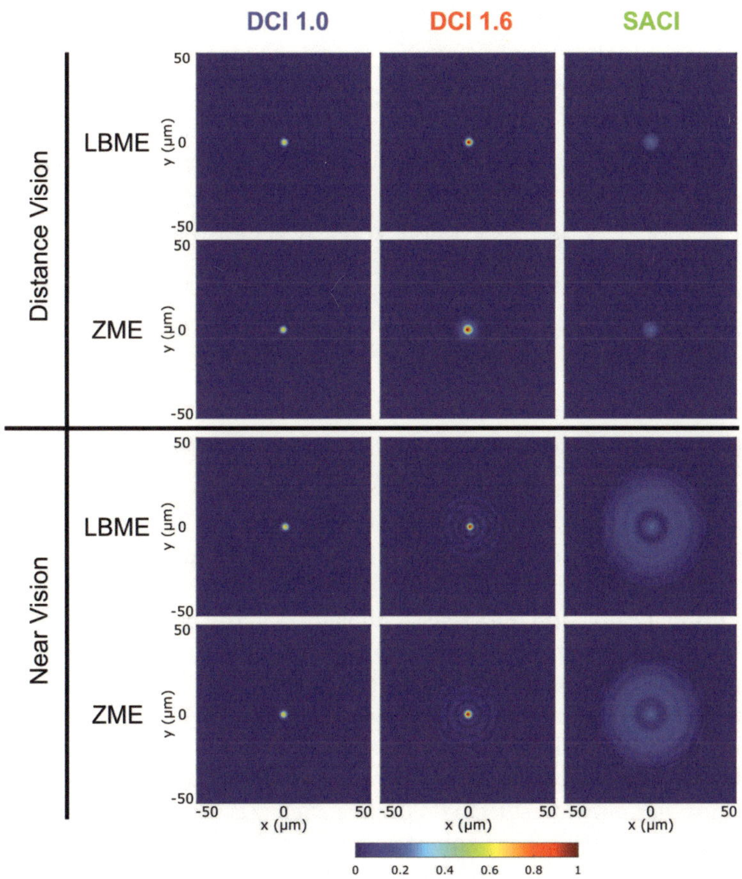

Figure 5.
PSFs normalized to the maximum of each triplet of CIs for pupil of 3.0 mm in distance vision (top) and near vision (bottom).

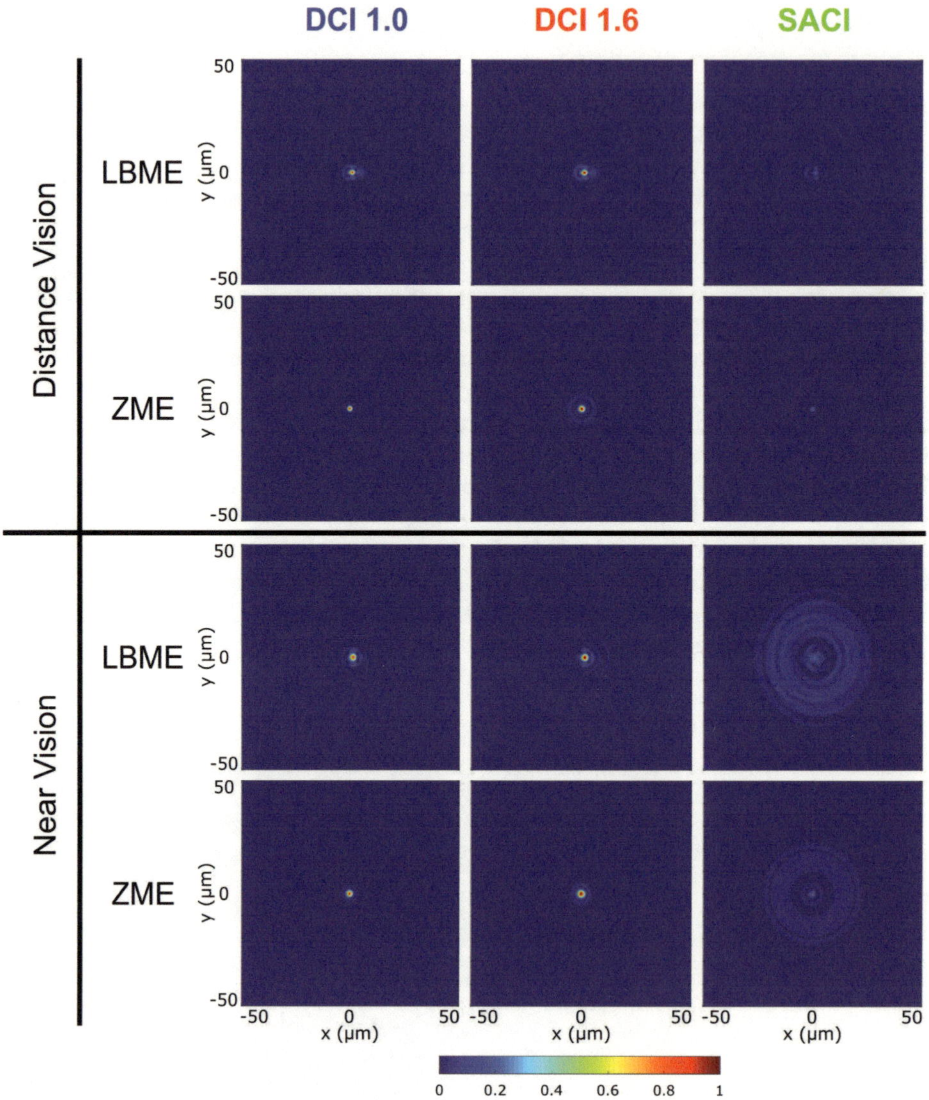

Figure 6.
PSFs normalized to the maximum of each triplet of CIs for pupil of 4.5 mm in distance vision (top) and near vision (bottom).

Figure 5 shows that, for both the LBME and the ZME in distance vision, DCI 1.6 has a more intense focus than the other two CIs, but it has a slightly wider peak than DCI 1.0. In near vision the same trend is shown, the maximum of the DCI 1.6 is higher than that of the other two CIs, but its surrounding halo is also more extended. Note that the SACI has an even greater halo. For 3.0-mm pupil at near vision, the first impression is that the PSF for DCI 1.6 is better than the one for DCI 1.0 PSF # 1; however, it should be borne in mind that, while the maximum value of the first one is the unity, the energy is very dispersed (the halo). In DCI 1.0, although the maximum is less than 0.802, the energy is more concentrated, and therefore the PSF is better. The explanation of why the PSF of DCI 1.6 is globally better is simple: the diffraction efficiency of DCI 1.6 is better, focusing more light on the near-vision focus. On the other hand, as expected, for 3.0-mm pupil diameter, the CIs' performance is similar in both eye models.

Figure 6 shows the same composition as **Figure 5** but with the 4.5-mm pupil. As we explained before, by increasing the pupil diameter, the influence of SA is higher on each eye model. On the one hand, a focal shift is produced, as already shown in **Figure 3c**, and on the other hand, the shape and height of the PSF are also affected. The comparison of the performance of both eye models for 4.5-mm pupil diameter shows more noticeable differences than those observed with the small pupil. In all cases, the LBME has more extended and asymmetrical halos than ZME. This is due to the influence of the SA and also, to the asymmetry of the LBME.

Finally, after the quantitative comparison of the merit functions for the three CIs, images of an optotype chart have been simulated. To this end, the PSFs obtained from ZEMAX were normalized to their respective maximum values and then weighed by the axial irradiances of each IC calculated in Section 3. These normalized and weighted PSFs were convolved with Landolt C optotypes corresponding to three different values of VA: 0.4 logMAR, 0.2 logMAR, and 0.0 logMAR.

Figures 7 and **8** show simulated images for 3.0 and 4.5-mm pupil diameters, respectively. For 3.0-mm pupil, it can be seen that, while the DCIs have a greater contrast than the SACI, the resolution of the three ICs is similar because the extension of the corresponding PSFs are almost the same (see **Figure 5**). At the near focus, it is observed that there is no focus on SACI, but in DCI 1.0 although the contrast is lower, the resolution is higher, and the halo is smaller than for DCI 1.6. When comparing the performance of the eye models, as already mentioned, there are no significant differences because when using a small pupil, the influence of high-order aberrations is minimal.

The simulated images for 4.5-mm pupil are shown in **Figure 8**. It can be seen that the differences between the eye models are most noticeable, mainly in the halos in near vision. The halos of the ZME are symmetrical, while those of the LBME are not. Despite these differences, the behavior of the three CIs maintains the same trend. The images at the foci for both DCIs are comparable in contrast

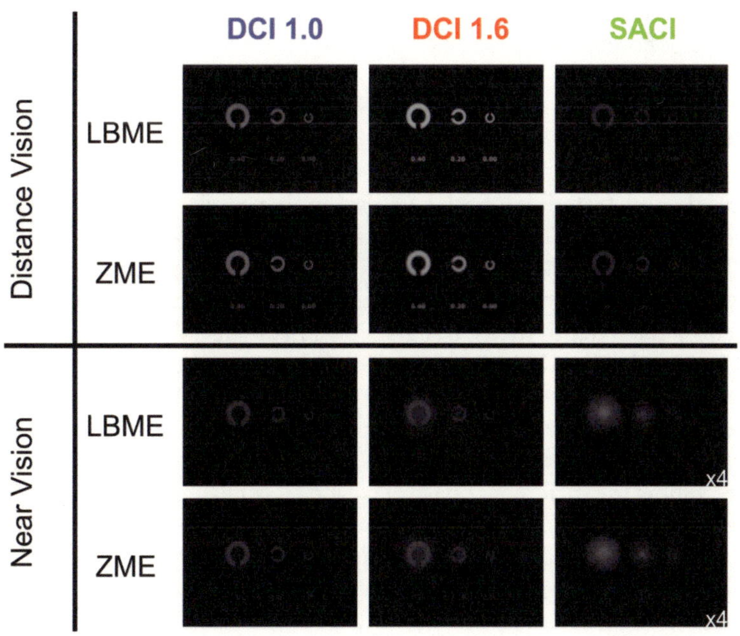

Figure 7.
Image simulation for 3.0 mm of pupil in distance vision (top) and near vision (bottom) for the three Cis in the two model eyes. The intensity of the image simulation of SACI in near vision has been multiplied 4×.

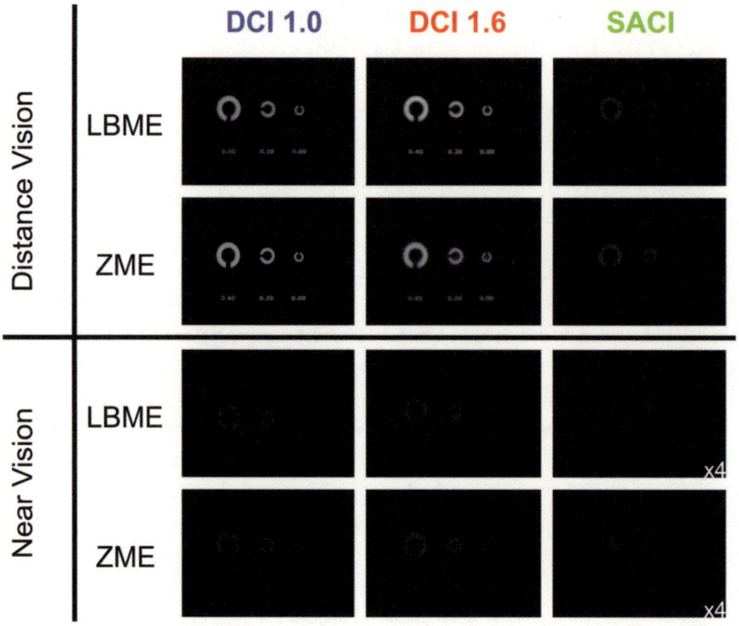

Figure 8.
Image simulation for 4.5 mm of pupil in distance vision (top) and near vision (bottom) for the three Cis in the two model eyes. The intensity of the image simulation of SACI in near vision has been multiplied 4×.

and definition. The reason that they resemble for distance vision is because with a large pupil, a part of the light that passes outside the inlays (external diameter of 4.15 mm) goes to the far focus. Therefore, the intensity ratio between the far and near foci increases and is similar for both DCIs.

By comparing both pupils, the best foci in the distance are for the DCIs with 4.5-mm pupil. The best focus for near vision is the DCI 1.0 since it presents more diffractive rings contributing to the near focus.

6. Conclusions

We have demonstrated that both DCI designs have a clearly bifocal profile due to their diffractive nature. Moreover, they also have better MTFs and AMTFs than the SACI (see **Figures 3** and **4**). The results presented in this chapter confirm the versatility of the DCI design because, opposite at what happens for the SACI which only presents a fixed depth focus, the distribution of the holes in the DCI can be modified (customized) to alter the relationship between the far- and near-vision foci. It is also verified that while for the 3.0-mm pupil, the three CIs have a similar behavior in both eye models, for 4.5 mm the differences are more due to the high-order aberrations of each model.

The PSFs show the differences between each CI for each situation; on the one hand, the DCIs generally show higher peaks and a high energy concentration and less extension of the PSF, but higher than SACI. These results can be clearly appreciated in the simulated images shown in **Figures 7** and **8**.

In summary, the DCI is a diffractive CI that combines the principle of operation of the small-aperture inlay, for the central hole, with the diffraction generated by the micro-holes in the ring to generate a focus in near vision. The micro-holes allow the construction of a single-piece inlay able to be inserted into the corneal stroma allowing nutrients to pass through it. The results show that the light throughput of the DCI is higher than the SACI, in addition to better PSFs and simulated images. In addition, we have demonstrated the differences that can be obtained in the results (light distribution between the foci) depending on the design of a DCI allowing to customize the CI for each patient based on their visual needs.

However, since it is a numerical simulation work with a ray tracing program, studies in an optical bench and clinical trials with contact lenses, which include the structure of the DCIs, should be carried out in the future.

Acknowledgements

Funding: Ministerio de Economía y Competitividad (DPI2015-71256-R); Generalitat Valenciana (PROMETEO/2019/048).

D. Montagud-Martínez and V. Ferrando acknowledge the financial support from the Universitat Politècnica de València, Spain (fellowships FPI-2016 and PAID-10-18, respectively).

D. Montagud-Martínez acknowledges the financial support from the Universitat Politècnica de València, Spain (fellowship FPI-2016).

Conflict of interest

The authors declare no conflict of interest.

Author details

Diego Montagud-Martínez[1*], Vicente Ferrando[1], Salvador Garcia-Delpech[2], Juan A. Monsoriu[1] and Walter D. Furlan[3]

1 Universitat Politècnica de València, Valencia, Spain

2 Hospital Universitari i Politècn ic La Fe, Valencia, Spain

3 Universitat de València, Valencia, Spain

*Address all correspondence to: diemonma@upvnet.upv.es

References

[1] Arlt EM, Krall EM, Moussa S, Grabner G, Dexl AK. Implantable inlay devices for presbyopia: The evidence to date. Clinical Ophthalmology. 2015;**9**:129-137

[2] Charman WN. Developments in the correction of presbyopia II: Surgical approaches. Ophthalmic & Physiological Optics. 2014;**34**:397-426

[3] Lindstrom RL, Macrae SM, Pepose JS, Hoopes PC. Corneal inlays for presbyopia correction. Current Opinion in Ophthalmology. 2013;**24**(4):281-287 Flexivue solo

[4] Limnopoulou AN, Bouzoukis DI, Kymionis GD, et al. Visual outcomes and safety of a refractive corneal inlay for presbyopia using femtosecond laser. Journal of Refractive Surgery (Thorofare, N.J.: 1995). 2013;**29**(1):12-18. DOI: 10.3928/1081597X-20121210-01

[5] Moarefi MA, Bafna S, Wiley W. A review of presbyopia treatment with corneal inlays. Opthamology and Therapy. 2017;**6**(1):55-65

[6] Garza EB, Gomez S, Chayet A, Dishler J. One-year safety and efficacy results of a hydrogel inlay to improve near vision in patients with emmetropic presbyopia. Journal of Refractive Surgery (Thorofare, N.J.: 1995). 2013;**29**(3):166-172. DOI: 10.3928/1081597X-20130129-01

[7] KAMRA Inlay Restores Reading Vision [Internet]. [cited 14 August 2019]. Available from: https://kamra.com/

[8] Yilmaz ÖF, Bayraktar S, Agca A, Yilmaz B, McDonald MB, van de Pol C. Intracorneal inlay for the surgical correction of presbyopia. Journal of Cataract & Refractive Surgery. 2008;**34**(11):1921-1927

[9] Wating GOVI. Correction of presbyopia with a small aperture corneal inlay. Journal of Refractive Surgery. 2011;**27**(11):842-845

[10] Vilupuru S, Lin L, Pepose JS. Comparison of contrast sensitivity and through focus in small-aperture inlay, accommodating intraocular lens, or multifocal intraocular lens subjects. American Journal of Ophthalmology. 2015;**160**(1):150-162

[11] Vukich JA, Durrie DS, Pepose JS, Thompson V, van de Pol C, Lin L. Evaluation of the small-aperture intracorneal inlay: Three-year results from the cohort of the US Food and Drug Administration clinical trial. Journal of Cataract & Refractive Surgery. 2018;**44**(5):541-556

[12] Gilchrist J, Pardhan S. Binocular contrast detection with unequal monocular illuminance. Ophthalmic and Physiological Optics. 1987;**7**(4):373-377

[13] Plainis S, Petratou D, Giannakopoulou T, Radhakrishnan H, Pallikaris IG, Charman WN. Small-aperture Monovision and the Pulfrich experience: Absence of neural adaptation effects. PLoS One. 2013;**8**(10):e75987. DOI: 10.1371/journal.pone.0075987

[14] Castro JJ, Ortiz C, Jiménez JR, Ortiz-Peregrina S, Casares-López M. Stereopsis simulating small-aperture corneal inlay and Monovision conditions. Journal of Refractive Surgery. 2018;**34**(7):482-488

[15] Machado FJ, Monsoriu JA, Furlan WD. Fractal light vortices. In: Chapter from the Book Vortex Dynamics and Optical Vortices. 1st ed. Intech; 2017. 257 p. DOI: 10.5772/66343

[16] Kipp L, Skibowski M, Johnson RL, Berndt R, Adelung R, Harm S, et al.

Sharper images by focusing soft X-rays with photon sieves. Nature. 2001;**414**:184-188

[17] Menon R, Gil D, Barbastathis G, Smith HI. Photon-sieve lithography. Journal of the Optical Society A. 2005;**22**(2):342-345

[18] Andersen G. Large optical photon sieve. Optics Letters. 2005;**30**(22):2976-2978

[19] Giménez F, Monsoriu JA, Furlan WD, Pons A. Fractal photon sieve. Optics Express. 2006;**14**(25):11958-11963

[20] Artal P. Handbook of Visual Optics, Volume One: Fundamentals and Eye Optics. 2nd ed. CRC Press; 2017. 437 p. ISBN 9781482237856DISEÑO

[21] Furlan WD, García-Delpech S, Udaondo P, Remón L, Ferrando V, Monsoriu JA. Diffractive corneal inlay for presbyopia. Journal of Biophotonics. 2017;**10**(9):1110-1114. DOI: 10.1002/jbio.201600320

[22] Liou HL, Brennan NA. Anatomically accurate, finite model eye for optical modeling. Journal of the Optical Society A. 1997;**14**(8):1684-1695

[23] Zemax OpticStudio Knowledgebase—Zemax [Internet]. [cited 14 August 2019]. Available from: https://customers.zemax.com/os/resources/learn/knowledgebase/zemax-models-of-the-human-eye

Section 2

Glaucoma and Blindness: Risk Assessment and Pathophysiology

Chapter 4

Intraocular Forced Convection Mechanism Defect as Probable Cause of Normal-Tension Glaucoma

Humberto D. Silva, Eduardo D. Silva, Maria Tamires D. Silva, Cristiana P. Dória and Cristiane P. Dória

Abstract

This paper describes several pathologies associated with pathological movements that can cause physical effort on the optic nerve and damage to vision. The accumulation of intraocular metabolic residues increases ocular globe mass and can change its position in the orbit, as well as increase the cornea and crystalline, accommodation resistance, in addition to being able to increase the aqueous humor output resistance. A series of discreet pathologies may result in optic nerve impairment: cyclotorsion and saccadic movement, position in the orbit, and increased intraocular pressure. The cyclotorsion movements can be stimulated by the superior visual field restriction, due to the metabolic residue accumulation in the light transmission regions of this visual field, preventing correct fusion of the images.

Keywords: binocular motion physiology, refraction error, ocular hypertension, retinal diseases, cataract, saccadic eye movements, photosensitive epilepsy, headache, anterior uveitis, cyclotorsion

1. Introduction

To recover a visual deficiency, the first author, who will be called the patient, began his research in 1996. The patient had no cataract, but had had eyelid ptosis in both eyes for over 10 years. He was wearing corrective lenses NV, OD +0.25 and OS +0.75, and had visual acuity OD 6/10 and OS 9/10 without corrective lenses when the first symptoms of presbyopia appeared. Thus, the patient was stimulated to look for a solution, since, besides hating the use of corrective lenses, he suffered from vision on the way home after using a computer for 4 hours in a row; by the time he arrived home, however, his vision was recovered. The patient assumed that this visual variation was associated to the degradation of the oculomotor movement. The strengthening of the oculomotor muscles was expected to control the quality of the visualized image. Exercises alternately focusing on near and far objects, called here the work, however, were interrupted due to recurrence of anterior uveitis in the left eye because of an unknown cause, 2 years after the second crisis. In this crisis, the patient delayed seeking professional help, and his intraocular pressure reached 40 mmHg. Many other crises have occurred. The patient was able to consult with an ophthalmologist before each uveitis crisis, when he felt a crisis coming on with pain in the left eye upper nasal position, perceived by pressing the eye with the eyelid closed. As the specialist consulted did not treat the uveitis as such, but only the associated pain, the patient began to use a drop of uveitis medicine one time in a day, and sometimes the next day, in order not to prejudice his health. In 2000, after working toward relaxation of the oculomotor musculature, the patient returned to the exercises. Around 5 years later, the patient began a search for more information in the literature, after visual perception of the light colors as lighter, and the dark, darker. This is a sign of a significant increase in intraocular transparency.

From 2009, the patient formed a study team, with the objective of gaining new knowledge and discussing the symptoms. Thus, in 2010, the works, initially empirical, passed to scientific form, with participation, in Paris, in the scientific conferences, sixth DSL and fourth ACE-X, with their respective publications [1, 2]. In 2011, authorized by the Universidade Federal de Pernambuco (UFPE) (Federal University of Pernambuco), the research group "Mass transfer in flexible porous medium" was created in the Conselho Nacional de Desenvolvimento Científico e Tecnológico (CNPq) (National Council for Scientific and Technological Development). The CNPq is an agency of the Ministério da Ciência, Tecnologia, Inovações e Comunicações (Ministry of Science, Technology, Innovation and Communications), of the Federal Government of Brazil. Physically, a flexible porous medium may be compared to a cleaning sponge but also serves as a model for demonstrating mass transfer movement by forced convection into the cornea, the lens, the trabecular meshwork, the retina, as well as in the muscles.

Currently the patient uses corrective lenses DV, OD -1.50 -1.25×85 and OS -2.75 -1.00×85, and presents visual acuity DV 20/400 OD and OD 20/400 and with corrective lenses 20/50 OU. In [3] it is shown that the prescribed corrective lens are not important for treatment evaluation of the elimination of intraocular metabolic residues.

This paper shows how ocular pathologies can physically affect the optic nerve, as it is known that some ocular pathologies are acquired as a result of an accumulation of dehydrated metabolic residues because of a deficiency in the intraocular mass transfer by forced convection [1–11]. The treatment of these pathologies is based on recovery of the intraocular metabolic residue by rehydration and drainage processes.

2. Nomenclature, function, and analysis

Visual field: Visual spatial array produces or reflects the visual rays of the image transmitted to the brain.

Right visual field (RVF): Visual spatial array that produces or reflects the visual rays of the image transmitted to the brain's left hemisphere.

Left visual field (LVF): Visual spatial array that produces or reflects the visual rays of the image transmitted to the brain's right hemisphere.

Central fixation point (P): The visual field point that is projected into the fovea centralis in both eyes.

Binocular visual field: The space region producing the projection visual rays image in the temporal retina.

Peripheral visual field: The space region producing the projection visual rays image in the nasal retina.

Visual axis: Imaginary straight line passing through the central fixation point and the fovea centralis or intersection of visual plane with vertical meridian plane.

Visual plane: Defined by the two visual axes.

Horizontal meridian plane: The ocular bulb intersection plane, in the horizontal meridian perimeter line.

Vertical meridian plane: The plane of intersection of the ocular bulb, in the perimeter line vertical meridian.

Rectus muscles: These maintain the central fixation point projection in the fovea centralis.

Superior oblique muscle: This controls the corneal accommodation to adjust the projected image on the nasal fovea horizontal meridian perimeter line to the image projected on the contralateral temporal fovea horizontal meridian perimeter line, admitted as fixed. It commands the forced convection system extrinsic muscle action. Its action includes an incyclotorsion physical effort.

Inferior oblique muscle: This has an excyclotorsive physical effort and is antagonistic to the superior oblique muscle physical effort, to avoid the pathological incyclotorsive movement.

Ciliary muscle: This controls lens accommodation to obtain the best-projected image on the temporal fovea and view objects at varying distances.

Corneal accommodation: The cornea curvature adaptation to compensate for the deformations of the conical projections through two distinct foci using image fusion.

Optic disc (OD): Oval region of the eye nasal retina without cones and rods.

Blind spot (BS): A visual field oval region that is projected onto the optical disc of ipsilateral eye.

Optical disc neural correspondent (NC): A visual field oval region, this is projected on the phototransducers, of the contralateral eye temporal retina, which has its periphery as the neural correlates of the phototransducers neural from optic disc periphery of the ipsilateral eye to the visual field.

Forced convection mechanism: The eye has two independent systems of forced convection: one under the extrinsic muscle action and the other under the intrinsic muscle action. The extrinsic muscles move the mobile mass in the cornea, trabecular meshwork, and retina, and the intrinsic muscles move the mobile mass in the lens and Schlemm's canal [4].

Iris: Main functions. Reduces the light diffusion in the projected image in the retina and prevents aqueous humor return when the pressure in the anterior chamber is greater than in the posterior one during the cornea accommodation process [2, 3]. After cataract surgery, there may be reflux of aqueous humor from the anterior chamber to the posterior chamber during the period of adaptation to the artificial lens, and metabolic residue contaminates the artificial intraocular lens causing posterior capsular opacification.

2.1 Main vision characteristics

Figure 1 shows a components schematic diagram necessary for image formation, image transmission to the brain, and how image fusion occurs. At the top of the diagram is shown the visual field. From this region, light rays are emitted or reflected to be projected into the retina. The projected image inversion projected onto the retina is a physical form of the selection of light rays that form the image of an object or body situated in the visual field. The physical principle can be best verified by a pinhole camera. The central fixation point "P" divides the visual field into the right (RVF) and left (LVF) visual fields, which are transmitted to the contralateral brain hemispheres. The visual field can also be divided into the binocular visual field, the region seen by both eyes, and the peripheral visual field, the region seen by one eye. Then, on the temporal retina, the image produced in the contralateral

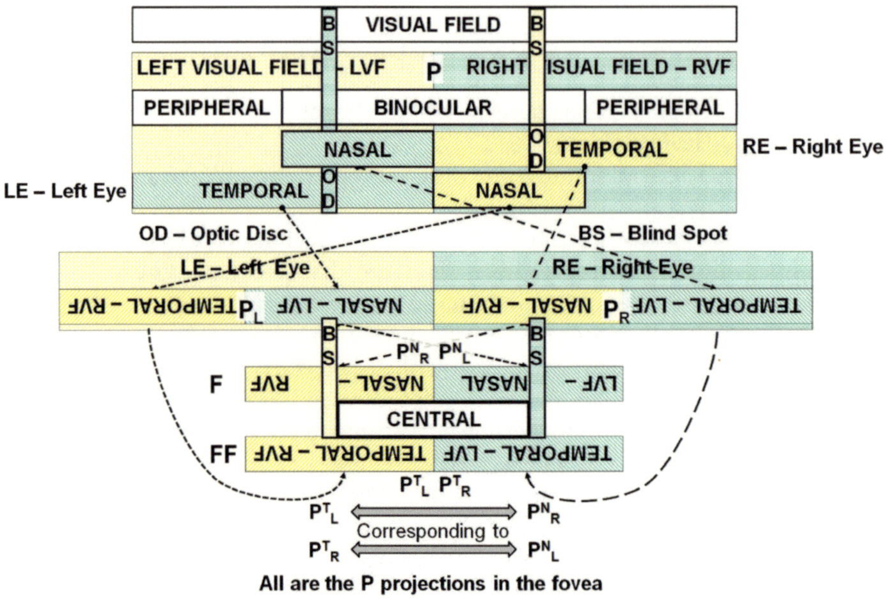

RETINA	CEREBRAL HEMISPHERE	CONTROL	MUSCLE	FUNCTION
Temporal	Ipsilateral P^T_R P^T_L	FF Focusing	Ciliary	Visual Focusing
		FF Fixation	Rectus	Visual Fixation
		Antagonistic	Inferior oblique	Torsional motion antagonist
Nasal	Contralateral P^N_R P^N_L	F Fusion	Superior oblique	Visual Fusion

Figure 1.
Main vision characteristics.

visual field (eye nasal visual field) is projected, and on the nasal retina, the image produced in the ipsilateral visual field (eye temporal visual field) is projected. The projected image to an optical disc region without photoreceptors cannot be transmitted to the contralateral cerebral hemisphere. The projected image in the temporal retina is transmitted to the brain's ipsilateral hemisphere, and the projected image in the nasal retina is transmitted to the brain's contralateral hemisphere.

2.2 Binocular vision physiology

In the summary, below, as shown in **Figure 1**, the binocular vision main controls are described. The projected image in the temporal retina is transmitted to the cerebral ipsilateral hemisphere, which controls the rectus muscles movement, to improve eyeball position fixation and controls the ciliary muscle movement to accommodate the lens and improve focusing. The image projected on the nasal retina is transmitted to the contralateral cerebral hemisphere, which controls the superior oblique muscle movement, changing the cornea curvature to adjust the projected image size in the nasal retina to the projected image in the contralateral temporal retina.

Figure 2 shows the fusion process of the retinal nasal image with the contralateral eye temporal image. Of course, a single movement by the oculomotor muscle reflects the movement of all the other muscles and consequently causes changes in these images. These changes, however, have not been taken into consideration here,

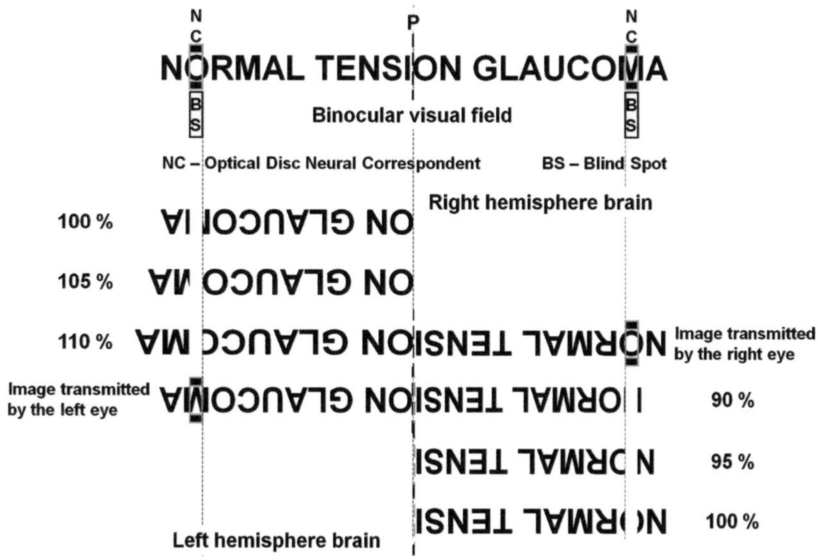

Figure 2.
Image fusions (superior oblique muscle action).

as to emphasize the action of the superior oblique muscle action on the nasal images received by the brain. In binocular vision, the "NC" and "BS" regions are coincident and have identical perimeter images. For example, if we take the written title of a work in the binocular visual field, three regions can be seen: the "P" fixation point, the "BS" regions that are projected in the ipsilateral eyes nasal retinas, and the "NC" regions that are projected in the contralateral eye temporal retinas (when the binocular visual gaze is in the lateral limit the nose profile protrudes through the ipsilateral dashed line). **Figure 2** shows how these images are transmitted to the brain. The image transmitted by the temporal retina is the reference image in the fusion of images, so it does not have primary changes related to the fusion of images. The image transmitted by the nasal retina is presented with an increase of 10% for the right eye and a 10% reduction for the left eye. In the brain, the neural region related to the optic disc (OD) region of the retina corresponds to the "BS" region of the visual field and is the corresponding neural region "NC." Note that the variation of 10% causes in the visual field the displacement of the "BS" regions to the left, so the two regions are not in the location shown in **Figure 2**. In the fusion of images, the brain commands the superior oblique muscle of the contralateral eye so as to adjust the projected image in the nasal retina to the projected image in the temporal retina of the ipsilateral eye. **Figure 2** shows the merger performed in two steps. Any change in the temporal image corresponds to a displacement of the "NC" region in the visual field. The image projected in the temporal retina is the main one because, in addition to being a reference in the fusion of the images, it is transmitted to the ipsilateral hemisphere to control the contralateral limbs and the movement of the ipsilateral eye. Given this, the reason for lateral dominance may be admitted as a genetic or acquired deficiency.

Lens accommodation and of the cornea are the two independent intraocular mass transfer movements, by forced convection. To eliminate metabolic residues without storing them, it is necessary to maintain the concentration of metabolic compounds uniform throughout the mobile mass, so that the simple draining of the mobile mass removes the metabolic residues without leaving accumulations. In order to standardize the concentration of metabolic residue produced, it is necessary to equalize the mobile mass movement in all intraocular regions. Over many years, these accumulated residues are agglutinated and form droplets that grow with the adjacent droplets to modify image projections on the retina and consequently modify the dimensions and position of the eyeballs as well as the ocular movements. Because of these ocular changes, the patient begins to suffer and to present the symptoms and signs of various ocular pathologies. As a result, the elimination of agglutinated residues through the anterior chamber can become lodged in the trabecular meshwork and increase the aqueous humor passage resistance, resulting in increased intraocular pressure.

2.3 Focusing, fixation, and fusion

Binocular vision is based on fixation by the eyes on an object of the visual field (rectus muscle action). To fix the eyes on an object, it is necessary that the eyes are able to focus the object (ciliary muscle action), so this action must be faster than the fixing action. When focusing and fixing on an object it, is necessary to adjust the binocular images to compensate, between them, for the distortions produced by the conical projections due to the horizontal distance between the eyes (superior oblique muscle action). Thus, action must be slower than the fixation action. In the appendix, a first-order linear model is used to analyze, by comparison, the rapidity effects among the changed muscular actions of state in the focalization, fixation, and fusion of the images, for binocular vision. Here, 0% is the initial state and 100% is the final state. The analytical equation that establishes the transition between the equilibrium states (initial and final) depends on the parameter τ (time constant). Thus, three time constants are required: τ_C (ciliary muscle), τ_R (rectus muscles), and τ_S (superior oblique muscle). For this, the relation among the time constants is given by Eq. (1).

$$\tau_C < \tau_R < \tau_S \tag{1}$$

3. Vision physiology, symptom, and sign analysis

Binocular motion physiology: In **Figure 3a** we have "F" as the fixation point in the visual field, as projected onto the fovea of the respective eyes. "I," the point of interest in the lateral visual field, has its projections on the nasal and temporal retinas of the respective ipsilateral and contralateral eyes. "M," the movable fixation point, maintains its projections on the fovea of the respective eyes as it moves along

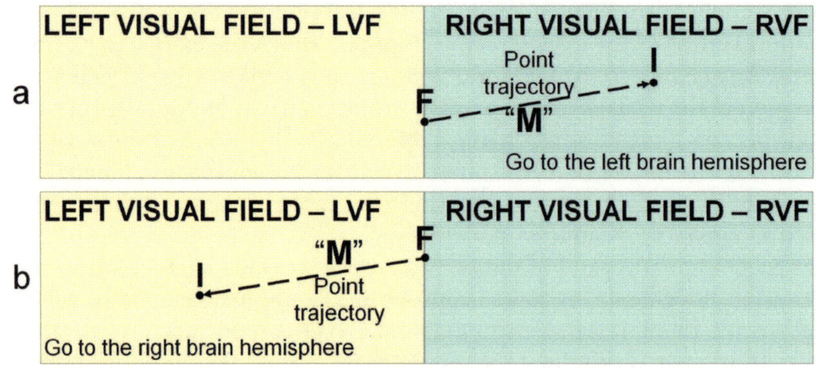

Figure 3.
Two possibilities of eye movements. (a) Eye shift in the right visual field. (b) Eye shift in the left visual field.

an visual field surface imaginary line, when the eyes travel the smallest angular displacement between the "F" and "I" points.

When the ocular direction shifts from point "F" to point "I," point "M," the contralateral eye visual axis intersection with the surface of the visual field (initially coincides with point "F"), is shifted to point "I." The "M" point moves across an imaginary line on the surface of the lateral visual field with the smallest angular displacement of the axial axis of the contralateral eye. In this trajectory, the contralateral eye maintains its focus at the "M" point because the ciliary accommodation time constant, τ_C, is much less than the ocular displacement time constant, τ_R (rectus muscles). Therefore, relative to the visual field laterality, the image projected on the contralateral ocular temporal retina is the primary image because it is the image used by the brain to control eye movement. The image projected on the nasal retina of the ipsilateral eye is the secondary image, because it is the image used by the brain to control the cornea accommodation movement, a slower movement, due to the time constant of the cornea accommodation, τ_S (superior oblique muscle), which is much longer than the ocular displacement time constant, τ_R (rectus muscles). Therefore, in this eye movement, the dominant eye is contralateral to the laterality of the "I" point visual field, and the auxiliary eye is ipsilateral because its movement depends on the fusion of the images to keep the projection onto its fovea, the "M" point.

On the return trajectory, **Figure 3b**, the current fixation point "F" is the previous "I" point, and the current interest point "I" is the previous "F" point; hence the current movable fixation point "M" will have an ipsilateral trajectory to the anterior trajectory of "M." Then, the dominant and auxiliary eyes will be contralateral in the anterior trajectory, so eye dominance is circumstantial.

Refraction error: Eyesight adaptation to dark is the common pathological symptom that precedes refractive error (see [3]). In 1619 Scheiner, *apud* [12], proved in his experiments, made with holes in a card, that an object is seen in each direction at a different distance. You can reproduce the effects perceived by Scheiner, by fixing the gaze on a distant object, through a pinhole in a paper pressed against the eyelid. When you move the paper without removing it from the eyelid, you can perceive the image of the object jumping from one position to another or moving its shape. The jump indicates the same pathology observed by Scheiner, and the change in form is another presentation of the same pathology [2]. This pathology can be acquired by the dehydrated accumulation of intraocular metabolic residues agglutinated in the form of drops. These drops form lenses that can produce overlapping images (causing blurred vision, floaters, monocular polyopia, and photopsia with and without photochromatic dispersion) and, depending on their transparency, make light transmission difficult. In the postoperative period of cataract surgery, patients report having a clearer view through the operated eye (greater light transmission in the artificial lens). Patients may report blurred vision and secretions released from the anterior surface of the cornea (corneal accommodation variation) and floaters (the metabolic mass stored in the lens prevented their viewing). In Ref. [2] the different symptoms of myopia, hypermetropia, astigmatism, and presbyopia are shown as visual disturbances of the same origin, the intraocular accumulation of dehydrated metabolic secretions.

Ocular hypertension: This can be caused by an imbalance in the production, concentration, and drainage of eye movable mass. Increased mass transfer resistance across the trabecular meshwork is an important impediment to aqueous humor drainage. Corneal accommodation movement failure hinders its mass transfer movement, thus being the major factor in the metabolic residue storage in the cornea [5]. The cornea stored metabolic residue elimination process consists in the movement of its curvature, in order to recover its healthy accommodation. In this process, the residues leave the two surfaces and are eliminated by dilution or suspension. On the anterior surface, the lacrimal fluid drags the residues, and on the posterior surface, the residues are dragged by the aqueous humor. If an important tear drag occurs when the patient is sleeping in the supine position, it may cause nostril obstruction, throat irritation, and hoarseness. Drainage of aqueous humor with suspended residues can impregnate the trabecular meshwork with the residues and increase resistance to outflow causing ocular hypertension. In the postoperative period of cataract surgery, the patient eliminates metabolic residues on both cornea surfaces, due to fusion of images and corneal accommodation; thus metabolic residues may impregnate the trabecular meshwork and cause ocular hypertension. It is possible, by a natural process, for the intraocular pressure return to its previous value.

Retinal mass transfer defect

- *Negative afterimage*: Common pathology in which retinal forced convection mechanism failure reduces the metabolic residue outflow may cause deposits in the choriocapillaris. The residue accumulation metabolic in the choriocapillaris makes it difficult for the retina's mobile mass to flow, thus increasing the time constant for the outflow to meet the new operating requirements. Then the phototransducers will take longer to react to color changes, and the observer will notice the complementary color during the transient state.

- *Retinal detachment*: Metabolic residues stored in the retina reduce its flexibility and create regions with different rigidity. The radius variation of retina curvature, due to fusion of the images, can cause physical efforts between the regions with different rigidity and cause its break, besides modifying the characteristics of the vitreous humor, due to the contact with the affected region.

- *Macular degeneration*: Transfer deficiency of retinal nutrients caused by metabolic residue accumulation leads to histotoxic hypoxia. Hypoxia stimulates angiogenesis and results in wet macular degeneration [6].

Lens mass transfer defect

- *Amblyopia*: The insufficient mechanism of forced convection of the lens prevents the healthy renewal of the moving mass in its interior, so the metabolic residue is agglutinated into particles and kept in suspension. The suspended particles refract, in diffused light, the incident light rays; thus the brain loses control over the ciliary muscle, for lack of clear image [5]. The amblyopic eye can project images through a small slit, because in this way the intraocular light scattering is reduced.

- *Cataract*: This pathology can be acquired by dehydrated accumulation of metabolic residue produced by the lens and agglutinated in droplet form. These droplets also cause refractive error that interferes with lens mass transfer movement control. As the metabolic residue is cloudy, its dehydration causes opacity (See [3, 8]). Cataract surgery extinguishes ciliary muscle movements and, consequently, affects the forced convective mass transfer mechanism in the Schlemm canal, which may cause metabolic residue accumulation that may increase intraocular pressure.

Pathological eye movements and related symptoms

- *Cyclotorsion* [13]: Common pathological movement resulting from the cornea accommodation difficulty. This pathology can produce movement perception in static images or graphic montages, make it difficult to count elements of an equal character set without the use of a pointer, and cause dizziness and nausea (incyclotorsion, excyclotorsion).

Saccadic eye movements: Common pathological movements caused by the metabolic residue accumulation stored in drops (forming small lenses with different transparencies, sizes, and viscosities) in the cornea and lens [7]. The rectus muscles perform these movements and are antagonistic to the instantaneous displacements of image projection on the temporal retina caused by the change of droplets in the passage of light rays. See Scheiner's experiment, *apud* [12]. Vergence eye movements are only observed if saccadic movements exist.

- *Photosensitive epilepsy*: This is triggered by resonant neural impulses caused by visual stimuli [2]. Resonant impulses may be formed by antagonistic responses to eye control stimuli. Antagonistic responses can be constructed by image transmissions through alternations between the metabolic residue droplets stored in the cornea and lens. Droplet alterations may be produced as result of lens accommodation. Then, when the accommodation process begins, the droplets are physically repositioned causing changes in the size and position of the image projection on the retina, which can be interpreted by the brain as a change in distance from the fixation point. The change in distance forces the brain to send a new neural stimulus to accommodate the lens, in many cases antagonistic, modifying the position of the droplets. Frequent recurrence of these actions can trigger resonant neural impulses. Therefore, the eye that holds the interest point in its temporal retina controls the movement of the eyes, as shown in *binocular motion physiology*. But, because refractive error occurs in both eyes, the point of interest may either be projected on the temporal retinas or on both nasal retinas. (Note: in normal vision, the point of interest is projected on the temporal retina of one eye and on the nasal of the other.) Projecting the interest point on the temporal retinas causes the brain to generate conflicting commands in both eyes. By projecting the interest point on the nasal retinas, the brain loses its command sense.

- *Anterior uveitis*: This may be caused by superior oblique muscle overuse. It is symptomatically characterized by pain caused by a slight pressure on the muscle through the eyelid. In the patient, this always occurred in the left eye upper nasal region.

- *Pterygium*: Excessive movement of the rectus muscle may cause this, in order to compensate for a jump in image as a result of the formation of metabolic residual drops as observed by Scheiner's experiment, *apud* [12].

- *Fixation instability*: This is easily observed in a dark environment, through the light path projected on the retina resulting from the head oscillatory rotation when the gaze fixed on a luminous LED. Motion perception in still images [14], stereoscopic depth, as well as the need for a pointer to count a large set of equal characters are some of the symptoms resulting from this pathology. Imperfections of the anterior surface of the cornea can be an important indicator of this serious pathology.

- *Tendinitis*: The occurrence was observed during manual activities with the near fixation point, during the removal of intraocular metabolic residues; however, the pathology may be combined with the *fixation instability*.

- *Disequilibrium*: This may occur because of pathological cyclotorsional movement. It may or may not be discreet. It can even form a dry callus [3].

- *Bruxism*: When trying to eliminate binocular diplopia, the patient may feel forced to contract other muscles (head and limbs). Because the jaw is the only moving bony part of the head, the patient may, "as an aid," contract the chewing muscles during eye correction exercises. Repetition of this contraction during sleep may be the cause of the condition.

- *Headache*: In eye treatment, the patient should not use analgesic. Headache is a nerve compression symptom that can be treated with eye alignment, and the pain disappears immediately [7].

- *Superior eyelid ptosis*: May be voluntarily stimulated to reduce light entry through the cornea because of intraocular light diffusion [4, 11].

- *Auditory perception*: In 2003, in the routine examination, the patient was first diagnosed with the absence of 6 kHz frequency perception in the left ear, and then the patient noticed the ipsilateral permanent presence of noise. Several otorhinolaryngologists have examined, and no cause has been diagnosed. The patient realizes that the noise intensity varies during eye exercises and there are occasions when the noise disappears [3].

4. Results analysis

4.1 Storage and evacuation processes of intraocular metabolic residue

This paper presents four states of metabolic residue accumulation during the process of stimulating eye movements for rehydration and drainage. In the first state, metabolic residues form droplet agglutinations without significant variations of their forms. In the second state, metabolic residue forms agglutinations in droplets with important variations in their forms. In the third state, metabolic residues are in suspension. In the fourth state, metabolic residues form films impregnated in the intraocular layers.

In the first state, the residue droplets maintain their different dimensions (constant volume), shapes, refractions, opacities, and high viscosities, so they form small lenses that can project the same image to the retina in different regions, with different dimensions, shapes, and intensities. This pathology was first observed in Scheiner's experiments in 1619, *apud* [12]. The drops, depending on their positions and shapes, in relation to incident light can cause chromatic scattering. The moving medium circulation between the drops can rehydrate them and transfer them to the second state.

In the second state, the droplets of the residues keep their different volumes fixed but vary their dimensions, shapes, opacities, and viscosities, so they form small, variable refractive lenses that can project radial beams with periodic expansions and reductions. These movements have different frequencies, depending on the movements of different drops, and can cause chromatic dispersion, depending on their shapes and positions, in relation to the incident light. Depending on the circulation of the moving medium, there may be dehydration of the droplets, and they may lose their movement, that is, move to the first state, or there may be rehydration of the droplets, and they may pass to the third state in suspension.

In the third state, the metabolic residues are in suspension. The residues in suspension diffuse the intraocular light. Intraocular diffusion can cause visual discomfort if there is pupillary constriction, a tendency in older people. Stimulated mydriasis enhances this discomfort. Miosis and prolonged stay of suspended residues stimulate upper eyelid ptosis to reduce the opening for light penetration. Depending on the circulation of the mobile medium, the suspended residues may become dehydrated or rehydrate. If dehydrated, the viscosity increases and is agglutinated into droplets, passing to a second state (droplets in different shapes). If rehydrated, the viscosity is reduced and eliminated through the nasal and oral routes or by the trabecular mesh. Elimination through the nasal and oral routes may cause tearing, burning in the cornea, obstruction of the nostril, and mild inflammation in the throat. The trabecular route can obstruct and increase intraocular pressure. From this state there may be migration to the first state through thin-layer deposits on the cornea or lens layers. This is the initial state of the metabolic residue storage process as well as the final state in the drainage process, depending on the moving medium circulation.

In the fourth state, the metabolic residues are stored as films in the intraocular layers. Symptoms can be perceived through the visualized sinuosities while moving the eye, observing a flat visual field. The mere circulation of the mobile medium is insufficient to rehydrate the metabolic residue films and transform them into aqueous suspension of the third state. To rehydrate the metabolic residue in this state requires an impulsive movement of the mobile mass.

The four states of intraocular storage are always present, but there are alternations between symptoms, although they may appear together. Thus visual acuity depends on the state predominance, the amount, and the way metabolic residue is accumulated. The rehydration exercises and drainage of metabolic residue depend on the symptoms.

4.2 Influence of bilateral upper eyelid blepharoplasty on cornea curvature

Table 1 shows, chronologically, the patient's intraocular pressure, on several dates, and, in addition, important information to show the situations experienced by the patient during the time while drainage work of intraocular metabolic residues was being analyzed. To renew the driver's license using corrective lenses in February 2014, the patient had to exercise his left eye for 10, 2 days apart, and then rest for 2 days, because there was little chance of approval, mainly because of the left eye. On the day of the exam, the left eye was fine, but the contralateral eye was in minimal approval condition. When an eye improves, the contralateral worsens. Five years later, in March 2019, the patient's driver's license was renewed with corrective lenses without any special attention, but 133 days later the patient's acuity was assessed with DV 20/50 OR, wearing corrective lenses. Visual acuity is not an important parameter to assess the drainage status of accumulated intraocular metabolic residue.

The patient noticed that his eyelid opening was compromised by corneal topography in April 2016, **Figure 4a**. The patient had never worn contact lenses. In May 2017 a bilateral upper blepharoplasty was performed. **Table 1** shows the highest pressure in the series was recorded in June, 2017, 49 days after surgery. 135 days later, lower intraocular pressure values were recorded. Upper blepharoplasty allows the light incidence in the region hidden by the upper eyelid ptosis and stimulates rehydration of metabolic residue stored in the region hidden by upper eyelid ptosis. Rehydration of a large volume of stored residue causes significant increase in drainage of metabolic residue through the oral and nasal routes, as well as through the trabecular meshwork. Intense passage of residue through the trabecular meshwork may obstruct the passage of aqueous humor and increase pressure. With the continuity of the exercises, obstruction can be removed from the trabecular meshwork and intraocular pressure reduced. Increased intraocular pressure should be observed in many patients after cataract surgery. Cataract reduces the light incidence on the retina and favors metabolic residue accumulation. A cataract surgery allows a higher light incidence in the retina, thus contributing to the rehydration

Pachymetry - 0.542 mm OD, 0.544 mm OS			
Calendar date	**IOP mmHg OD**	**IOP mmHg OS**	**Observation**
November 28, 2007	18	17	Uveitis OS Discreet PSC OU
October 31, 2008	16	16	Lens id.
April 27, 2009	16	16	Lens id.
November 30, 2009	16	15	Incipient cataract PSC OU Little most evident OS
August 30, 2010	17	14	Cataract id.
December 21, 2011	---	---	Uveitis OS
February 14, 2012	16	16	Cataract (+) OD, (+/++) OS
February 24, 2014	**---**	**---**	**Eye exam for new driver's license**
July 14, 2014	16	14	Cataract (+/++) OD, (++) OS
April 9, 2015	14	14	Cataract id.
September 14, 2015	17	16	Cataract id. (OS increased)
March 10, 2016	16	14	Cataract (++) OU (PSC OE)
April 5, 2016	**---**	**---**	**1st corneal topography**
September 29, 2016	16	14	Cataract (++) PSC OU (OS increased)
May 8, 2017	**---**	**---**	**Upper eyelid blepharoplasty - OU**
June 26, 2017	18	17	Cataract id.
September 4, 2017	**---**	**---**	**2nd corneal topography**
November 9, 2017	15	14	Cataract id.
March 5, 2018	**---**	**---**	**3rd corneal topography**
October 23, 2018	**---**	**---**	**4th corneal topography**
November 29, 2018	15	15	Cataract id.
March 18, 2019	**---**	**---**	**Eye exam for new driver's license**
July 29, 2019	15	15	Cataract (++) OD, (+++) OS, (OD increased) VA DV 20/400 OD, 20/400 DS With corrective lens 20/50 OU

Table 1.
Chronological presentation of medical examinations and surgery.

of an important volume of metabolic residue that can obstruct the trabecular meshwork and increase intraocular pressure. Since cataract surgeries and upper blepharoplasty are not followed by orthoptic exercises, in the postoperative period, it is important to develop a trabecular meshwork cleaning procedure to resolve cases in which intraocular pressure does not return to preoperative levels. Intraocular pressure should always be evaluated during residue drainage work, as well as in the postoperative period of cataract surgery and upper blepharoplasty.

Figure 4 shows, in four corneal topographies, the evolution of the anterior corneal surface curvature recovery, produced by the rehydration and drainage exercises of intraocular metabolic residues. The rehydration and drainage of intraocular metabolic residue can solve different pathologies related to anterior surfaces of the cornea. Although not the best way to evaluate the eyelid opening, this was the way available to the authors, in search of parameters that could evaluate the evolution of the work. The ocular region was recorded in the same laboratory on the dates presented in **Table 1** and **Figure 4**. The diameters, horizontal and vertical, were found for each mapping, in relation to their own scales. **Figure 4** shows, with dashed lines, how scales and diameters were evaluated. **Table 2** shows that the horizontal diameters of the two eyes did not show significantly different percentages (OD 14.3%,

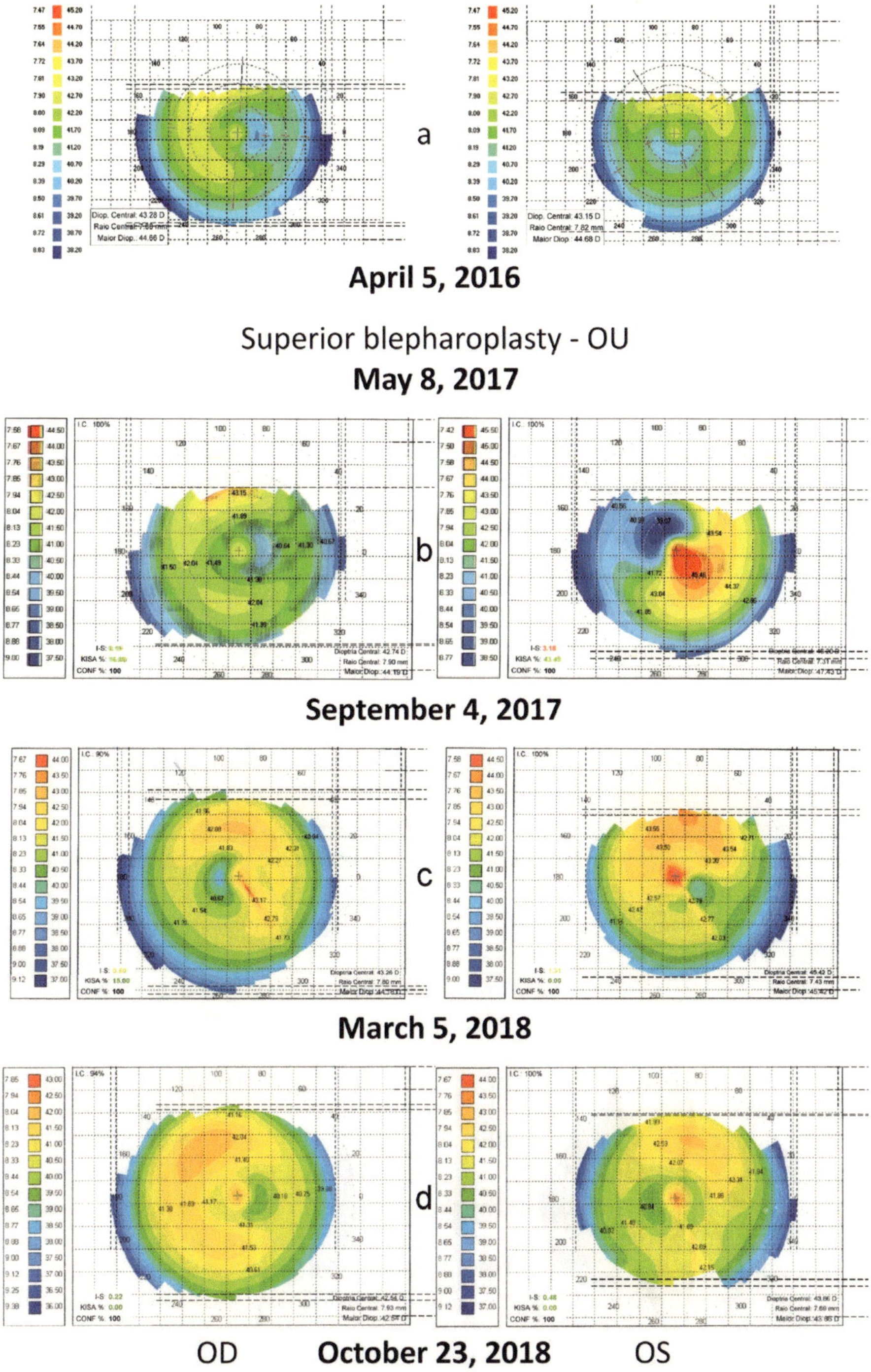

Figure 4.
Four corneal topography exams from the same patient. (a) On April 5, 2016 (before superior blepharoplasty - OU, on May 8, 2017). (b) On September 4, 2017. (c) On March 5, 2018. (d) On October 23, 2018.

month / year		a - 4 / 2016		b - 9 / 2017		c - 3 / 2018		d - 10 / 2018	
Eye	Position	Ø	ε	Ø	ε	Ø	ε	Ø	ε
OD	HORIZ	9,85	15,8%	10,07	13,9%	9,87	15,7%	10,02	14,3%
	VERT	6,91	34,8%	6,91	34,8%	8,92	15,8%	8,39	20,9%
OS	HORIZ	9,27	20,8%	9,74	16,8%	9,81	16,2%	9,89	15,5%
	VERT	6,75	36,3%	7,02	33,8%	7,54	28,9%	7,39	30,2%
Corneal diameter reference [6]				HORIZ	11,7			VERT	10,6

Table 2.
Diameters and errors relative to a pattern.

OS 15.5%) but the vertical diameters of the two eyes show significantly different percentages (OD 20.9%, OS 30.2%), that is, their evolution had not yet stabilized. The vertical diameter of both eyes exposed to the instrument was reduced because of simultaneous eyelid ptosis. The percentage error was calculated using as default the values cited in [6]. The percentage value is a referential error, serving only to compare the respective eye diameters. As such, the vertical diameter of the left eye is still far from the dimension of the collateral eye, i.e., the vertical limits had not yet fully recovered. The evolution shown in **Figure 4** shows the need for orthoptic exercises after upper eyelid blepharoplasty to recover eyelid opening and probably after cataract surgery.

4.3 Current state of intraocular cleansing

Although the results presented do not seem encouraging, there are interpretations that minimize the apparent divergence of the successful progress of the work. At the beginning of the study, the patient had presbyopia, had had eyelid ptosis in both eyes for over 15 years, and had no cataract. Blepharoplasty in both eyes was performed in 2017, when the cataract was at an advanced stage. This shows that the patient spent 17 years trying to rehydrate and drain metabolic residue with serious upper visual field constraints [8]. That is, the patient did not have the opportunity to recover the mechanisms of intraocular mass transfer by forced convection and, as a result, developed cataracts. Cataract is the storage of dehydrated metabolic residue in the lens due to a defect in the mechanism of mass transfer in the lens by forced convection [3, 8]. Even so, it was possible to recover from some pathologies described in the works [9, 14]. Rehydration of intraocular metabolic residue is a slow and difficult process to perform because it does not require any external physical effort or any agent that reduces the viscosity of dehydrated residue. It does, however, require changes in habits and a lot of sleep, and success may depend on acquired physiology, congenital and hereditary, as well as diet, among others. The intermediate stages of intraocular cleaning indicate that rehydration of the concentrated metabolic residue reduces its concentration and viscosity due to the increase in mobile mass added to the stagnant residue. Thus increasing its stagnant volume may represent an increase in the extent of the stagnant area, resulting in cataract evolution, if any, but with lower density and viscosity, which are not evaluated. Due to the rehydration and drainage process, the patient showed signs in the cycle of improving and degrading visual acuity. The patient did not have access to any test that evaluated the storage of intraocular metabolic residue. **Figure 4** shows the evolution of corneal curvature in several tests. The patient has already overcome two pathologies, dark adaptation, for which there is no measurement standard and can read a text right after looking at the sun. It is important to know that activities in the dark stimulate rehydration of intraocular metabolic residue (sleeping in the dark), fixation instability favors dehydration of intraocular metabolic residue, and eyelid ptosis impairs the mechanism of intraocular mass transfer by forced convection. It is worth noting that headache and its immediate recovery through eye alignment, without medication, are symptoms of suffering caused in the oculomotor support system of the eyeball and an important sign of displacement in its support base, due to the disposition intraocular storage of metabolic residues.

5. Conclusion

With much simplification, the eye can be described as having three power supplies and four excretory paths, controlled by two forced convection systems [10]. There are three sources of food: tear fluid (feeds the corneal epithelium and excretes through the nasal and mouth cavities as well as the digestive system), aqueous humor (feeds the lens and corneal stroma and excretes through the venous system), and through Bruch's membrane (the circulatory system feeds and excretes the retina). There are two systems of forced convection, the intrinsic muscles (the crystalline and Schlemm canal) and the extrinsic muscles (cornea, trabecular mesh, and retina), which drive mass transfer. The physical properties of a cleaning sponge can be used as a metaphor for four greatly simplified mass transfer models. The four adaptations are these: a cleaning sponge to represent bidirectional movements on its sides, for the feeding and excretion of the lens; a cleaning sponge with its closed sides, to represent the bidirectional movements on its two other sides for feeding and excretion of the retina (Bruch's membrane) [6]; a cleaning sponge with closed sides to represent the unidirectional passage on both sides for the passage of aqueous humor and metabolic residue (trabecular meshwork) [1, 11]; and finally, two cleaning sponges, juxtaposed to closed flat surfaces, to represent bidirectional movements on their free sides for feeding and excretion of the epithelium and corneal stroma (epithelium, Bowman's membrane, and stroma) [1, 6]. Intraocular metabolic residues are stored when mass transfer mechanisms are insufficient to maintain constant, concentration, and agitation of dissolved or suspended metabolic residue components in the moving mass. An insufficiency of these mechanisms causes the mobile mass to stagnate in both forced convection systems and to store the metabolic residue due to dehydration. Dehydrated residues are stored simultaneously in the cornea, trabecular mesh, Schlemm's canal, lens, and retina. Vicious and frequent habits can cause mobile mass stagnation.

Metabolic residue is released if there is a physical work of forced convection systems capable of excreting concentrated metabolic residue in solution or suspension in the mobile medium. The release of fixed metabolic residue depends on its rehydration to transform it into a solution or suspension. The cornea, trabecular mesh, lens, Schlemm's canal, and retina simultaneously excrete accumulated residues. Orthoptic exercises can stimulate the physical effort to excrete metabolic residue, as well as rehydrate the fixed residues; these, however, cause sleep. Cataract surgery stimulates the forced convection system because it unbalances the efforts of the extrinsic muscle due to increased light transmission and change in refractive power resulting from intraocular lens implantation. Therefore, postoperative symptoms caused by cataract surgery are similar to those caused by orthoptic exercises that excrete intraocular metabolic residue.

When stimulated, stored metabolic residues can be rehydrated and simultaneously expelled from all intraocular regions. The accumulated metabolic residues in the corneal epithelium can be expelled through the cavities, nasal and mouth, as well as through the digestive system. Through the nasal cavity, they can plug up the nostrils as well as become dehydrated and form a deposit in the nasal passages. Through the oral cavity, they can be expelled but, even without fever, can cause cough and inflammation of the throat and vocal cords, which makes swallowing difficult and often produces a hoarse or muffled voice. Through the digestive system there is nothing observed. Accumulated metabolic residue in the corneal, crystalline, and retinal stroma can be expelled through the venous system and cause slight body aches (feeling unwell, malaise) without fever. Corneal and crystalline residues cross the anterior chamber, trabecular meshwork, and Schlemm's canal before reaching the venous system. In addition to these symptoms, there may be the production of tears and headache. The production of tears is linked to cleansing and may be a photoneural perception of impeding light transmission across the anterior surface of the cornea. A headache may be linked to physical exertion between the Zinn ring and the eyeball because the most efficient treatment is the alignment of the eyes to a fixation point. This alignment can correct the diopter difference between the eyes and acts much faster than the use of analgesic; if delayed, its application impairs its efficiency. Patients after cataract surgery also eliminate intraocular metabolic residue, so they should have the same symptoms, depending on the eliminated mass. However, symptoms may appear only 2 months after surgery, because metabolic residues rehydration is a slow process. On the other hand, the slight body aches do not last more than a day, but throat inflammation can last up to 5 days. Under these circumstances and without fever, if the patient ever seeks medical attention, it is not likely to return to the ophthalmologist unless the patient receives guidance.

The stored intraocular residues simultaneously cause some physical and symptomatic pathologies. Among the major ocular pathologies are the increase in eye mass and volume, and, consequently, the eyeball changes the shape, inertia moment, position in the eye socket, refractive disposition and error in intraocular light transmission, dislocation of its mass center, saccadic movements, cyclotorsion, fixation instability, and increased intraocular pressure. Refractive disposition and error in intraocular light transmission are consequences of the formation of metabolic residue droplets. Error in intraocular light transmission causes error in image transmission. Error in image transmission is image refraction in different dimensions, intensity, and locations when there is slight variation in lens accommodation or visual axis angular displacement. This pathology was verified in Scheiner's experiments in 1619, *apud* [12]. In response, to maintain the fixation point on the fovea, the rectus muscles receive a compensatory movement impulse, in the opposite direction to the unwanted displacement of image projection on the retina, which results in saccadic movement. Importantly, the saccadic pathological movement occurs in conjunction with two other pathologies, cyclotorsion and fixation instability, which can aggravate the consequences. Then the initial thrust and final deceleration of saccadic movement occurs in a structurally unbalanced system, so it can produce physical effort between the attachment points of the eyeball. The eyeball has three fixation points on the superior orbital fissure (posterior orbit), the trochlea of superior oblique, and maxillary bone (origin of the inferior oblique muscle). Frequent acceleration and deceleration of saccadic movement can cause frequent and important impulsive physical efforts in the anteroposterior axis and in the opposite direction, causing frequent variations in intraocular pressure. Frequent impulsive physical efforts and variations in intraocular pressure can slowly damage the optic nerve. If this situation is combined with the patient's high intraocular pressure, it would be very difficult to control the pressure alone by reducing the production of aqueous humor.

Acknowledgements

The English text of this paper has been revised by Sidney Pratt, Canadian, MAT (The Johns Hopkins University), RSAdip-TESL (Cambridge University). There was no public or private financial participation for publication in this work.

Appendix

A. Dynamic comparison of the state change agility between the activities of focusing, fixation, and images fusion

Figure 5 shows three graphs of Eq. (2), which is the analytical solution of state change in a first-order linear model. The graphs were obtained by replacing the time constant (τ) by the time constants (τ_C, τ_R, and τ_S) according to Eq. (3). The relation was defined from the numerical analysis compatibility, associated with the agility for object visualization.

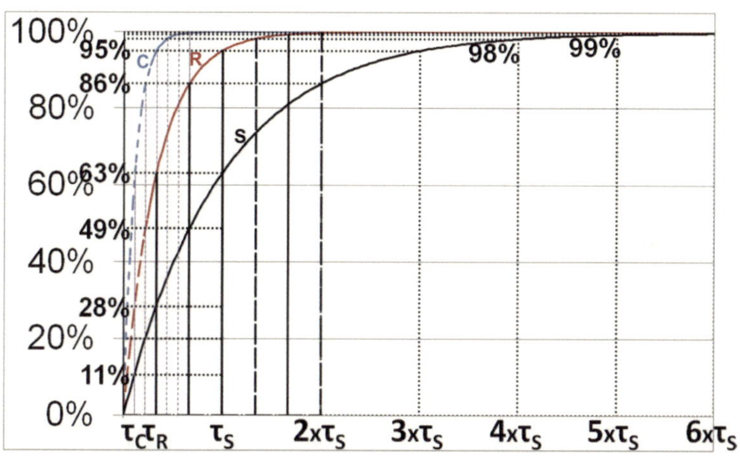

Figure 5.
Muscle contraction percentage graph, Eq. (2), (C) Ciliary muscle contraction (time constant τ_C). (R) Rectus muscle contraction (time constant τ_R). (S) Superior oblique muscle contraction (time constant τ_S).

$$f(t) = 100 \times (1 - e^{-t/\tau}) \quad (2)$$

$$3\tau C = \tau R = \tau S/3 \quad (3)$$

A.1 Analysis of the relationship $\tau_C = \tau_R/3$

Voluntary action, in order to observe an object of interest, requires the movement of the eyes toward it, under the rectus muscles control (τ_R). For this, it is necessary, in the first place, to focus on the object (τ_C) at the moment of its projection in the fovea. Therefore, focalization agility is then considered to be three times higher than fixation agility. The effect of the variation of the projection of the image on the retina, due to the accommodation of the lens, occurs more rapidly than the effect of the angular displacement of the eyeball, because the amount of mass displaced by the eyeball is much larger than the amount of mass that is moved to crystalline accommodation. Graph 3 shows that at time $t = \tau_C = \tau_R/3$, the focus had completed 63% of the work, while the displacement is 28%. That is, the numerical result is compatible with the associated analysis between the focus and fixation agility.

A.2 Analysis of the relationship $\tau_R = \tau_S/3$

People who have the perfect vision feel safer with binocular viewing than with monocular viewing. However, it is necessary that there is the nasal image fusion with the contralateral eye temporal image. In this way, the brain corrects the conical deformations caused by the distance between the eyes foci and uses twice as many neurotransmitters to interpret the received image, producing mathematically more than twice the accuracy than obtained with the monocular visualization. However, when the distance between the foci of the eyes is negligible in relation to a distant object under observation, the accuracy between the binocular and monocular visualizations is negligible; however, it is necessary to always use the binocular visualization to avoid habitual use of the same eye and thus stimulate ocular dominance.

Fusion of the images is the last step in the binocular visualization process, i.e., when the eyes are concluding their targeting on to the fixation point, fusion of images is at its beginning. Based on this, it was concluded that the time constant of the cornea accommodation (τ_S) is equal to three times the time constant for the eye fixation in the direction of the object (τ_R). Graph 3 shows that at time $t = \tau_R = \tau_S/3$, the fixation has 63% of the work completed, while the image fusion is 28%; that is, the numerical result is compatible with the associated analysis between the agility of the fixation and the accommodation of the cornea. Fusing images stabilizes the eye fixation direction.

Author details

Humberto D. Silva[1*], Eduardo D. Silva[1], Maria Tamires D. Silva[2], Cristiana P. Dória[2] and Cristiane P. Dória[2]

1 Universidade Federal de Pernambuco, Recife, Brazil

2 Independent Professional, Recife, Brazil

*Address all correspondence to: hdoria@ufpe.br

References

[1] Silva HD, Dória LCP, Dória CP, Dória CP, Silva MCTD, Silva HD Jr, et al. Nutrients and metabolic secretions transfer in cornea. Defect and Diffusion Forum. 2011;**312-315**:737-742. DOI: 10.4028/www.scientific.net/DDF.312-315.737

[2] Silva HD, Dória LCP, Dória CaP, Dória CeP, Silva MCTD, Silva HD Jr, et al. Simulation of the errors of refraction in the human eye. In: Öchsner A, da Silva LFM, Altenbach H, editors. Analysis and Design of Biological Materials and Structures. Advanced Structured Materials Book Series V. 14. Berlin, Heidelberg: Springer: 2012. p. 185-185. DOI: 10.1007/978-3-642-22131-6_15

[3] Silva HD, Silva ED, Silva MTD, Dória CP, Dória CP. Analysis of the disturbances caused by intraocular forced convection mechanism failure. In: Zilfyan A, editor. Difficulties in Cataract Surgery. London: IntechOpen; 2018. pp. 45-64. DOI: 10.5772/intechopen.72248

[4] Silva HD, Silva ED, Silva MTD, Dória CP, Dória CP. Movimento oculomotor e algumas patologias. In: Maravieski SP, editor. Teorias e Métodos da Biofísica book. Ponta Grossa (PR): Atena Editora; 2019. pp. 36-42. Available from: https://www.atenaeditora.com.br/wp-content/uploads/2019/03/E-book-Teorias-e-Metodos-da-Biofisica-2.pdf

[5] Silva HD, Dória LCP, Dória CaP, Dória CeP, Silva MCTD, Silva HD Jr, et al. Analysis of failure mechanism of forced convection in the cornea of the human eye. In: Öchsner A, da Silva LFM, Altenbach H, editors. Analysis and Design of Biological Materials and Structures. Advanced Structured Materials Book Series V. 14. Berlin, Heidelberg: Springer: 2012. p. 217-226. https://doi.org/10.1007/978-3-642-31470-4_16

[6] Silva HD, Silva ED, Dória LCP, Dória CP, Dória CP, Silva MCTD, et al. Forced convection mechanism failure in the eye can cause macular degeneration. Defect and Diffusion Forum. 2013;**334-335**:230-234. DOI: 10.4028/www.scientific.net/DDF.334-335.230

[7] Silva HD, Silva ED, Dória LCP, Dória CP, Dória CP, Silva MCTD, et al. Forced convection mechanism failure in the eye can cause cataract. Defect and Diffusion Forum. 2013;**334-335**:225-229. DOI: 10.4028/www.scientific.net/DDF.334-335.225

[8] Silva HD, Silva ED, Silva MTD, Dória CP, Dória CP. Consequences of upper visual field restriction. Brazilian Journal of Development. 2019;**5**(8):11288-11293. DOI: 10.34117/bjdv5n8-011

[9] Silva HD, Dória LCP, Dória CP, Dória CP, Silva MCTD, Silva HD Jr, et al. Mass transport mechanism in the retina of the human eye. Defect and Diffusion Forum. 2012;**326-328**:18-23. DOI: 10.4028/www.scientific.net/DDF.326-328.18

[10] Silva HD, Silva ED, Dória CP, Silva MTD, Dória CP. Forced convection intraocular system modeling. Brazilian Journal of Development. 2019;**5**(7):10541-10551. DOI: 10.34117/bjdv5n7-200

[11] Silva HD, Dória LCP, Dória CaP, Dória CeP, Silva MCTD, Silva HD Jr, et al. Simulation of variation of intraocular pressure. In: Öchsner A, da Silva L, Altenbach H, editors. Characterization and Development of Biosystems and Biomaterials. Advanced Structured Materials Book Series V. 29. Berlin, Heidelberg: Springer: 2012. p. 235-253. Available from: https://link.springer.com/chapter/10.1007%2F978-3-642-31470-4_18

[12] Werner L, Trindade F, Pereira F, Werner L. Physiology of accommodation and presbyopia. Arquivos Brasileiros de Oftalmologia. 2000;**63**(6):487-493. DOI: 10.1590/S0004-27492000000600011

[13] Bicas HEA, Jorge AAH. Oftalmologia: fundamentos e aplicações. 1st. ed. Tecmedd editor: São Paulo, SP; 2007

[14] Murakamia I, Kitaokac A, Ashida H. A positive correlation between fixation instability and the strength of illusory motion in a static display. Vision Research. 2006;**46**:2421-2431. DOI: 10.1016/j.visres.2006.01.030

Chapter 5

Training Reading Skills in Central Field Loss Patients: Impact of Clinical Advances and New Technologies to Improve Reading Ability

Coco-Martin MB, J. Herrera Medina, J. Oliveros López, N.C. Platero Alvarado and L. Leal Vega

Abstract

The primary goal of patients with central field loss attending to visual rehabilitation (VR) offices is to get adapted to daily life activities in near vision, mainly looking for recovering their ability to read again. The disparity in the functionality of these patients, due to the new advances in medical treatment and the increasing number of new apps and technological devices in the market, implies a heterogeneity in the reading training programs to be applied, and consequently a variability in the results obtained. Currently, with the increasing access to information and communication technologies and social networks, the opportunities for improving their access to information and communication is taken an important role. For this reason, the basis of ad-hoc evidence-based reading training programs is needed to standardized the clinical practice in reading rehabilitation for visual impaired and blind patients. This chapter will go in depth into these topics offering an exhaustive state of the art of reading rehabilitation for central field loss patients that will be useful for clinicians dedicated to the rehabilitation of visual impaired and blind people.

Keywords: visual rehabilitation, age-related macular degeneration, central field loss, eccentric fixation, saccades, optical aids, reading training, reading speed

1. Introduction

Reading is an extraordinarily sophisticated task that involves the synthesis of a number of different motor, sensory and cognitive functions [1]. Its proper performance largely depends on the state of the macula lutea and the optical pathway and visual cortex. Conditions affecting these areas such as age-related macular degeneration (AMD) and acquired brain injury (ABI) are frequent in the elderly and can compromise the reception or the conduction and processing of central visual information, with the consequent impairment of this ability, of great importance for the vocational, educational and daily life of the individual. Consequently, in low vision rehabilitation services, reading is the most common clinical complaint, as well as the primary goal for patients with central vision loss [1–3], whose prevalence is expected to increase in the coming years, as well as the diseases continues to rise in line with the aging of the population. Thus, improvement of reading performance in central vision loss patients is nowadays considered as one of the main objectives pursued by neuro-vision rehabilitation (NVR).

When the vision in the center of the visual field decreases, reading speed declines and oculomotor pattern differs compared with normal reading, showing an increase in the mean fixation duration and in the number of saccades [4, 5]. It is known that many of these individuals may eventually adopt one or more locations on the retinal periphery to serve as the preferred retinal locus (PRL). Therefore, for these patients, visual function is still malleable and able to adapt to unfavorable conditions [6, 7].

2. Development of visual rehabilitation and training in brief

When you hear the word blind or low vision, Braille system and the inability for the person to perform everyday tasks such as moving around comes to your mind [7].

If we trace a low vision timeline backwards in history, we can find that it is known that Marco Polo discovers elderly Chinese people using magnifying glasses for Reading (1270), and the first magnifying aid for visual defects attributed to Rene Descartes in 1637 [8]; But it is not until the nineteenth century that the LVR receives attention. In 1850, Amsterdam separately counts the number of inhabitants with impaired vision, Hermann von Helmholtz invents the ophthalmoscope (1851) and, in 1897, Charles Prentice invents the typoscope [8]. The beginnings of the current era can be said to have begun at the first international congress in low vision, sponsored by the American Foundation for the Blind, in 1986. In 1996, International Society for Low-vision Research and Rehabilitation (ISLRR) officially incorporated in Amsterdam [8]. By the mid-twentieth century, the first manuals including information on methods of visual rehabilitation were published. E. Faye was the first person to coin the term low vision.

In 1973, the first Low Vision Diplomate program established was registered within American Academy of Optometry first diplomate awarded Western Michigan University (USA) offers first required low vision course as part of orientation & mobility program Low Vision Clinical Society founded in the United States [8].

Currently, a person with distant visual acuity (VA) 0.3 or less (20/60 Snellen notation), a visual field of 10° from the point of fixation, and with reduced functionality is considered low vision [7]. This definition was not always universal, previously low vision was defined by a VA of 20/70 or less, however, it did not include the degree of functional defect. The subject's functionality may be affected (even in VAs greater than 20/70) by problems of loss of contrast sensitivity (CS) and glare [9].

In 2018, the International Classification of Diseases separated visual impairment into two groups: far and near. Thus, the near vision impairment is an VA lower than N6 or N8 at 40 cm with the existing correction. There are signs that worldwide the World Health Organization estimates that there are 1300 million people with visual impairment [10].

It should be noted that visual rehabilitation requires multidisciplinary work, which includes ophthalmologists, optometrists and visual therapists, in most cases psychologists and social workers work together.

The work of psychologists is important in those patients who are in a state of depression. Depression can be detected by optometrists or ophthalmologists through anamnesis and the use of questionnaires. Studies have found that people with vision loss have four times more depression than a person without visual impairment [11]. One of the main objectives of the visual rehabilitation service is to improve the functional capacity of each subject and the action plan must be adapted individually [12].

Visual rehabilitation, apart from improving the quality of life of subjects by increasing their functionality, avoids a series of events that can be triggered by their visual impairment. Among the events are: falls, being people with low vision more likely to suffer [13] and depression, which more than 30% of these subjects develop and show an improvement in VR by eliminating it [14].

3. Reading as one of the objectives of visual rehabilitation

Visual rehabilitation seeks to regain the skills of a person with visual impairment. This recovery is done gradually, using optical and non-optical aids, in addition to the strategies proposed by the visual therapist. The action of reading necessarily implies using the central retina. Therefore, a visual disability due to an ophthalmological pathology that affects the central visual field will significantly affect to the action of reading.

Several studies indicate that reading is one of the most important actions that visually impaired people want to recover [15, 16]. This task is usually the main objective in the elderly, children and adolescents with low vision.

Being referred to low vision service implies a loss of vision that can generate loss of functionality, and consequently the subject may be perceived as not very competent, which will influence his mental state. Such a state can influence the outcome of rehabilitation, which in turn can contribute to changing the way in which the subject views himself.

3.1 How do we read?

Every time we read, the eyes perform a sequence of movements. The ocular movements by which these jump from one stimulus to another are called *saccadic* movements. Normally in the reading process, they go from left to right, but sometimes there are movements in the opposite direction to change lines or to return to what was read, in which case they are called *regression* movements [17].

We call *fixation* to the pause between a saccadic movement and another, in which moment the information is extracted. The amount and duration of this fixation calculates the reading capacity of the subject. The reading speed serves to evaluate the reading ability of the subject; in a subject in normal vision, recognize from 7 to 11 characters in the fovea during fixation in the right half but four or five characters in the left half. In other words, it is called *visual span* to the number of letters that can be recognized without moving the eyes [17].

3.2 How does reading performance work in AMD patients?

In a subject with low vision restoring its functionality and independence has a lot of meaning. Reading is also important for those children or adolescents who suffer from low vision, these subjects need to continue schooling or simply enjoy reading as a leisure, remaining functional, independent and psychologically motivated. Our world has been designed for the reader, for those people who are able to interpret all the information that surrounds us. Reading is an activity that affects all the orders of daily life, from access to the content of a letter or a medicine label, to the buy of a product or the information that we can find in the street or in a public building.

The Johns Hopkins Wilmer Eye Institute study showed that 60% of patients referred to low vision report that the main reason for consultation is the difficulty to read, other studies such as, see [18, 19] give similar results. There are also studies on age-related macular degeneration (AMD), the most common pathology that causes severe disability in the western world, where they mention the increase in emotional state, cognitive and quality of life of patients by improving the speed of reading [20].

When a person cannot use the fovea, all eye movements involved in the reading process are affected and as a consequence performance decreases considerably; other daily activities are also affected. Understanding that there are ophthalmological pathologies that affect the central field of vision, it is necessary to use the peripheral retina. Subjects use a region of para-central retina, normally less than 20° from the damage fovea [21]. This retinal place to use is known as preferential retinal locus (PRL). This PRL gives the ability to perform the function of the damaged central retinal area, can be trained and used for activities such as reading. In short, it is necessary to evaluate the PRL, know its location, characteristics (a microperimeter offers a precise method for this action) and from then on use optical and non-optical aids to rehabilitate the reading. Studies show that the use of microperimetry for rehabilitation generates improvements in visual acuity, fixation stability and reading speed.

When central field loss (CFL) is present, saccadic movements are erratic, with constant regression movements; fixation is very unstable and, as a consequence, perceived information is scarce and partial. All this affects two fundamental aspects for a satisfactory reading: reading speed and reading comprehension. In order to assess reading ability, these aspects must be measured. One of the goals of visual rehabilitation is to help the subject establish their own PRL as well as learn to use it efficiently. Sometimes the person has more than one PRL, and may even use it consciously or unconsciously.

Other aspects that affect the reading process and are involved in rehabilitation are the effect of crowding, which together with the visual span, present a correlation that is clarifying; reducing crowding enlarge the visual span and can facilitate reading [22].

4. Medical and technological advances for patients with central field loss

4.1 Central field loss pathologies

Central field loss is associated with macular diseases. Examples of these diseases are age-related macular degeneration, macular hole, macular edema and diabetic retinopathy [23]. In general, patients with these pathologies have preserved peripheral vision. As central vision is affected, reading or face recognition are affected. Rehabilitation strategies and visual aids are focused on those tasks.

4.2 Therapeutic strategies

In atrophic diseases, there is not a specific treatment, so actions are directed to prevention and in advanced cases, rehabilitation. In exudative diseases such as exudative AMD, there has been a wide range of treatments, including laser, radiation and anti- vascular endothelial growth factor (VEGF) therapy [24].

Laser photocoagulation was the first treatment for exudative AMD from 1979 [24]. This treatment stopped neovascularization progression, but laser burned retinal tissue, so patients with macular neovascularization could not be treated [24, 25]. This technique consisted in impacting with a laser on the retina to produce heat and that the proteins coagulate in order to slow down the appearance of neovases [26].

Another therapeutic strategy is radiation. This procedure attempts to affect the angiogenesis of choroidal neovases either directly by destroying endothelial cells and cytokines or indirectly on genes that regulate the action of cytokines. It can be administered by brachytherapy directly on the affected tissue; or by teletherapy administering the isotope externally [24]. It can be combined with anti-VEGF therapy [27].

With photodynamic therapy a photosensitive substance is injected in vein in order to activate it with a laser at a choroidal vessels level. In 1999, the efficacy of photodynamic therapy to stop choroidal neovascularization was tested, as well as the maximum and minimum doses to achieve the desired effect, being 150 and 25 J/cm^2, respectively [24].

Repeated intravitreal injections of anti-VEGF drugs are currently the most widely used treatment in AMD. VEGF is an angiogenic and vasculogenic factor; that is, it is involved in the formation of new vessels from existing ones and in the formation of embryonic vessels; as well as in their reappearance [28]. Several drugs had been developed, such as pegaptanib, bevacizumab, ranibizumab and, recently aflibercept. However, these anti-VEGF drugs only are trying to slow down the progression, they are not able to reverse the effect of the disease [25].

4.3 Optical coherence tomography (OCT): advances in screening technology

OCT is a diagnostic and control technology based on the principle of Michelson interferometry whereby light is divided into two optical pathways to the eye and a mirror. Thanks to this we can analyze the posterior retina, the macula, the papilla and the relations they have with the vitreous and the choroid [29]. The OCT Macular Cube 512 × 128 strategy allows, in addition to the analysis of macular layers, comparison with different measures in the same patient and comparison with the OCT database to establish whether the values are within normal or not, analyzing the macula in nine areas, being a central and two rings with four layers each (**Figure 1**). By means of this strategy, an area of 6 × 6 mm is measured using 128 A-Scans with 512 B-Scans.

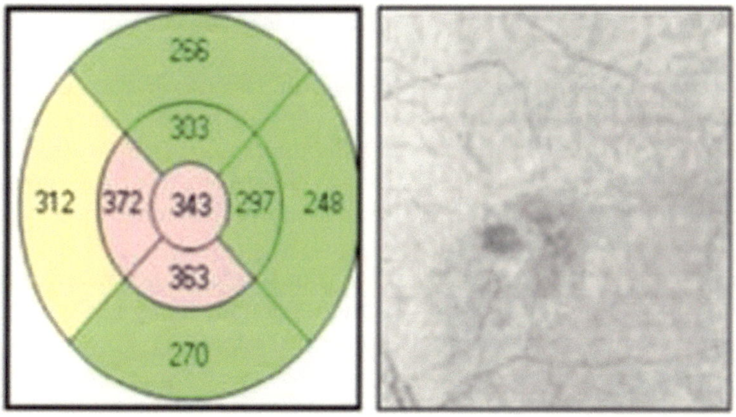

Figure 1.
An example of the nine analysis areas of macular cube strategy (from https://www.ncbi.nlm.nih.gov/pmc/articles/PMC4478143/).

5. Terminological problems

The term low vision was coined in the 1950s to convey the idea that vision can vary between the extremes of sighted and blindness [30]. Low vision generally refers to any chronic form of visual impairment that cannot be corrected with eye glasses, contact lenses, medical treatment or surgery and that negatively affects daily function of the individual [31, 32]. Although there is no universally accepted definition of "low vision," it is globally conceived as visual acuity of less than 0.3 (6/18) but equal or better than 0.05 (3/60) and/or visual field loss of less than 20 degrees in the better eye with the best possible correction [33].

This is based on the 10th revision of International Classification of Diseases derived from a World Health Organization Study group on the Prevention of Blindness that was convened in 1972 to provide a standardized definition to facilitate the data collection of population on prevalence of vision impairment and blindness.

Traditionally, low vision has been known by other numerous names such as partly sighted or subnormal vision, concepts that have already been outdated.

In 2002 at the 29th International Congress of Ophthalmology, the International Council of Ophthalmology (ICO) adopted a resolution where the following terminology was recommended [33, 34]:

- Blindness: to be used exclusively for total vision loss and for conditions where individuals have to rely predominantly on vision substitution skills.

- Low vision: to be used for lesser degrees of vision loss, where individuals can be helped significantly by vision enhancement aids and devices.

- Visual impairment: to be used when the condition of vision loss is characterized by a loss of visual functions, such as visual acuity or visual field, at the organ level since "impairment" is defined as any loss or abnormality of psychological, physiological or anatomical structure or function. Many of these functions (for example, visual acuity) can be measured quantitatively and in each eye separately.

- Visual disability: to be used when the condition prevents the undertaking of specific visual tasks, for example, loss of ability to read, since "disability" is defined as any restriction or lack resulting from an impairment of the ability to perform an activity in a manner or within a range considered normal.

- Visual handicap: to be used when the condition is described as a barrier to social participation (for example, loss of a driving license), since handicap is defined as a disadvantage for a given individual resulting from a disability or impairment that limits or prevents the fulfillment of a role that is normal for that individual (depending on age, sex and cultural factors).

- Functional vision: to be used when the vision loss is defined in terms of the individual's abilities with regard to activities of daily living (ADL). Thus, it applies to the individual and not to the visual system.

6. Current situation and its problems

Several research pieces have attempted to improve reading performance in people with central vision loss. Some authors have proposed to determine the mode of text presentation that offers these patients the fastest reading speed [35, 36] while others have suggested to examine whether simple manipulations of text typography or text typesetting (such as increasing letter or line spacing) could enhance this ability [37, 38]. Unfortunately, most of these studies did not found statistically significant differences in reading speed for different text presentations or when text typography or text typesetting were modified.

To date, only measures that have led to modest gains in reading speed among this group of people have been magnified font size, increased lighting and contrast conditions and the provision of optical magnifiers [39–41]. More recently, some works have established that reading performance on retinal periphery may benefits from perceptual learning based on certain tasks that include training in reading or identifying random letters sequences at various points across the visual field, although considerable individual variability was found in the results obtained from these investigations [42, 43].

As well as until the 1970s of the last century, people with low vision were rehabilitated as people with blindness, it is from that moment on that the magnification of texts and especially the use of optical and electronic aids allowed the development of the specific field of visual rehabilitation. The introduction of microscopes, magnifiers, telescopes and filters, together with the use of lecterns and adequacy of lighting, have allowed the development of a complete body of knowledge concerning to the new skills implemented when the person with CFL reads. The same can be said of electronic aids such as close-circuit television (CCTV) magnifiers and electronic magnifiers, which provide improved contrast and magnification that common optical aids of this type. These tools can be available mounted on a stand, head-mounted or hand-held.

As technological progress advances, numerous software apps and tech devices emerge to meet the reading needs of low-vision population. The production and distribution of digital documents was the beginning of harnessing technological advances for the visually impaired and brought new opportunities for reading improvement by allowing customization of lighting, contrast and font size variables to optimize the text display on the screen [44].

We are talking about software that magnify and provide contrast improvements or text to speech reproductions, compatible with computers and tablets, as well as the tablets and electronic books themselves, which thanks to the options they offer of brightness control, contrast, selection of type and font size, have been an important progress for people with AMD, and has enabled them to have free access to information.

At present, high-tech digital image enhancement programs are under study to provide better visualization for central vision loss patients. They represent an important challenge due to the change of model that they offer in the intervention in visual rehabilitation. It is necessary at this point to expand the reach and depth of research related to the use of these devices and software for reading.

A very relevant innovation is retinal implants; this is a prosthetic system that performs a process that captures the image, processes it and transforms it into electrical impulses and stimulates the retina's ganglion cells (RGCs) [45]. It appears to increase vision with acceptable safety profiles, even though the amelioration of functional vision generated by the prosthesis nowadays remains limited [46]. But it is still hopeful and promising in degenerative retinal diseases, and will surely bring a major challenge in the rehabilitation of these persons.

7. Theory of reading performance

Comprehensive reading is a tremendously complex activity. Although for skillful readers, it is a task that does not seem to offer too many difficulties, and proof of this is the speed with which it is read (between 150 and 400 words per minute), the truth is that in such a short time several cognitive operations have to be carried out [47].

Reading is only possible if a good number of cognitive and visual operations function properly. It has been verified that the reading system is made up of several separable, relatively autonomous modules, each of which oversees carrying out a specific function. Specifically, four modules or processes are distinguished: perceptual processes, lexical processing, syntactic and semantic [48].

7.1 Perceptual processes

The first step for the reading is the perception of the text, the recognition of the word, opening here a question: is each letter identified separately or is the word identified in its entirety? Already in 1972, Gough found that it was easier to find or recognize a letter when it was part of a word than when it was isolated in a random series of letters [49]. On the other hand, it is possible that both theories have their share of reason and that using the letter or the global word as a processing unit depends on the task, the context, the characteristics of the word and the reader's skill [50]. Also, spacing is important in reading speed. It has been proved that increasing letter spacing has a negative effect on reading speed in experienced adult readers;

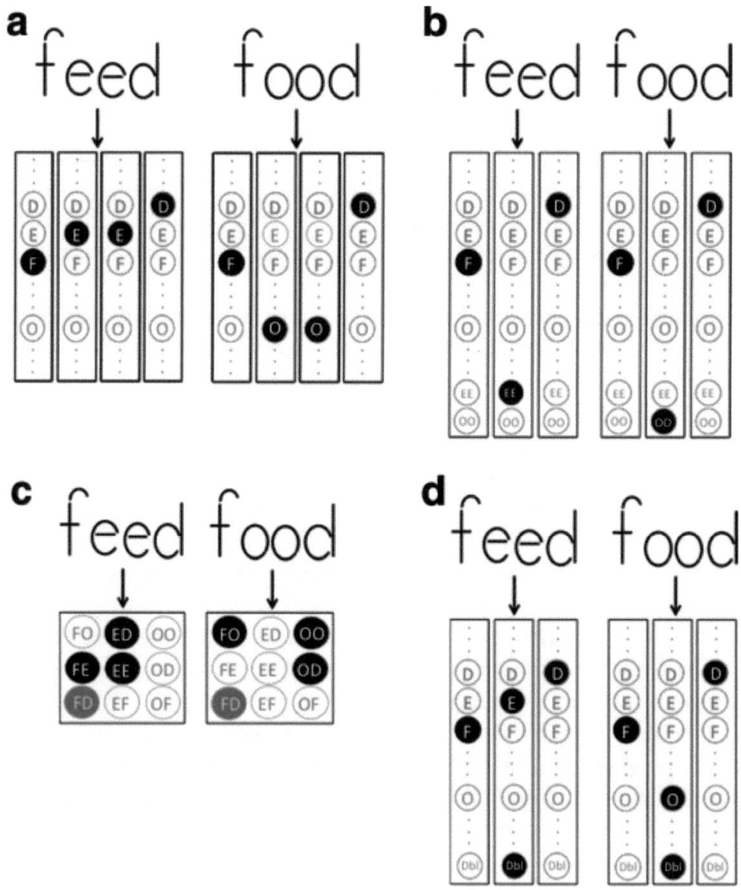

Figure 2.
Orthographic representations in various theories of visual word processing of the words feed and food [52]. (a) Representation of letter identify and order theories. (b) Theory of grapheme identification. (c) Open bigram theory. (d) Separation of letter identity and letter doubling information theory (from https://link.springer.com/article/10.3758%2Fs13423-016-1149-8).

while in children has no effect [51]. On the other hand, Fischer-Baum researched word identification, taking special focus on double letters [52]. He also noticed that a patient with acquired dyslexia used to spell words in a similar way as a previous spelt word, including double letters [53]. He found that letter identity and double letters are separately represented in written language, showing a complex reading capacity and a common orthographic representation of reading and writing (**Figure 2**).

Eye movements and fixations are involved in the perceptual process. The information we extract passes into iconic memory, of great capacity but short duration. The information is transferred from iconic memory to short-term visual memory, which allows it to be maintained for a longer period of time and is now retained as linguistic material. Finally, a comparison is made with the long-term memory to check whether the word is stored [47].

7.2 Lexical processing

The next step is the recognition of the meaning of the word, a process that can be done in two ways. One of them is to compare the spelling of the word with a series of representations stored in the memory to see which one fits. All that is needed is the existence of a word store or mental lexicon in which all the words known to the reader are represented [53]. Reading by this route involves several operations: the visual analysis of the word that is transmitted to a store of orthographic representations of words called "visual lexicon", where it is identified by comparison with the units stored there. This in turn will activate the corresponding phonological representation, located in another lexical warehouse, the so-called "phonological lexicon", and from here it will be deposited in the "pronunciation warehouse" ready to be issued. This route is known by the name of lexical route or also visual route [53].

7.3 Syntactic processing

We talk about the process of understanding how words are interrelate to each other. Isolated words do not convey any new information, but it is in the relationship between them that the message is found [54]. Once the words of a sentence have been recognized the reader must determine how they are related to each other. The parsing process therefore comprises three main operations [55], by means of which the areas to which the words correspond are labeled, the relationship between the components is established and a structure is constructed according to the hierarchy of its components.

7.4 Semantic processing

In this process, once the meaning of the sentence has been extracted, it is integrated and compared with previous knowledge; therefore, the richness of the person's vocabulary and previous experience will be decisive. The process ends when extracted meaning is integrated into memory, with the rest of the reader's knowledge. During this process, the reader makes certain inferences, makes deductions about the information and adds non-explicit information. This last phase of the process is the most complex but it is not carried out independently of the previous ones, but all the processes interact with each other [47].

When assessing reading comprehension, sometimes independent phrases are used, outside of a story or context. If there are no given part, the sentences could not be understood as we do not know what facts they refer to. If, on the other hand, there are no new parts, they would not provide any knowledge other than that which is already possessed [49].

8. Updated reading skills development strategies

8.1 Introduction

Reading is one of the most important visual activities, requiring complex cognitive processes. One of the most important reading skills is reading speed, being critical to understand the reading text. But achieving an adequate reading speed for compression requires mastery of the various eye skills and movements described above. The stimulus required for an optimal reading is also important. Its parameters are: characters size subtending 0.3–2°; field size up to 4 characters independent of character size; bandwidth up to 2 cycles/degree independent of character size; and 1 spatial-frequency channel suffices for reading [3]. Visual spam requires 7–11 characters to be recognized at the fovea for normal reading rates during fixation [56]. It is well-known that the maximum visual acuity is located in the fovea and decreases directly with eccentricity [57].

In a meta-analytic study, reading skills components were evaluated to determine their importance on reading comprehension in healthy adults. Results showed a great relationship between comprehension and the following skills: morphological awareness, language comprehension, fluency, oral vocabulary knowledge, real word decoding and working memory [58].

This section will address the assessment of cognitive skills in a rehabilitation program, the eccentric viewing training, the optical correction and other training techniques such as oculomotor control and perceptual training.

8.2 Cognitive skills

Assessment of cognitive skills is the step prior to the development of a visual rehabilitation program. Several tests are used for cognitive skills evaluation, such as MoCA, MMCT or CDT [59] or the scale COGEVIS, which is specially designed for low vision patients [60]. Also, it is essential to evaluate the level of literacy of the patient before visual and reading evaluation. If the patient is illiterate or has a low level of reading comprehension, it may be useful the tumbling E test for visual acuity [3].

8.3 Eccentric viewing training and preferred retinal loci (PRL)

Eccentric viewing consists of using a non-central part of the retina for viewing. In this method of vision, given when central retina is damaged, the eye uses an eccentric retinal location, known as preferred retinal loci (PRL) [61]. It is common for many patients with eccentric viewing not to realize that they are fixing in that way. According to Jeong and Moon, no improvements were found in best corrected visual acuity after 2 weeks of self-training; however, there were significant improvements in reading speed and satisfaction scores [61].

Nowadays, microperimeters can evaluate the visual field and the PRL even in patients without fixation, correlating the exact retinal locations with the visual field [62]. There are two microperimetry techniques: static and dynamic. The first of these can detect mild scotomas and defining their shape, with no movement of the stimulus. In dynamic microperimetry, the stimulus moves from the periphery towards the point of fixation, presenting difficulties in identifying the relative scotomas [7].

Sometimes PRL is not located in an appropriate area and it should be relocated in a better retinal location, closer to the fovea so visual acuity will be the best [7]. Some studies have shown that patients trend to develop the PRL at the left side of the atrophy [63]. However, Greenstein et al. evaluated several patients with macular disease such as AMD and Stargardt disease, founding a majority of PRL located above the atrophic lesion [64]. A superior or inferior location of the PRL is better than a left location for reading because scotoma does not interfere much in continuous reading.

In some patients, oculomotor deficits can reduce reading skills, so training methods with using eye movements are needed for these patients. It is the case of Rapid Serial Visual Presentation (RSVP) training, which allows PRL training without eye movements to read. The words of the sentence are presented one by one at the center of the screen, allowing reading without eye movements because fixation with the PRL is maintained on the screen [3].

8.4 Optical correction and the use of prisms

Optical correction plays a very important role to make the most of patients' vision. Nevertheless, optical correction is not only optical lenses with the correction of patients' refractive error, but also adds power for reading distance and prisms if necessary [65].

As a field defect, prisms can be used for AMD patients. Several studies have been conducted to determine the benefits of repositioning the retinal image in its PRL, the area of the retina where the subject looks and replaces the pitting, using prisms in patients with macular degeneration. Three different studies evaluated the use of prisms in subjects with AMD, shifting the image from the visual field to the PRL predetermined by the subject for rehabilitation [66–68]. Visual acuity was assessed with the best correction, obtaining significant values of improvement with the use of prisms. In addition, the PRL preferred by patients was mostly in the upper retina and showed conformity and adaptation to the use of prisms in the three studies. This indicates that the use of prisms, with good PRL delimitation, may be an appropriate rehabilitation option for patients with AMD.

8.5 Training materials and devices

First of all, we must make a distinction between optical devices and non-optical devices for low vision patients. An optical aid is an optical system made up of high-powered lenses that help people with reduced vision make the most of their remaining vision. On his behalf, a non-optical aid, such as light flexes or lecterns, is a complement to help make the most of vision. For reading, spectacles magnifiers and hand and stand magnifiers are the most classical optical aids used; while macro types, lecterns and an appropriate illumination are the non-optical aids most important for central vision loss patients [7]. Filters are used in patients suffering from photophobia and glare and they have a great visual impact in macular disease patients [7]. Over the years several studies have shown the effects of filters on glare, but there is no global filter prescribing protocol for each disease [69–71]. One of those studies found that with a blue-violet filter, patients with central and peripheral scotoma improved visual acuity, contrast sensibility and glare better than the yellow filter [71].

Contrast plays an important role on training reading skills. Reading materials should have a 100% black and white contrast and reading conditions should reduce the amount of glare, specially created by short wavelength light. Also, light position is a crucial point to be considered, being recommendable that light source is placed above or behind the patient [3]. Finally, text font is also important. In a Canadian research with patients with AMD, Courier text font was found as the most recommendable font for these patients, whereas Arial was found as the worst for reading smaller print [72].

8.6 Oculomotor control training

It is necessary to train eye movements, saccades and fixation stability in order to rehabilitate reading performance. The flashlight technique is useful to train oculomotor movements and fixation stability on distance targets. The patient holds a flashlight and, keeping their head still, follows the light with their eyes. A test variation uses a laser pointer directed to the wall as a stimulus, which allows the patient to detect relative scotomas [3]. The King-Devick test (KDT) for low vision patients is an advanced training of fixation stability, saccades and tracking eye movements. It is based on performance of rapid number naming. In a 6 weeks research with KDT training in first and second grade children, the treatment group improved significantly compared with the control group in reading fluency and reading comprehension, with efficient eye movements [73].

8.7 Perceptual training

Perceptual training is the last step of the rehabilitation program. Then, an example of a protocol is shown [3]:

- Start with large print: it is important to start with large print and, to decrease the size as the patient improves his or her reading skills. If it is possible, the ideally size is comparable with a newspaper print (size 1 M).

- Start reading single letters: its aim is to get the patient to recognize each letter and number detail with eccentric vision for, then, explore simple words. At the end of this process, the patient may be capable of reading a continuous text.

- Use training to improve comprehension: this can be possible by providing the patient reading material with higher levels. Improving reading speed a comprehensive rehabilitation can be achieved.

- Transfer acquired reading skills into daily life activities.

9. Assessment and individual reading rehabilitation plan

Visual impaired patients require an individualize assessment and rehabilitation plan due to the affectation by their pathology varies from one patient to another. This fact makes it difficult to develop a standardized attentional plan for these patients. However, several assessment guidelines for central vision loss patients can be recommended.

Firstly, fluent reading requires a minimal visual acuity of 20/50, a visual field at least of 2° to the right and the left and a holding position of 250 ms between saccades [74].

Nowadays, microperimetry is one of the most important tests in patients with central vision loss. The origin of microperimetry is due to the need to evaluate the visual field in people with unstable or extrafoveal fixation problems or because of problems in the macula. Conventional perimetry is based on the fixation of the subject. If the fixation is extrafoveal and/or unstable, the visual field will not be correct, with values displaced from their true location and incorrect scotoma sizes [75]. Microperimetry allows the points of the visual field to be correlated with the exact retinal location; at the same time, the fundus of the eye can be visualized while visual stimuli are projected [62] (**Figure 3**). It allows also eccentric fixation training.

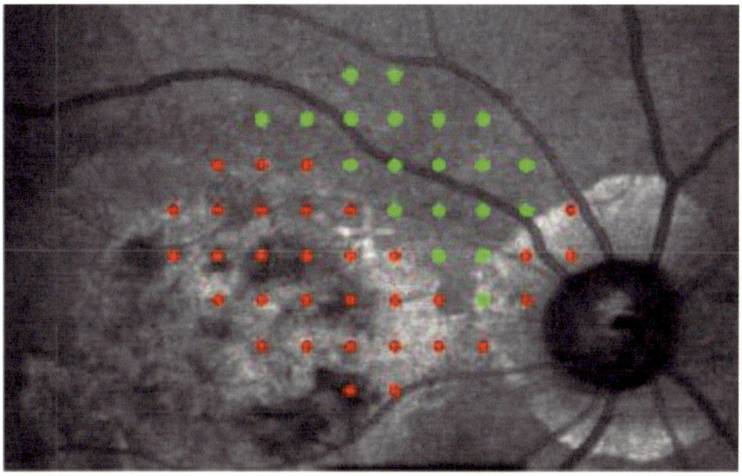

Figure 3.
Microperimetric image in which the evaluated points and the anatomical situation in the fundus of the eye are observed (from https://www.canadianjournalofophthalmology.ca/article/S0008-4182(13)00209-3/fulltext).

In macular abnormalities, microsacadic movements are greater than in a normal eye, affecting fixation stability [76]. Due to poor fixation stability, the reading speed is affected and reduced [77]. This fixation stability can be improved by training, and microperimetry is essential for such training.

An important consequence of central vision loss in some patients is depression, which has a prevalence of 2–5% [78]. Low-vision rehabilitation aids have shown to improve reading speed but no effects on depression have been reported in AMD patients [79]. If traditional rehabilitation protocols do not show a great impact on depression, prevention of depression may be an appropriate action. The sum of visual rehabilitator, behavioral activation and occupational therapist has shown an effective effect on depression.

An improvement on quality of life and reading has been seen in AMD patients who already use magnifying aids, after a computer-based reading training at home [78]. On that randomized and controlled trial, patients were divided into two groups: primary reading training group and control group with placebo training. Control group started with reading training after 6 weeks of placebo, which consist of crossword puzzles. Reading speed was measured with the German version of the International Reading Speed Texts (IReST), eye movements were measured with a scanning lases ophthalmoscope (SLO); and degree of depression, cognition and quality of life were measured with Montgomery-Asberg Depression Rating Scale (MADRS), dementia detection test (DemTect) and Impact of Vision Impairment (IVI) questionnaires, respectively. Reading speed improved in training group, as well as emotional status. Such results were not given in the control group [78].

10. Innovative reading rehabilitation strategies and devices: assistive devices and technology

With the development of technology, a new field of rehabilitation opened up, beginning with the first electronic aids. Tablets and iPads are currently widely used, even in elderly AMD patients. It has been shown in these patients that they read faster on iPad with larger text sizes when compared with paper. Also, patients reported to have the best clarity with it [80]. Moreover, it has been proved to improve reading speed in low vision patients, as well as other low vision devices such as closed-circuit television (CCTV); being the previous experience with an iPad decisive in order to obtain greater reading speeds [81].

10.1 Head-mounted display

Another technological aids can be a virtual bioptic telescope and a virtual projection screen, implemented in a head-mounted display (HMD) [82]. In this research, two new magnification strategies were developed: a virtual bioptic telescope and a projection screen presented in virtual reality. The first one consists of a user-defined region of a wide-field binocular head-mounted display where the image can be magnified (**Figure 4**). With this system, visual function was significantly improved, including reading. The minimum clinically important difference (MCID) frequency in reading task was 85.7% of participants [82], which shows an appropriated visual aid for central vision loss patients.

10.2 Intra-ocular telescopic implants

Intra-ocular telescopic implants are commercially invasive aids for low vision patients. Dunbar and Shawahir-Scala review showed the different implants available on the market for patients with AMD [83]. These implants consist of intra-ocular lens combined in order to create an optic system. Lipshitz mirror implant (LMI) is a modified conventional intra-ocular lens (IOL) with two miniature mirrors in a combination that creates a dual optical system in a similar way to multifocal IOL. The central part of the IOL magnifies the image while the peripheral portion remains unmagnified. Quality of life improved and single letter near acuity with early treatment diabetic retinopathy study (ETDRS) near vision chart at 20 cm improved [84]. With the same optical basis of a multifocal IOL, the Scharioth Macula Lens (SML) has a central optic zone with +10.00 D addition. Compared with a +6.00 D spectacle lens for near vision, SML reported 2.1 lines better visual acuity at 15 cm than the spectacle lens at 1 month [85]. Similar results to those of LMI were obtained with IOL-AMD after 4 months. This implant consists of a Galilean telescope in one eye with two hydrophobic IOLs, one negative and one positive [83]. Finally, the intra-ocular miniaturized telescope (IMT) takes advantage of corneal optical power. It is implanted in one eye, used for near vision, while the other eye is used for distance vision. At 1 year, 3.2 lines of improvement in near vision acuity in ETDRS was reported compared with baseline, remaining after 5 years of surgery [83, 86].

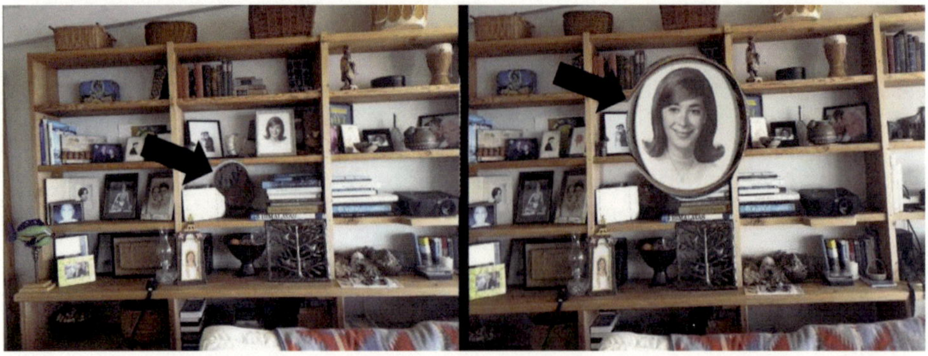

Figure 4.
Example of the user-defined region or "bubble" where image can be magnified [82] (from https://tvst.arvojournals.org/article.aspx?articleid=2725386).

10.3 Gaming and electronic devices

Relying on the development of technology, games have also undergone a revolution. Today, there are multiple games that can be played on iPad. AMD patients in a large percentage use personal electronic devices for playing games [87]. Due to these results, gaming could play an important role in earlier detection of AMD. Video games had been used to train visual acuity, fixation pattern and retinal sensitivity in patients with Stargardt disease [88]. Patients of this study played action video-game during 1 h per day each eye with alternate patching. Results showed an improvement of these visual functions, which opens a new option of rehabilitation based on video-games.

11. Conclusions

Reading involves the participation of different perceptive and cognitive processes. When a person suffers a pathology such as AMD, the vision in the central visual field is reduced and all the processes are altered, being necessary a rehabilitative intervention that determines the scope of the visual loss, helps to establish a new point of visual fixation and trains in the ocular movements, so that the reading becomes fluid and comprehensive. In this rehabilitative process, it is necessary to implement optical and non-optical aids that improve the visual functioning of the person affected by AMD. New electronic devices and access to digital information are producing changes in the visual rehabilitation strategies of people with AMD.

Conflict of interest

None of the authors have any conflict of interest on the devices or technology described in this chapter.

Abbreviations

ABI	acquired brain injury
ADL	activities of daily living
AMD	age-related macular degeneration
CCTV	close circuit television
CFL	central field loss
CS	contrast sensitivity
CVF	central visual field
ETDRS	early treatment diabetic retinopathy study
HMD	head-mounted display
ICO	International Council of Ophthalmology
IOL	intra-ocular lens
IMT	intra-ocular miniaturized telescope
IReST	International Reading Speed Texts
ISLRR	International Society for Low-vision Research and Rehabilitation
IVI	impact of vision impairment
KDT	King-Devick test
LMI	Lipshitz mirror implant
LVR	low vision rehabilitation
MADRS	Montgomery-Asberg Depression Rating Scale

MCID	minimum clinically important difference
NVR	neuro visual rehabilitation
OCT	optical coherence tomography
PRL	preferred retinal locus
RSVP	rapid serial visual presentation
RGCs	retinal ganglion cells
SLO	scanning laser ophthalmoscope
VEGF	vascular endothelial growth factor
VA	visual acuity

Author details

Coco-Martin MB[1*], J. Herrera Medina[2], J. Oliveros López[1], N.C. Platero Alvarado[1] and L. Leal Vega[1]

1 Clinical Neurosciences Research Group, Neurology Department, Vision Rehabilitation, Faculty of Medicine, University of Valladolid, Valladolid, Spain

2 University of Valladolid/ONCE (Spanish National Organization for the Blind), Spain

*Address all correspondence to: mbegococom@gmail.com

References

[1] Kanonidou E. Reading performance and central vision loss. Hippokratia. 2011;**15**:103-108

[2] Chung ST. Enhancing visual performance for people with central vision loss. Optometry and Vision Science. 2010;**87**:276-284. DOI: 10.1097/OPX.0b013e3181c91347

[3] Markowitz M, Daibert-Nido M, Markowitz SN. Rehabilitation of reading skills in patients with age-related macular degeneration. Canadian Journal of Ophthalmology. 2018;**53**:3-8. DOI: 10.1016/j.jcjo.2017.10.042

[4] Rainer K. Eye movements in reading and information processing: 20 years of research. Psychological Bulletin. 1998;**124**:372-422

[5] Bullimore MA, Bailey IL. Reading and eye movements in age-related maculopathy. Optometry and Vision Science. 1995;**72**:125-138

[6] Crossland MD, Culham LE, Kabanarou SA, Rubin GS. Preferred retinal locus development in patients with macular disease. Ophthalmology. 2005;**112**:1579-1585. DOI: 10.1016/j.ophtha.2005.03.027

[7] Coco Ma B, Herrera J. Manual de Baja Visión y Rehabilitación Visual. Madrid: Médica Panamericana; 2015

[8] Goodrich G, Arditi A, Rubin G, Keeffe J, Legge G. The low vision timeline: An interactive history. In: International Low Vision Conference (ISLRR); 7-11 July 2008; Montreal, Canada: Visual Impairment Research. 2008. pp. 67-75

[9] World Health Organization. Consultation on development of standards for characterization of vision loss and visual function [Internet]. 2003. Available from: https://apps.who.int/iris/bitstream/handle/10665/68601/WHO_PBL_03.91.pdf;jsessionid=8AD5F022F7989A5B11635CD79330BE0D?sequence=1 [Accessed: 05 June 2019]

[10] World Health Organization. Ceguera y discapacidad visual [Internet]. 2018. Available from: https://www.who.int/es/news-room/fact-sheets/detail/blindness-and-visual-impairment [Accessed: 05 June 2019]

[11] NIH Consensus Development Conference. Diagnosis and treatment of depression of late life. JAMA. 1992;**268**:1018-1029

[12] Dagnelie G. Age-related psychophysical changes and low vision. Investigative Ophthalmology & Visual Science. 2013;**54**:88-93. DOI: 10.1167/iovs.13-12934

[13] Shen SH, Huang KC, Tsai YH, Yang TY, Lee MS, et al. Risk analysis for second hip fracture in patients after hip fracture surgery: A nationwide population-based study. Journal of the American Medical Directors Association. 2014;**15**:725-731. DOI: 10.1016/j.jamda.2014.05.010

[14] Nollett CL, Bray N, Bunce C, Casten RJ, Edwards RT, et al. Depression in visual impairment trial (DEPVIT): A randomized clinical trial of depression treatments in people with low vision. Investigative Ophthalmology & Visual Science. 2016;**57**:4247-4254. DOI: 10.1167/iovs.16-19345

[15] Coco-Martin MB et al. Design and evaluation of a customized reading rehabilitation program for patients with age-related macular degeneration. Ophthalmology;**120**(1):151-159. DOI: 10.1016/j.ophtha.2012.07.035

[16] Owsley C, McGwin G Jr, Lee PP, Wasserman N, Searcey K. Characteristics of low-vision rehabilitation services

in the United States. Archives of Ophthalmology. 2009;**127**:681-689. DOI: 10.1001/archophthalmol.2009.55

[17] Legge GE, Cheung SH, Yu D, Chung T, Lee HW, et al. The case for the visual span as a sensory bottleneck in reading. Journal of Vision. 2007;7:1-15. DOI: 10.1167/7.2.9

[18] Crossland MD, Gould ES, Helman CG, Feely MP, Rubin GS. Expectations and perceived benefits of a hospital-based low vision clinic: Results of an exploratory, qualitative research study. Visual Impairment Research. 2007;**9**:59-66. DOI: 10.1080/13882350701643582

[19] Friedman SM, Munoz B, Rubin GS, West SK, Bandeen-Roche K, et al. Characteristics of discrepancies between self-reported visual function and measured reading speed. Salisbury eye evaluation project team. Investigative Ophthalmology & Visual Science. 1999;**40**:858-886

[20] Mielke A, Wirkus K, Niebler R, Eschweiler G, Nguyen NX, et al. The influence of visual rehabilitation on secondary depressive disorders due to age-related macular degeneration. A randomized controlled pilot study. Der Ophthalmologe. 2013;**110**:433-440

[21] Cheung SH, Kallie CS, Legge GE, Cheong AM. Nonlinear mixed-effects modeling of MNREAD data. Investigative Ophthalmology & Visual Science. 2008;**49**:828-835. DOI: 10.1167/iovs.07-0555

[22] He Y, Legge GE. Linking crowding, visual span, and reading. Journal of Vision. 2017;**17**:11. DOI: 10.1167/17.11.11

[23] Kanski J. Oftalmología Clínica. Vol. 13. Elsevier; 2006. pp. 413-427

[24] Lim JI. Age-Related Macular Degeneration. 3rd ed. Taylor & Francis Group; 2013

[25] Ryan SJ. Retina. Vol. 3. Elsevier; 2013. pp. 1213-1214

[26] Gómez-Ulla F, Rodríguez Cid MR, Marín E. Fotocoagulación del edema macular y retinopatía proliferante. In: Retinopatía Diabética. Sociedad Española de Oftalmología; 2006

[27] Rating P, Freimuth MA, Stuschke M, Bornfeld N. Adjuvant radiotherapy during anti-VEGF in neovascular age-related macular degeneration. Der Ophthalmologe. 2017;**114**:370-374

[28] Andrini LB. Expresión del factor de crecimiento del endotelio vascular (vegf) durante la regeneración hepática [thesis]. Universidad Nacional de La Plata; 2010

[29] Courtney RJ, McClintic JI, Ehlers JP. Comparison of spectral domain optical coherence tomography scan patterns and clinical review strategies in neovascular aged related macular degeneration. Retina. 2015;**35**(7):1315-1322. DOI: 10.1097/IAE.0000000000000478

[30] Colenbrander A, Fletcher DC. Low vision rehabilitation: Basic concepts and terms. Journal of Ophthalmic Nursing & Technology. 1992;**11**(1):5-9

[31] American Academy of Ophthalmology. What is Low Vision?. 2019. Available from: https://www.aao.org/eye-health/diseases/low-vision [Accessed: 03 June 2019]

[32] Acosta R, Bentley SA, Giacomelli G, Allcock C, Evans JR, Virgili G. Reading aids for adults with low vision. The Cochrane Database of Systematic Reviews. 2018;**4**:CD003303. DOI: 10.1002/14651858.CD003303.pub4

[33] European Council of Optometry and Optics. Low Vision (Position Paper). 2011. Avaiable from: https://www.ecoo.info/2011/03/10/position-paper-low-vision/ [Accessed: 07 June 2019]

[34] International Council of Ophthalmology. Visual Standards: Aspects and Ranges with Emphasis on Population Surveys. 2002. Available from: http://www.icoph.org/downloads/visualstandardsreport.pdf [Accessed: 07 June 2019]

[35] Presentation formats. Optometry and Vision Science. 2004;**81**(3):205-213

[36] Fine EM, Peli E. Scrolled and rapid serial visual presentation texts are read at similar rates by the visually impaired. Journal of the Optical Society of America. 1995;**12**(10):2286-2292. DOI: 10.1364/JOSAA.12.002286

[37] Chung ST. The effect of letter spacing on reading speed in central and peripheral vision. Investigative Ophthalmology & Visual Science. 2002;**43**(4):1270-1276

[38] Chung ST, Jarvis SH, Woo SY, Hanson K, Jose RT. Reading speed does not benefit from increased line spacing in AMD patients. Optometry and Vision Science. 2008;**85**(9):827-833. DOI: 10.1097/OPX.0b013e31818527ea

[39] Rubin GS, Feely M, Perera S, Ekstrom K, Williamson E. The effect of font and line width on reading speed in people with mild to moderate vision loss

[40] Bowers AR, Meek C, Stewart N. Illumination and reading performance in age-related macular degeneration. Clinincal & Experimental Optometry. 2001;**84**(3):139-147

[41] Christen M, Abegg M. The effect of magnification and contrast on reading performance in different types of simulated low vision. Journal of Eye Movement Research. 2017;**10**(2):5. DOI: 10.16910/jemr.10.2.5

[42] Chung STL. Improving reading speed for people with central vision loss through perceptual learning. Investigative Ophthalmology & Visual Science. 2011;**52**(2):1164-1170. DOI: 10.1167/iovs.10-6034

[43] Chung STL, Legge GE, Cheung SH. Letter-recognition and reading speed in peripheral vision benefit from perceptual learning. Vision Research. 2004;**44**(7):695-709. DOI: 10.1016/j.visres.2003.09.028

[44] Legge GE. Reading digital with low vision. Visible Language. 2016;**50**(2):102-125

[45] Bloch E, Luo Y, da Cruz L. Advances in retinal prosthesis systems. Therapeutic Advances in Ophthalmology. 2019;**11**:1-16. DOI: 10.1177/2515841418817501

[46] Humayun MS, de Juan E, Dagnelie G. The bionic eye: A quarter century of retinal prosthesis research and development. Ophthalmology. 2016;**123**(10):89-97. DOI: 10.1016/j.ophtha.2016.06.044

[47] Cuetos VF. Psicología de la lectura. Madrid: Escuela Española; 2008

[48] Mitchell D. The Process of Reading. Chichester: John Wiley & Sons; 1982

[49] Gough PB. One Second of Reading. Cambridge: JF Cananaugh y IG Mattingly; 1972

[50] Just MA, Carpenter PA. A theory of reading: From eye fixations to comprehension. Psychological Review. 1980;**87**:329-354

[51] Weiss B, Knakker B, Vidnyánszky Z. Visual processing during natural reading. Scientific Report. 2016;**6**:26902

[52] Fischer-Baum S. The independence of letter identify and letter doubling in reading. Psychonomic Bulletin & Review. 2017;**24**:873-878

[53] Allport D. Components of the Mental Lexicon. London: P Kolers Ed; 1979

[54] Legge GE, Glenn A. Fry award lecture 1990: Three perspectives on low vision reading. Optometry and Vision Science. 1991;**68**:763-769

[55] Zurif EB, Caramazza A, Myerson R. Grammatical judgments of agrammatic aphasics. Neuropsychologia. 1972;**10**:405-417

[56] Legge GE, Mansfield JS, Chung STL. sychophysics of reading. XX. Linking letter recognition of reading speed in central and peripheral vision. Vision Research. 2001;**41**:725-743

[57] Chung STL, Mansfield JS, Legge GE. Psychophysics of reading. XVIII. The effect of print size on reading speed in normal peripheral vision. Vision Research. 1998;**38**:2949-2962

[58] TigheE,SchatschneiderC.Examining the relationships of component reading skills to reading comprehension in struggling adults readers: A meta-analysis. Learning Disability. 2016;**49**:395-409

[59] Killen A, Firbank MJ, Collerton D, Clarke M, Jefferis JM, Taylor JP, et al. The assessment of cognition in visually impaired older adults. Age and Ageing. 2013;**42**:98-102

[60] Meyniel C, Samri D, Stefano F, Crevoisier J, Bonté F, Migliaccio R, et al. COGEVIS: A new scale to evaluate cognition in patients with visual deficiency. Behavioural Neurology. 2018

[61] Jeong JH, Moon NJ. A study of eccentric viewing training for low vision rehabilitation. Korean Journal of Ophthalmology. 2011;**25**:409-416

[62] Fletcher DC, MacKeben M. Microperimetrycorrespondence.Everyday use of modern microperimetry in a low-vision service. Canadian Journal of Ophthalmology. 2013;**48**

[63] Rubin GS. Vision rehabilitation for patients with age-related macular degeneration. Eye. 2001;**15**:430-435

[64] Greenstein VC, Santos RAV, Tsang SH, Smith RT, Barile GR, Seiple W. Preferred retinal locus in macular disease: Characteristcs and clinical implications. Retina. 2008;**28**:1234-1240

[65] Markowitz SN. Principles of modern low vision rehabilitation. Canadian Journal of Ophthalmology. 2006;**41**:289-312

[66] Al-Karmi R, Markowitz SN. Image relocation with prisms in patients with age-related macular degeneration. Canadian Journal of Ophthalmology. 2006;**41**:313-318

[67] Markowitz SN, Reyes SV, Sheng L. The use of prisms for vision rehabilitation after macular function loss: an evidence-based review. Acta Ophthalmologica. 2013;**91**:207-211

[68] Reyes SV, Silvestri V, Amore F, Markowitz SN. Use of prisms for vision rehabilitation after macular function loss may impact oculomotor control. Canadian Journal of Ophthalmology. 2013;**48**:427-430

[69] Monés J, Gómez-Ulla F. Degeneración Macular asociada a la edad. Prous Science. 2005

[70] Bailie M, Wolffsohn JS, Stevenson M, Jackson AJ. Functional and perceived benefits of wearing coloured filters by patients with age-related macular degeneration. Clinical & Experimental Optometry. 2013;**96**:450-454

[71] Colombo L, Melardi E, Ferri P, Montesano G, Samir Attaalla S, Patelli F, et al. Visual function improvement using photochromic and selective blue-violet light filtering spectacle lenses in patients affected by retinal diseases. BMC Ophthalmology. 2017;**17**:149

[72] Tarita-Nistor L, Lam D, Brent MH, Steinbach MJ, González EG. Courier: A better font for reading with age-related macular degeneration. Canadian Journal of Ophthalmology. 2013;**48**:56-62

[73] Dodick D, Starling AJ, Wethe J, Pang Y, Messner LV, Smith C, et al. The effect of in-school saccadic training on reading fluency and comprehension in first and second grade students: A randomized controlled trial. Journal of Child Neurology. 2017;**32**:104-111

[74] Legge GE, Ahn SJ, Klitz TS, Luebker A. Psychophysics of reading—XVI. The visual span in normal and low vision. Vision Research. 1997;**37**:1999-2010

[75] Sunness JS, Schuchard RA, Shen N, Rubin GS, Dagnelie G, Haselwood DM. Landmark-driven fundus perimetry using the scanning laser ophthalmoscope. Investigative Ophthalmology & Visual Science. 1995;**36**:1863-1874

[76] MAIA. Centervue, Engineering Italian Creativity [Internet]. 2019. Available from: https://www.centervue.com/products/maia/ [2019/06/05]

[77] Rohrschneider K, Bültmann S, Springer C. Use of fundus perimetry (microperimetry) to quantify macular sensitivity. Progress in Retinal and Eye Research. 2008;**27**:536-548

[78] Kaltenegger K, Kuester S, Altpeter-Ott E, Eschweiler GW, Cordey A, Ivanov IV, et al. Effects of home reading training on reading and quality of life in AMD—A randomized and controlled study. Graefe's Archive for Clinical and Experimental Ophthalmology. 2019

[79] Hamade N, Hodge WG, Rakibuz-Zaman M, Malvankar-Mehta MS. The effects of low-vision rehabilitation on reading speed and depression in age-related macular degeneration: A meta-analysis. PLoS ONE. 2016;**11**

[80] Gill K, Mao A, Powell AM, Sheidow T. Digital reader vs print media: The role of digital technology in reading accuracy in age-related macular degeneration. Eye. 2013;**27**:639-643

[81] Morrice E, Johnson AP, Marinier JA, Wittich W. Assessment of the apple iPad as a low-vision reading aid. Eye. 2017;**31**:865-871

[82] Deemer AD, Swenor BK, Fujiwara K, Deremeik JT, Ross NC, Natale DM, et al. Preliminary evaluation of two digital image processing strategies for head-mounted magnification for low vision patients. Translational Vision Science & Technology. 2019;**8**:23

[83] Dunbar HMP, Dhawahir-Scala FE. A discussion of commercially available intra-ocular telescopic implants for patients with age-related macular degeneration. Ophthalmology and therapy. 2018;**7**:33-48

[84] Agarwal A, Lipshitz I, Jacob S, Lamba M, Tiwari R, Kumar DA, et al. Mirror telescopic intraocular lens for age-related macular degeneration. Journal of Cataract & Refractive Surgery. 2008;**34**:87-94

[85] Scharioth GB. New add-on intraocular lens for patients with age-related macular degeneration. Journal of Cataract and Refractive Surgery. 2015;**41**:1559-1563

[86] Boyer D, Freund KB, Levy MH, Garg S. Long-term (60-month) results for the implantable miniature telescope: Efficacy and safety outcomes stratified by age in patients with end-stage age-related macular degeneration. Clinical Ophthalmology. 2015;**9**:1099-1107

[87] Razavi H, Baglin E, Shatangan P, Caruso E, Tindill N, Griffin S, et al.

Gaming to improve vision: 21st century self-monitoring for patients with age-related macular degeneration. Clinical and Experimental Ophthalmology. 2018;**46**:480-484

[88] Ratra D, Rakshit A, Ratra V. Visual rehabilitation using video game stimulation for Stargardt disease. Therapeutic Advances in Ophthalmology. 2019;**11**:1-9

Chapter 6

Efficient Computer-Aided Techniques to Detect Glaucoma

Nataraj Vijapur and R. Srinivasarao Kunte

Abstract

A survey of the World Health Organization has revealed that retinal eye disease Glaucoma is the second leading cause for blindness worldwide. It is a disease which will steals the vision of the patient without any warning or symptoms. About half of the World Glaucoma Patients are estimated to be in Asia. Hence, for social and economic reasons, Glaucoma detection is necessary in preventing blindness and reducing the cost of surgical treatment of the disease. The objective of the chapter is to predict and detect Glaucoma efficiently using image processing techniques. We have developed an efficient computer-aided Glaucoma detection system to classify a fundus image as either normal or glaucomatous image based on the structural features of the fundus image such as cup-to-disc ratio (CDR), rim-to-disc ratio (RDR), superior and inferior neuroretinal rim thicknesses, vessel structure-based features, and distribution of texture features in the fundus images. An automated clinical support system is developed to assist the ophthalmologists to identify the persons who are at risk in the early stages of the disease, monitor the progression of the disease, and minimize the examination time.

Keywords: glaucoma, cup-to-disc ratio (CDR), rim-to-disc ratio (RDR), superior, inferior, neuroretinal rim, structure features, texture features

1. Introduction

According to the survey of the World Health Organization, over the last 10 years, cataract remains the highest leading cause of blindness worldwide covering 47.9% of overall blindness. It is a progressive and painless clouding of the internal lens of the eye. Similarly, the survey declares Glaucoma as the second leading cause for blindness worldwide. About 12.3% of patients in the world are suffering from Glaucoma [1]. It is a disease which will steal the vision of the patient without any warning or symptoms. Surveys conducted in North America and Europe revealed a significant proportion of new Glaucoma patients who were previously gone undetected. The proportion estimated for Glaucoma patients in Asia and developing countries is even larger [2]. This calls for the need for early Glaucoma detection, and we can prevent blindness and reduce the surgical cost involved in treating the disease. The fundus image of the eye, Glaucoma disease, structural changes in fundus image due to Glaucoma, and its diagnosis are presented in this section.

1.1 Fundus image of the eyes

The eye is the most complex organ of the human body with approximate dimension of 2.54 cm width, 2.3 cm height, and 2.54 cm deep [3]. The human eye acts like a camera [4] and processes the visual signals. **Figure 1** shows the front view of the eye fundus image consisting of the optic disc and optic cup. The optic nerves and blood vessels exit the retina from the optic disc. It is considered as one of the main features of a retinal fundus image and is located to the nasal side of the fovea. It is vertically oval, with an average dimension of horizontally 1.76 mm and vertically 1.92 mm. Inside the optic disc, there is a central depression, of variable size, called the optic cup.

The optic nerve head is the location where ganglion cell axons exit the eye to form the optic nerve. The changes in the shape and color or depth of the optic disc and optic cup are the indicators of various ophthalmic pathologies especially for Glaucoma and other eye diseases. Optic disc and cup are the brightest features of the normal fundus. The disc appears to be as a bright yellow or white region in colored fundus image.

1.2 Structural changes in fundus image due to glaucoma

The structure and appearance of the optic disc can reveal the presence of Glaucoma, and they are considered as very important features to assess the damage due to Glaucoma. The optic cup concentric enlargement, decrease in rim area, and other such patterns of glaucomatous damage are most commonly found. The ratio of area of optic cup to area of the optic disc is normally considered to evaluate the disease. Due to Glaucoma, in the retina the optic cup area enlarges and progresses toward the disc. This distinction can be seen between normal and Glaucoma-affected fundus images as shown in **Figure 2(a)** and **(b)**, respectively. This cup-to-disc area ratio (CDR) is used in ophthalmology to determine the progression of Glaucoma. If the CDR value is greater than 0.3, the patient has a threat of Glaucoma. The CDR of the image in **Figure 2(b)** is nearly 0.7, and it is a prominent case of Glaucoma.

The area present between the cup and disc boundary of the eye is termed as neuroretinal rim [5] as shown in **Figure 3(a)** and **(b)** for a sample of normal and Glaucoma eye, respectively. Thinning of the neuroretinal rim is also one of the symptoms of Glaucoma. Rim-to-disc area ratio (RDR) is also an indicator

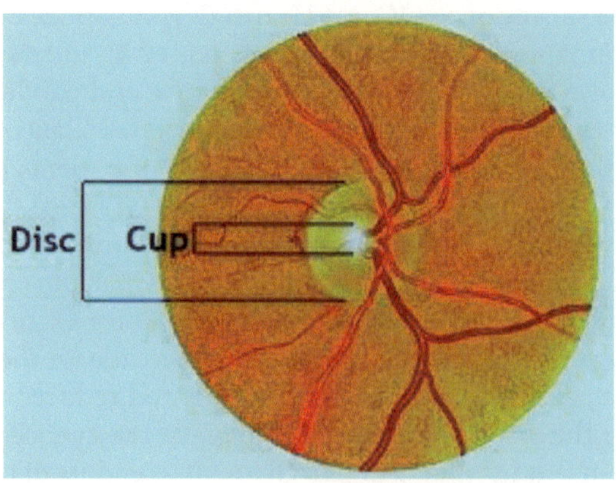

Figure 1.
Front view of the eye fundus image.

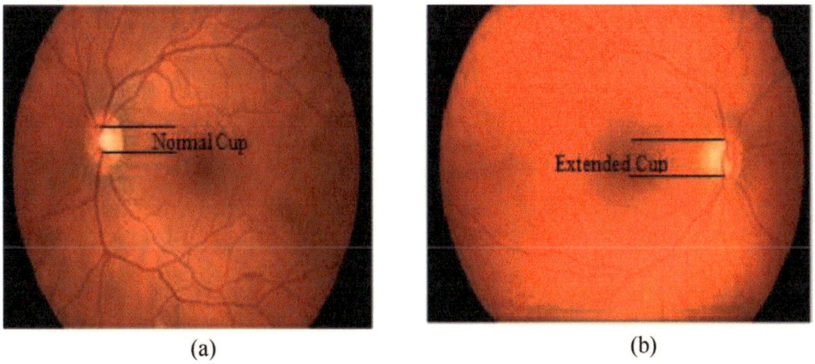

Figure 2.
Fundus images: (a) normal eye; (b) glaucoma eye.

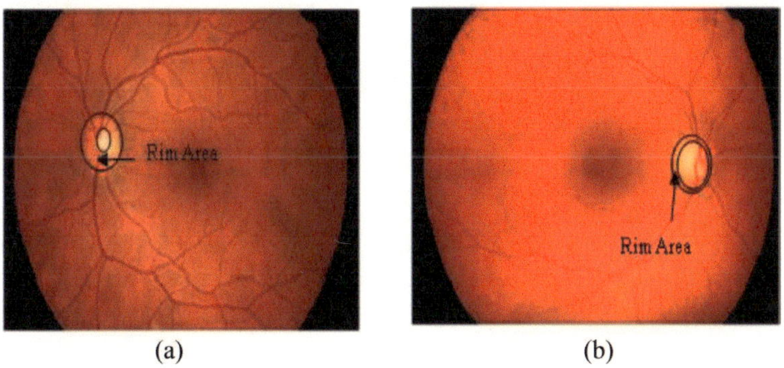

Figure 3.
Neuroretinal rim: (a) rim area in the normal eye; (b) rim area in the Glaucoma eye.

for Glaucoma. As seen from **Figure 3**, the normal eye has more RDR than the Glaucoma eye.

The retinal image shall be seen as composed of inferior, superior, nasal, and temporal regions as shown in **Figure 4(a)**. Due to Glaucoma, blood vessels covered by the nasal region increase, and the inferior–superior region decreases. Hence, the ratio of the area of the sum of blood vessels in the inferior–superior region to the sum of blood vessels in the nasal-temporal region (ISNT) decreases. This feature can also be used to detect Glaucoma more accurately [5, 6].

A study has revealed that the diameters of the retinal vessels have been seen to be significantly smaller in the glaucomatous eyes than the normal eyes [7, 8]. This reduction in vessel diameters can be continuously monitored, and the disease can be detected in early stages. Also, in the case of prominent cases of Glaucoma, there is a distortion observed in cup structure. Cup usually expands downward more toward inferior side. Therefore, disease can be detected by measuring the difference in neuroretinal rim thickness at the superior and inferior regions, which are referred as superior rim thickness and inferior rim thickness as shown in **Figure 4(b)**.

In the case of Glaucoma, thickness of the vessels around the disc goes on reducing due to lack of fresh aqueous humor. This also results in disappearance of small vessels around the disc. A normal eye contains a lot of very minute vessels like small branches of tree around the optic disc, which are absent in the Glaucoma eye as shown in **Figure 5**.

In the normal eye, peripheral vision is present fully. In the Glaucoma-affected eye, peripheral vision goes on reducing. As an illustration, **Figure 6(a)** shows the

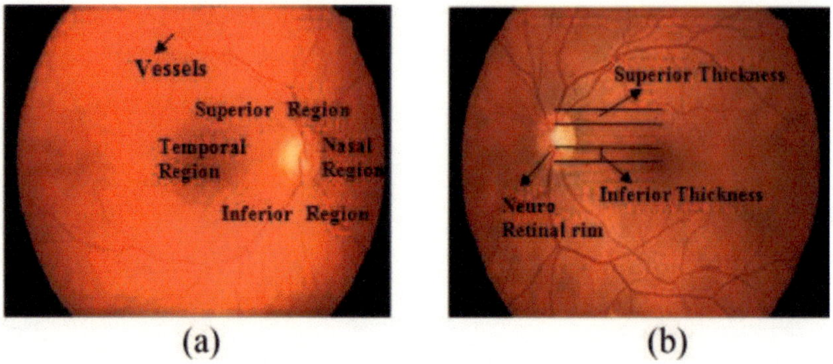

Figure 4.
Regions of fundus image: (a) ISNT regions and vessels, (b) neuroretinal rim and superior and inferior thicknesses.

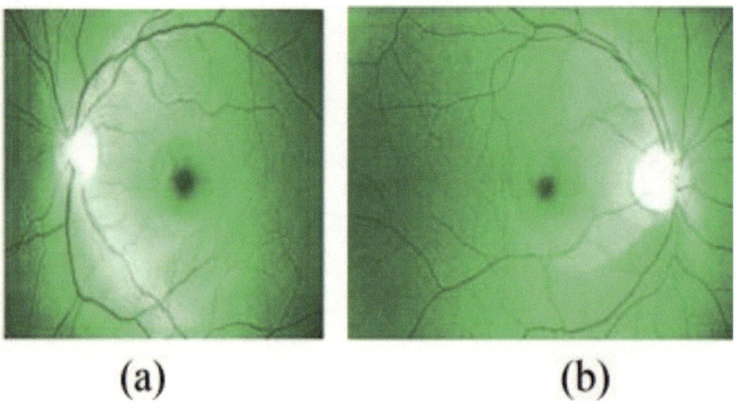

Figure 5.
Vessels in fundus image: (a) a normal eye as seen through the green filter; (b) a glaucoma eye in green filter.

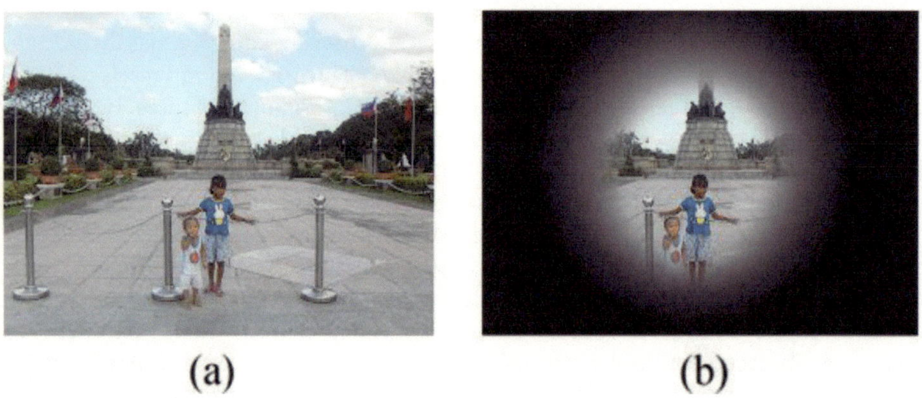

Figure 6.
Vision loss due to Glaucoma: (a) normal eye vision; (b) glaucoma eye vision (courtesy: http://www.caeps.org/).

vision of a sample picture as perceived by a normal eye, and **Figure 6(b)** shows the vision of the same picture as perceived by a Glaucoma eye.

1.3 Fundus features used for glaucoma detection

We have used the fundus features such as (i) CDR, (ii) RDR, (iii) superior rim thickness, (iv) inferior rim thickness, (v) structural features of vessels around the disc such as maximum vessel diameter, number of vessel segments, and total number of smaller diameters of vessels, and (vi) spatial textures to detect Glaucoma by the digital image processing techniques [9–12].

2. Proposed comprehensive efficient integrated glaucoma detection system

The block schematic of our proposed comprehensive efficient integrated Glaucoma detection system for Glaucoma identification using image processing techniques is shown in **Figure 7**.

The retinal image of the eye is captured using a fundus camera. The captured eye fundus image is subjected to various image processing techniques to extract different features of fundus image.

Our proposed system extracts and uses the following three different sets of fundus eye image features for detection of Glaucoma:

Fundus structure based features (CDR, RDR and Neuroretinal rim thicknesses), Vessel structural features and Textural features.

Structure-based features of fundus image are extracted using a template-based approach. A template aids the segmentation of the optic cup and disc from the fundus image. A template is correlated with fundus image using Pearson-r correlation for segmentation. Structure-based features such as CDR, RDR, and superior and inferior rim thicknesses are extracted.

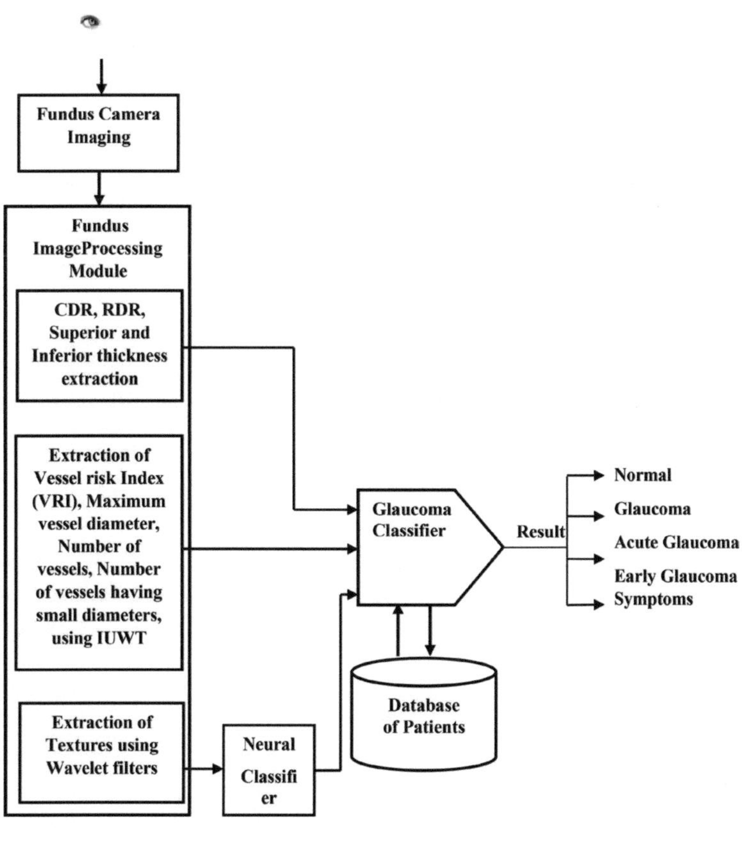

Figure 7.
Comprehensive efficient integrated glaucoma detection system.

Fundus images' vessel structure-based features such as vessel count, vessel diameters, maximum vessel diameter, and count of vessels having fewer diameters are extracted using isotropic undecimated wavelet transform (IUWT).

Fundus images' texture features are extracted using three families of wavelet filters: daubechies (db3), symlets (sym3), and biorthogonal (bio3.3, bio3.5, and bio3.7) wavelet filters. A trained neural classifier fed with the texture features classifies the given test image into a normal or Glaucoma image as the first stage of classification.

Based on the literature survey and suggestion of ophthalmologists, the ultimate Glaucoma classifier is developed. The above set of extracted features and neural classifier output are fed to the final classifier. It finally classifies the given test image as either (i) normal or (ii) Glaucoma or (iii) acute Glaucoma or (iii) early Glaucoma symptom image.

The extracted features like CDR, RDR, superior and inferior rim thicknesses, vessel count, vessel diameter, maximum vessel diameter, and count of vessels having fewer diameters are stored in a database meant for the patient. These features can be used to assess the progression of the disease during the next visit of the patient. This will assist the ophthalmologists for better monitoring of patients. Database will be very useful for mass screening programs and also plays an important role in detecting Glaucoma at an early stage in the case of risk patients who are having genetic background of Glaucoma.

2.1 Sources of image dataset used for the development of proposed glaucoma detection system

For our Glaucoma detection system experiments, analysis, and testing results, we have used the glaucomatous fundus image dataset and normal image dataset from the following sources:

High-Resolution Fundus (HRF) image dataset, available on the public domain https://www5.cs.fau.de/research/data/fundus-images/. This dataset has been established by a collaborative research group to support research and comparative studies on retinal fundus images [13, 14], which is used by many researchers for their experiments and testing results. This dataset comprises of a set of 15 Glaucoma and 15 normal images and fundus images available at KLE Dr. Prabhakar Kore Hospital, Belagavi, India, which have been captured using a Canon CF1 High-Resolution fundus camera with a 50° field of view. Each image was captured using 24 bits per color plane at dimensions of 2534 × 2301 pixels.

We are referring the above two datasets in our thesis as (i) HRF dataset and (ii) Hospital dataset, respectively.

2.2 Glaucoma detection using template

This chapter presents an efficient methodology developed for the automatic localization and segmentation of the optic cup and disc in retinal images followed by extraction of some structural features for Glaucoma detection. Localization of the optic disc in the retinal image and extraction of the features are done by correlating the fundus image with a newly developed template using Pearson-r correlation. Segmentation of the optic cup and disc is done on the basis of correlation levels [15–18].

2.2.1 Preprocessing

Our proposed methodology is based on correlating the fundus image with a designed template. The template is designed based on intensity distribution of the fundus image. Hence, it is required to determine the intensity component of the input image. The true color format of the fundus image captured by the fundus camera does not reveal the intensity component value directly, whereas hue, saturation, and intensity (HSI) format representation of an image directly provide the intensity component value of an image (refer to **Figure 8**). Therefore, the RGB format captured by the fundus image is converted into HSI format in the preprocessing stage.

Conversion from RGB to HSI is achieved using the following equations:

$$I(\text{intensity}) = \frac{R(\text{red}) + G(\text{green}) + B(\text{blue})}{3} \tag{1}$$

$$H(\text{hue}) = \cos^{-1}\left\{\frac{\frac{1}{2}[(R - G) + (R - B]}{[(R - G)^2 + (R - B)(G - B)]^{\frac{1}{2}}}\right\} \tag{2}$$

$$S(\text{saturation}) = 1 - \frac{3}{(R + G + B)}[\min(R, G, B)] \tag{3}$$

A sample RGB fundus image and its corresponding converted HSI image is shown in **Figure 8**.

2.2.2 Glaucoma detection using Pearson-r coefficient extraction

Further, the intensity component of the fundus image is correlated with a template designed using Pearson-r correlation to localize the optic disc in the image. The template is designed keeping in view the general structure of the optic disc and cup. The size of the optic disc varies significantly with the different fundus images. We observed that the optic disc widths varied from 60 to 100 pixels in the images of our dataset. The optic disc consists of a rim and cup. The intensity of the rim is higher than the rest of the image outside the rim, and the cup is the brightest part of the fundus image. We have designed a square-shaped image template to have a disc with a rim and cup as shown in **Figure 9(a)**. The cup will have the highest intensity, and intensity decreases toward the rim and other outer parts of the image similar to intensity distribution pattern of a fundus image. A Laplacian of Gaussian distribution is used to get this intensity distribution pattern. Pearson-r coefficients are extracted from correlating the template with the preprocessed image. The correlated image contains the information of optic cup and disc in the form of intensity variation with respect to template image from the fundus image. As seen from **Figure 8(b)** for a sample correlated image, the optic disc and cup can be very easily separated on an intensity plane.

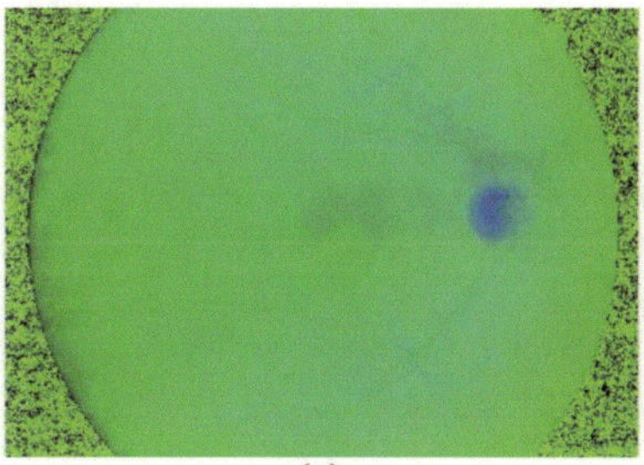

(a)

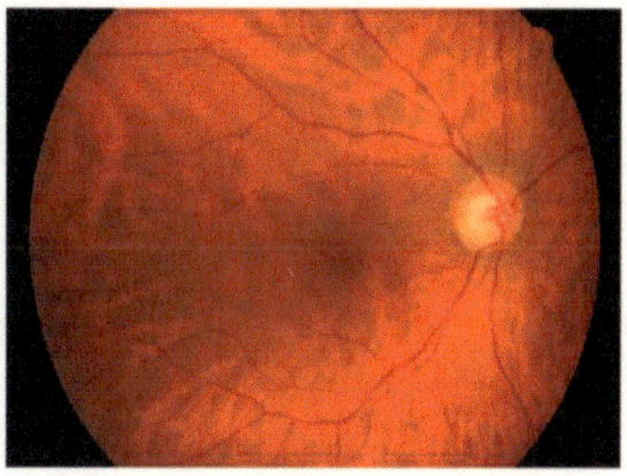

(b)

Figure 8.
Preprocessing stage: (a) input fundus RGB image; (b) converted HSI image.

Further, the optic cup and disc are easily segmented as they differ in their correlated magnitudes. Binary images of the segmented optic disc, cup, and rim are shown in **Figure 10**.

Figures 11 and **12** show the segmentation of optic cup and disc and neuroretinal rim in binary image for a sample image of Hospital dataset and HRF dataset, respectively.

The values of CDR, RDR, and superior and inferior rim thicknesses are calculated from the extracted image.

2.3 Glaucoma detection using vessel segmentation

According to the literature survey due to progression of Glaucoma, blood vessel diameter decreases [19–22], and smaller diameter vessels around the optic disc start diminishing and disappearing. We have employed these aspects of vessels as features to detect the Glaucoma at an early stage. **Figure 13** clearly shows these aspects. The region where these significant vessels of interest are present in a small area around the optic disc in the image for detection of Glaucoma is considered as region of interest (ROI).

2.3.1 ROI extraction

In previous section, we presented the methodology of segmenting the optic disc by correlating the input fundus image with designed template using Pearson-r

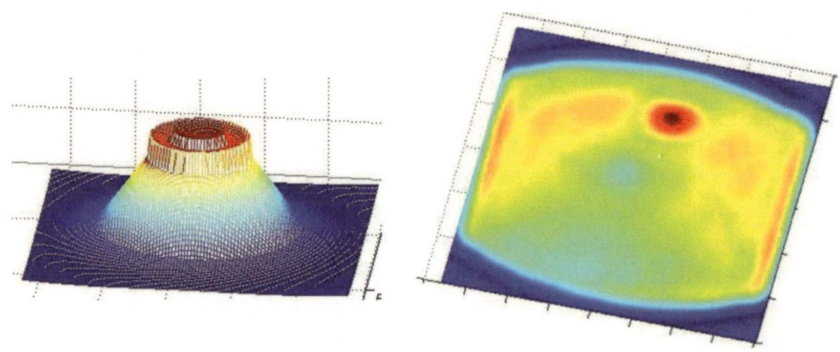

Figure 9.
Correlation: (a) correlation filter; (b) intensity distribution of correlated fundus.

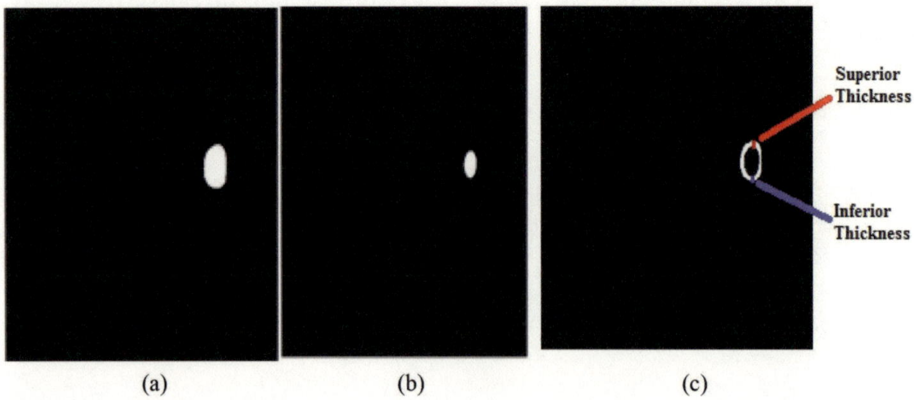

Figure 10.
Segmentation. (a) Segmented optic disc. (b) Segmented optic cup. (c) Neuroretinal rim thickness.

correlation. The value of Pearson-r correlation is maximum at the center of the optic disc which corresponds to the brightest spot in the fundus image. After segmenting the disc as discussed in Section 2.2.2, its boundary points on the top,

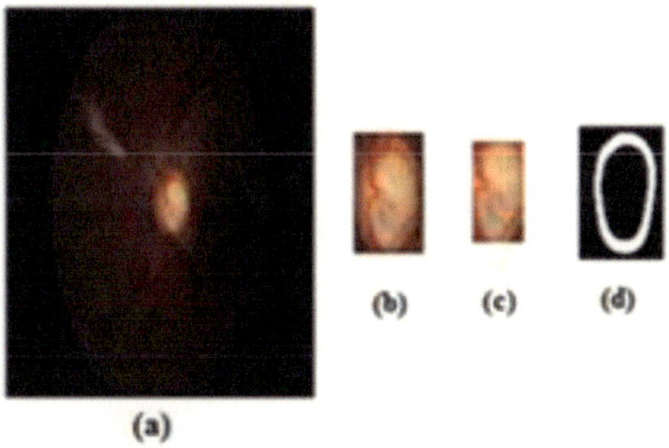

Figure 11.
Hospital dataset sample. (a) Original sample. (b) Segmented optic disc. (c) Segmented optic cup. (d) Binary image showing neuroretinal rim.

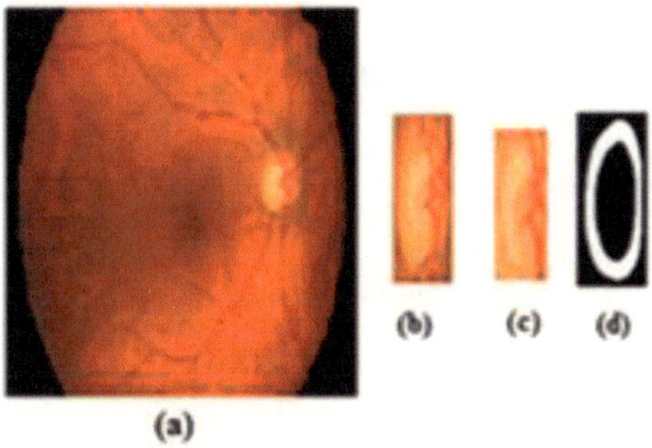

Figure 12.
HRF dataset sample. (a) Original sample. (b) Segmented optic disc. (c) Segmented optic cup. (d) Binary image showing neuroretinal rim.

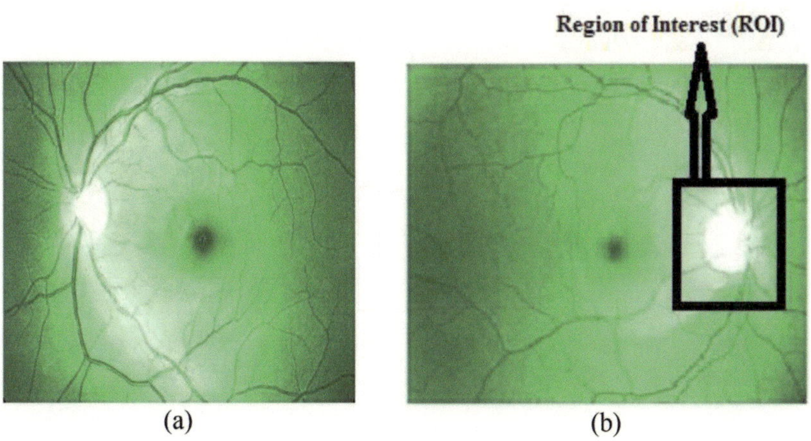

Figure 13.
Vessels in fundus image showing ROI: (a) vessels in the normal eye with smaller vessels around the optic disc; (b) the absence of smaller vessels around the optic disc in the glaucoma eye.

bottom, left, and right sides are identified, thus localizing it. A sample fundus image from our dataset and its corresponding identified ROI image part are shown in **Figure 14**.

In signal processing applications, analysis of signal in frequency domain is preferred over the time domain since they contain more information of the signal. This requires conversion of the signal from time domain to frequency domain. Fourier transform can be used to obtain the frequency contents of a signal. But it does not reveal which frequency component is present at what time instance of the signal. Wavelet transform, on the other hand, reveals this information and conveys more detailed information regarding the signal or the image. In image processing techniques such as segmentation, image decomposition using undecimated biorthogonal wavelet transforms is employed, as these transforms also facilitate reconstruction of the images [23]. For segmentation of astronomical and biological images where images contain isotropic objects, the isotropic undecimated wavelet transform (IUWT) can be applied for segmentation. In the fundus images, vessels are isotropic in nature. Hence IUWT can be used for segmentation of vessels. When ROI is subjected to IUWT, decompositions at different wavelet levels are shown in **Figure 15**.

2.3.2 Vessel localization

For further processing, an image with a wavelet level of 3 is considered. To obtain the centerline of each of the segmented vessels, they are subjected to a thinning process which converts a vessel into a thin vessel of one pixel thickness. The position of this thin vessel will be almost in the center of the vessel, and it represents the centerline of the vessel. A sample of segmented vessels of ROI is shown in **Figure 16(a)**. The output of the thinning process of the sample vessels is shown in **Figure 16(b)**, which depicts the thinned centerlines of vessels. **Figure 16(c)** depicts the identified thinned branches after removing the branch pixels. Each thin line in the image of **Figure 16(c)** represents a separate vessel. Now, each thin line in the image represents a separate vessel.

Using connected component technique, each line (vessel) in the image is indexed and can be accessed with that index. Further, using the index information, the coordinates of the centerline pixels of each vessel are determined, thereby localizing the vessels. Further, the vessel data structure is created and maintained

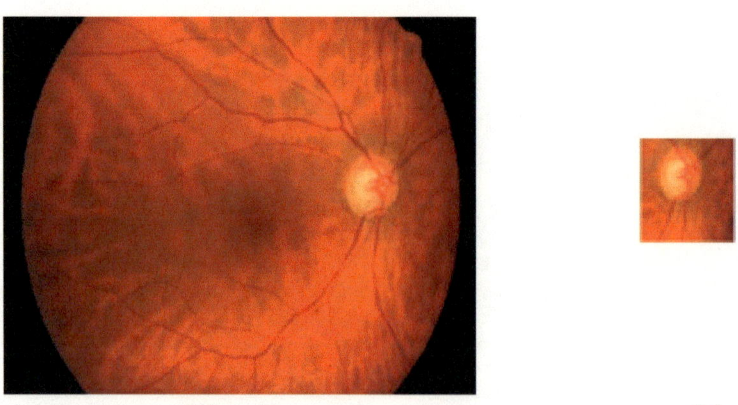

Figure 14.
(a) Input image. (b) Extracted ROI.

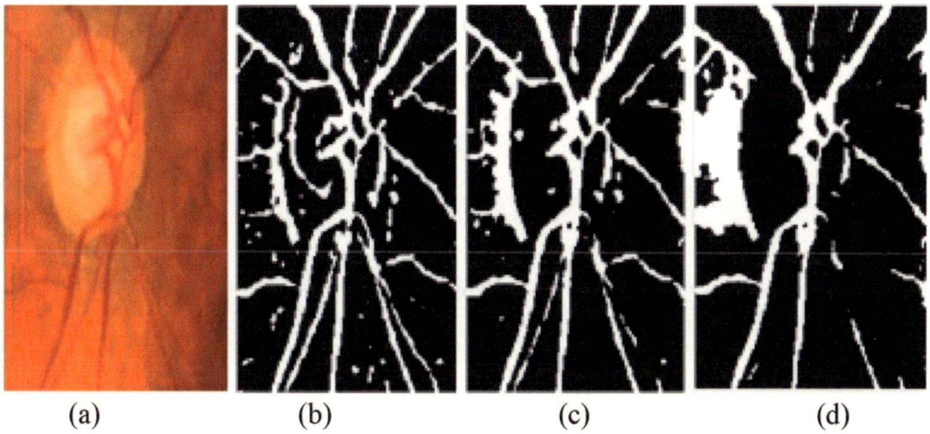

Figure 15.
(a) Extracted ROI. (b) Image with low wavelet level of 3. (c) Image with high wavelet level of 4. (d) Image with wavelet level of 5.

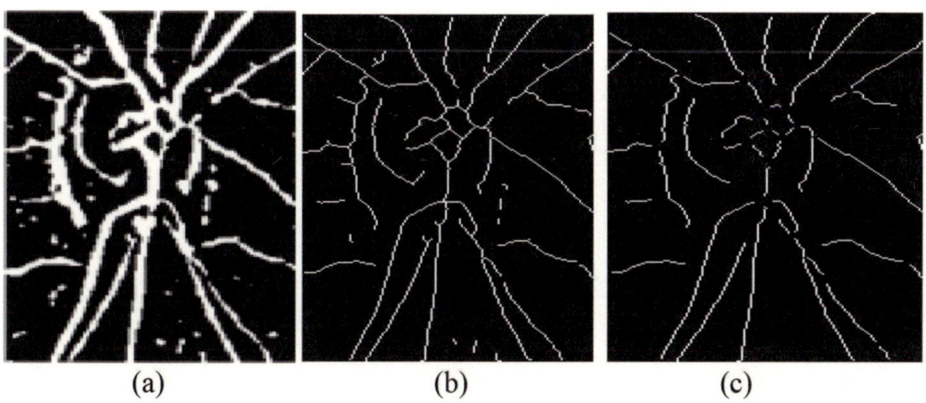

Figure 16.
(a) Vessels from the segmented image. (b) Thinned centerlines and (c) centerlines with branches separated.

which contains the entire information regarding the vessels. Vessel-based feature vessel risk index (VRI) is extracted from the information obtained in vessel data structure [18].

2.4 Glaucoma detection methodology using wavelet texture features

The block diagram of the methodology used is shown in **Figure 17**. The input fundus image is preprocessed for removal of background noise. Preprocessed image is decomposed by using wavelet filters to obtain the approximation and detail coefficients of the image. From these coefficients, texture features are generated. These texture features are fed to the ANN classifier to detect Glaucoma. In the preprocessing stage, arithmetic mean filter [20] is used to remove the background noise of the fundus image.

2.4.1 Image decomposition and texture feature extraction

The preprocessed image is decomposed by applying the wavelets. The set of 14 wavelet features' average and energy values are considered as the texture

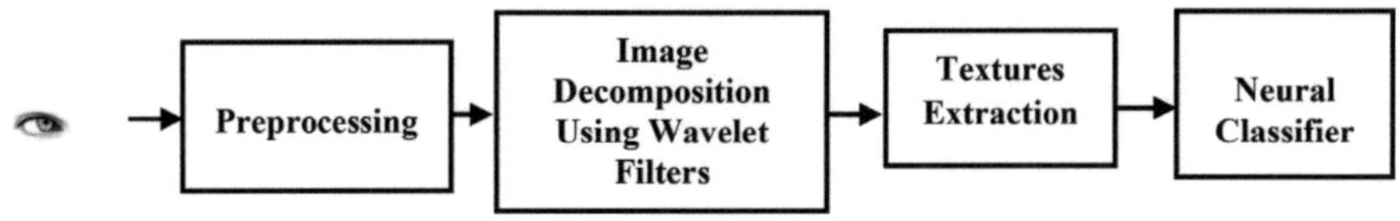

Figure 17.
Block schematic of glaucoma detection using texture features.

features of an image which can be used for classification of the image as normal or Glaucoma image.

We apply the three wavelets daubechies (db3), symlets (sym3), and biorthogonal (bio3.3, bio3.5, and bio3.7) separately for the fundus image and first obtain the approximation and the detail coefficients. Later, we compute the average and the energy values from these coefficients.

Among the average and energy values, we have used only average value of the horizontal information and energy of vertical information for all the wavelets (db3, sym3, bio3.3, bio3.5, and bio3.7). In addition, we have used the diagonal energy values for bio3.3, bio3.5, and bio3.7 and horizontal energy value for bio3.7, totaling to 14 texture values all together from all the wavelets. The other average and energy values are not used since their values for the normal and Glaucoma images lie in the same range, which has been verified by analyzing the values. This selection also has been reported in [24]. The texture values extracted from a fundus image are fed to the neural classifier for classification.

2.4.2 Neural classifier

Classification using ANN is the state-of-the-art technique employed for efficient classifications. We have used feedforward ANN with modified backpropagation training technique to implement the classifier. Feedforward multiple layer perceptron (MLP) neural networks are one of the important types of neural networks. They are widely used in recognition systems due to their good generalization property. MLPs consist of multiple layers as shown in **Figure 18**. It has one input and one output layer. One or more hidden layers are used in between input and output layers. The number of neurons in the input layer depends on the number of inputs to be fed to the network, and the number of neurons in the output layer depends on the number of outputs to be generated for the final classifier output. Hidden layers can have any number of neurons. Output of a neuron of input/hidden layer is connected to the input of all neurons in the next layer in fully connected network, as shown in **Figure 19**.

2.4.3 Glaucoma neural classifier architecture

We used a 4-layer MLP with input layer, two hidden layers, and output layer. For each input fundus image, 14 wavelet features are extracted. To feed these 14 features, input layer has 14 neurons. As the output result we want it to be either normal or Glaucoma indication, the output layer consists of only one neuron. We used two hidden layers with 14 neurons in each layer as we could get better results with two hidden layers than one. The architecture of the neural classifier used is shown in **Figure 18**.

Different training methods can be used to train the MLPs for classification. We employed the modified popular backpropagation training algorithm with the minimum

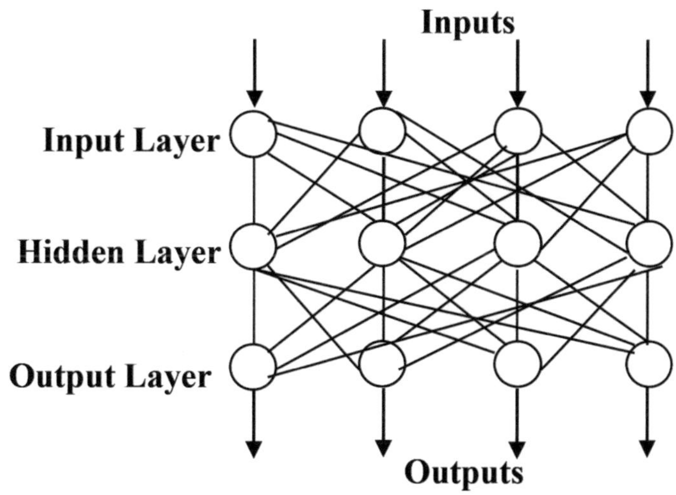

Figure 18.
Architecture of glaucoma neural classifier.

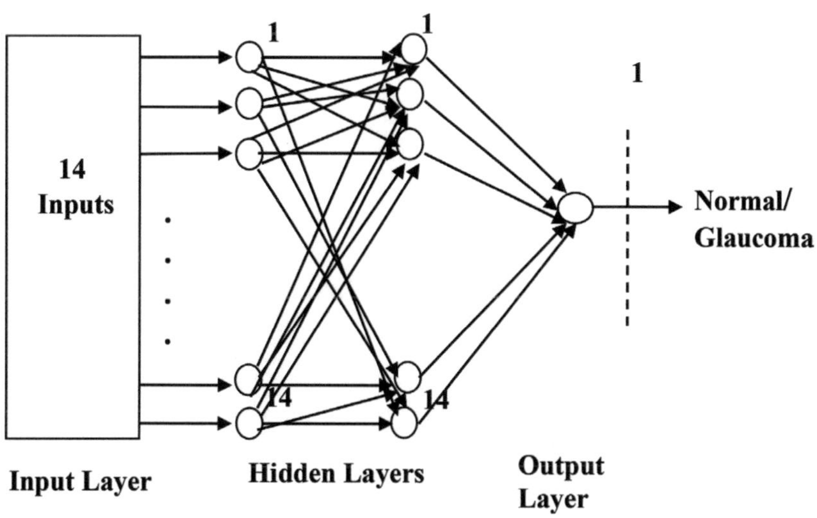

Figure 19.
Feedforward neural network.

mean square error performance as a function for training our neural classifier. Levenberg–Marquardt method [25, 26] of optimization is used to train the classifier.

3. Results and discussion

Our final proposed integrated Glaucoma classifier system considers all these proposed features for classification. The structural features are related to the optic disc and cup such as CDR, RDR, and superior and inferior rim thicknesses, which are extracted using template methodology. VRI, the vessel structural feature, and texture features are obtained by wavelet filters. This aspect of incorporating more features has led to improvement of the efficiency of Glaucoma detection which can be seen from comparison of results as shown in **Table 1**. Totally, 120 Glaucoma images and 60 normal images were used from the datasets for comparison.

Image type	Results of using vessel-based feature VRI	Results of feature extraction using NSK template	Results of using wavelets and neural classifier	Results of final integrated glaucoma classifier
Glaucoma dataset	85%	94%	95%	98.57%
Normal dataset	83%	90%	94%	94%

Table 1.
Results of glaucoma classifier.

4. Conclusions

Literature survey reveals that previous attempts were made to detect Glaucoma by extracting predominantly CDR or wavelet-based features. In our research work of Glaucoma detection, we have enhanced the efficiency of Glaucoma detection system by processing and analyzing additional fundus image features apart from the CDR or wavelet features leading to a hybrid approach.

We have also improved the efficiency of CDR-based Glaucoma detection system by a template for correlation with input fundus images. As seen from Results section, template correlation approach is better than intensity threshold techniques. Additional features, RDR and neuroretinal rim thickness, have improved the efficiency of the system.

We have introduced vessel-based features for Glaucoma detection which is a significant step toward Glaucoma detection. As seen in the literature, reductions in vessel diameters are the indication of Glaucoma. To detect this we have incorporated database where these significant features can be stored and monitored for regular visits of patients.

Wavelet-based strategy has also been used by us to increase the efficiency of the system. We have used feedforward neural networks to classify the input fundus images using wavelet-based textures.

Acknowledgements

We would like to express our sincere gratitude to Ophthalmology department of KLE Society's Dr. Prabhakar Kore Hospital & M.R.C., Belagavi, India, for providing us with necessary guidance and resources required for experimentation and special thanks to High-Resolution Fundus (HRF) Image Database available on the Internet [13]. We would like to thank Research Center, E & C Department of Jawaharlal Nehru National College of Engineering, Shivamogga, India, and Electronics and Communication Department, KLE Dr. M.S. Sheshgiri College of Engineering and Technology, Belagavi, India, for technical guidance and resources, without which venture would not have been possible.

Author details

Nataraj Vijapur[1]* and R. Srinivasarao Kunte[2]

1 KLE Dr. M.S. Sheshgiri College of Engineering and Technology, Belagavi, Karnataka, India

2 Sahyadri College of Engineering and Management, Mangalore, Karnataka, India

*Address all correspondence to: nvijapur@gmail.com

References

[1] Raychaudhuri A, Lahiri SK, Bandyopadhyay M, Foster PJ, Reeves BC, Johnson GJ. A population based survey of the prevalence and types of glaucoma in rural West Bengal. The West Bengal Glaucoma Study. The British Journal of Ophthalmology. 2005;**89**(12):1559-1564

[2] Song X, Song K, Chen Y. A computer-based diagnosis system for early glaucoma screening. In: Proc. IEEE Engineering in Medicine and Biology 27th Annual Conf. 2005. pp. 6608-6611

[3] Eye Anatomy. Available from http://www.optos.com/en-US/Patients/Healthy-sight/Eye-anatomy/ [Accessed: 15 December 2016]

[4] Guyton AC, Hall JE. Textbook of Medical Physiology. 9th ed. Elseveir Saunders; 1996

[5] Nath MK, Dandapat S. Techniques of glaucoma detection from color fundus images: A review. International Journal of Image, Graphics and Signal Processing. 2012;**4**:44-51

[6] Mishra M, Nath MK, Nirmala SR, Dandapat S. Image processing techniques for Glaucoma detection. Communications in Computer and Information Science: Advances in Computing and Communications: Springer. 2011;**192**:365-373

[7] Jonas JD, Nguyen XN, Naumann GOH. Parapapillary retinal vessel diameter in normal and glaucoma eyes: Morphometric data. Investigative Ophthalmology & Visual Science. 1989;**30**(7):1599-1603

[8] Hall JK, Andrews AP, Walker R, Piltz-Seymour JR. Association of retinal vessel caliber and visual field defects in glaucoma. American Journal of Ophthalmology. 2001;**132**(6):857-859

[9] Dua S, Acharya UR, Ng EYK. Computational Analysis of the Human Eye with Applications. World Scientific Press; 2011

[10] Nayak J, Rajendra Acharya U, Bhat PS, Shetty N, Lim T-C, et al. Automated diagnosis of glaucoma using digital fundus images. Journal of Medical Systems. 2009;**33**:337-346. DOI: 10.1007/s10916-008-9195-z

[11] Vijapur N, Chitins S, Kunte RSR. Improved efficiency of glaucoma detection by using wavelet filters, prediction and segmentation method. International Journal of Electronics, Electrical and Computational System. 2014;**3**(8):1-13

[12] Uhm KB, Lee DY, Kim JT, Hong C. Peripapillary atrophy in normal and primary open-angle glaucoma. Korean Journal of Ophthalmology. 1998:37-50

[13] Budai A, Odstrcilik J. High-Resolution Fundus (HRF) Image Database. Available from: https://www5.cs.fau.de/research/data/fundus-images/

[14] Odstrcilik J, Kolar R, Budai A, Hornegger J, Jan J, Gazarek J, et al. Retinal vessel segmentation by improved matched filtering: Evaluation on a new high-resolution fundus image database. IET Image Processing. 2013;**7**(4):373-383. DOI: 10.1049/iet-ipr.2012.0455

[15] Lowell J, Hunter A, Steel D, Basu A, Ryder R, Fletcher E, et al. Optic nerve head segmentation. IEEE Transactions on Medical Imaging. 2004;**23**(2):256-264

[16] Real Statistics Using Excel: Correlation: Basic Concepts, Available from: http://www.real-statistics.com/correlation/ [Accessed: 22 February 2015]

[17] Nataraj A Vijapur, R. SR Kunte. Glaucoma detection by using Pearson-R correlation filter. In: Proc. 4th IEEE International Conference on Communication and Signal Processing (ICCSP'15). 2015; 1194-1198. DOI: 10.1109/ICCSP.2015.7322695

[18] Vijapur NA, Kunte RSR. Sensitized glaucoma detection using a unique template based correlation filter and undecimated isotropic wavelet transform. Journal of Medical and Biological Engineering. 2017;**37**:365. DOI: 10.1007/s40846-017-0234-4

[19] Nyúl LG. Retinal image analysis for automated glaucoma risk evaluation. In: Liu J, Doi K, Fenster A, Chan SC, editors. Medical Imaging, Parallel Processing of Images, and Optimization Techniques. Vol. 7497. 2009. pp. 74971C-1-74971C-9. DOI: 10.1117/12.851179

[20] Xu Y, Xu D, Lin S, Liu J, Cheng J, Cheung CY, et al. Sliding window and regression based cup detection in digital fundus images for glaucoma diagnosis. LNCS. 2011;**6893**:1-8

[21] Patton N, Aslam TM, MacGillivray T, Deary IJ, Dhillon B, Eikelboom RH, et al. Retinal image analysis: concepts, applications and potential. Progress in Retinal and Eye Research. 2005:99-127

[22] Lee SB, Hong KBUC. Retinal vessel diameter In normal and primary open angle glaucoma. Korean Journal of Ophthalmology. 1998;**12**:51-59

[23] Starck J-L, Fadili J, Murtagh F. The undecimated wavelet decomposition and its reconstruction. IEEE Transactions on Image Processing. 2007;**16**(2):297-309

[24] Dua S, Acharya UR, Chowriappa P, Sree SV. Wavelet-based energy features for glaucomatous image classification. IEEE Transactions on Information Technology in Biomedicine. 2012;**16**:80-87. DOI: 10.1109/TITB.2011.2176540.

[25] Levenberg K. A method for the solution of certain non-linear problems in least squares. Quarterly of Applied Mathematics. 1944;**2**:164-168

[26] Auer P, Burgsteiner H, Maass W. A learning rule for very simple universal approximators consisting of a single layer of perceptrons. Neural Networks. 2008;**21**(5):786-795

Chapter 7

Risk Assessment of Ocular Hypertension and the Use of Medication

Claire Chow and Poemen Pui-man Chan

Abstract

Ocular hypertension (OHT) is the only known modifiable risk factor of glaucoma development. Intraocular pressure (IOP)-lowering therapy reduces the risk of glaucoma development. The 5-year risk of glaucoma conversion is <10% for untreated OHT patients. Cost-effectiveness analyses suggested that it is not cost-effective to treat all patients with OHT. Treatment should be targeted towards the higher-risk group—namely, patients with older age, a higher level of IOP, a thinner central corneal thickness (CCT), a larger vertical cup-to-disc ratio (VCDR) and a smaller pattern standard deviation (PSD) value on visual field (VF) test. These risk factors were established by the Ocular Hypertension Treatment Study (OHTS) and the European Glaucoma Prevention Study (EGPS). However, there is significant variability in the measurement of the currently known risk factors, especially if the assessment is taken from a longitudinal perspective. This can lead to overtreatment or under-treatment: the former exposing the patient to unnecessary side effects of IOP-lowering eye drops and the latter putting the patient at risk of developing glaucoma. The advancement of new VF algorithm and ocular imaging can lead to the identification of new approaches to risk stratification and, thus, more specific treatment for OHT patients.

Keywords: ocular hypertension (OHT), glaucoma 5-year risk calculator, vertical cup-to-disc ratio (VCDR), intraocular pressure (IOP)

1. Introduction

Glaucoma is a leading cause of irreversible blindness worldwide [1]. Subjects with ocular hypertension (OHT) are known to have a higher risk of glaucoma development. OHT is defined as a mean intraocular pressure (IOP) ≥24 mmHg from two separate consecutive measurements without structural and functional evidence of glaucoma [2]. Patients with OHT are usually treated with IOP-lowering therapy based on the effectiveness of reducing the risk of glaucoma development according to the result of the Ocular Hypertension Treatment Study (OHTS) [3], which demonstrated a cumulative probability of 9.5% of developing primary open-angle glaucoma (POAG) in 5 years in the untreated OHT patients, compared with 4.4% in the treated group (patients who received IOP-lowering therapy). Hence, the incidence of POAG could be reduced by about 50% with adequate IOP reduction. In clinical practice, it is not uncommon that we adopt a treatment approach of liberally prescribing IOP-lowering medication based on the study results.

On the other hand, the result of the OHTS also reflects that only <10% of the untreated OHT patients developed glaucoma in 5 years, compared to the 4.4% of the treated group. Hence, the number needed to treat to prevent one glaucoma development is 20. Indeed, it has been shown that treating all patients with OHT is not cost-effective [4, 5]. The estimated incremental cost of treating all OHT patients to prevent one subject from developing glaucoma was US$89,072 [4]. This is considered not cost-effective according to the standard of The National Institute for Health and Care Excellence (NICE), which classified a treatment as cost-effective at the level of risk when the incremental cost-effectiveness ratio (ICER) is equal to or less than US$50,000 [6]. Furthermore, long-term treatment with IOP-lowering medications can impose significant inconvenience and undesirable side effects to patients, such as ocular surface disease. For instance, a study that involved 537 OHT and POAG patients showed that side effects from medication can independently contribute to health-related quality of life scores, which could be as worse as 0.11 [7]. This is equivalent to the utility loss of patients with early to moderate stage of glaucoma [8, 9]. Therefore, selective and targeted use of medication is not merely a health economic issue; unnecessarily treating low-risk OHT patients would expose them to undesirable medication side effects without beneficial gain.

2. Risk stratification and cost-effectiveness of treating ocular hypertension

A more cost-effective approach is to treat OHT subjects who have higher risk of developing POAG—namely, an older age, a higher level of IOP, a thinner central corneal thickness (CCT), a larger vertical cup-to-disc ratio (VCDR) and a smaller pattern standard deviation (PSD) value on visual field (VF) test. These are risk factors of POAG development according to the joint data of the OHTS [2] and the European Glaucoma Prevention Study (EGPS) [10]. These are the two major multicentre, randomised control trials (RCTs) that involved patients with OHT. Stewart et al. suggested that it is cost-effective to treat patients with older age (≥76 years old), higher intraocular pressure (≥29 mmHg), thinner central corneal thickness (≤533 μm) and wider vertical cup-to-disc ratio (≥0.6) [4]. Kymes et al. suggested that treating OHT patients with IOP ≥24 mmHg and a ≥ 2% annual risk of glaucoma development is likely to be cost-effective [5]. Weinreb et al. suggested a risk stratification strategy: observation for patients with lower than average risk of POAG conversion (5-year risk of <5%), collaborative treatment decision between doctor and well-informed patient for those with moderate risk (5-year risk of 5–15%) and treatment for all subjects with higher than average risk (5-year risk of >15%) [11]. Based on this risk stratification strategy, it was demonstrated that nearly half (43.9%) of low-risk OHT eyes could safely have their medications reduced over 1 year, realising substantial savings [12]. In this study, only 1 out of 107 eyes (0.93%) developed a repeatable VF defect in the first year [12].

The 5-year risk of POAG development can be calculated using the available risk calculator, which was developed based on a predictive model that utilised the joint data of OHTS and EGPS [13]. The calculation is based on the risk factors as mentioned—age, IOP, CCT, VCDR and PSD value of VF. It has the advantage of integrating multiple risk factors into one quantitative, estimated percentage risk of glaucoma development in OHT subjects. This can facilitate treatment decision because high-risk subjects can be identified based on simultaneous and quantitative consideration of all these available risk factors; thus, allows a more straightforward and cost-effective approach of treatment; and reduces unnecessary patient exposure to medication side effects.

3. Variability of risk factor measurement and the effects on risk assessment

It is important to note that, similar to most multivariate prediction models derived from prospective studies [14], we are making several assumptions when we apply the 5-year risk calculator to guide treatment decision: [1] we assume that the baseline variables that were measured are the most predictive of the risk of glaucoma development, [2] the model also assumes that the risk of glaucoma progression is linear, and [3] patients who are being assessed have similar clinical characteristics as the participants in the OHTS and EGPS.

However, the variability of baseline risk factor measurements is a known phenomenon. IOP is well known to vary from visit to visit [15], which can be due to regression to the mean phenomenon, diurnal variation as well as order of IOP measurement [15]. This variability is also observed in the performance of VF, hence the PSD value [16]. Results of VF examination can be affected by patients' subjectivity and the substantial test-retest variability. The PSD value is a weighted standard deviation of the differences between the measured and normal reference visual field at each test location. A higher PSD value merely suggests a more irregular 'hill of vision', which can contribute to variability in patients' responses and/or areas of focal loss. Given that, by definition, OHT subjects do not have glaucomatous VF defect, the PSD value tends to be low. Therefore, a slight variability in patients' responses can contribute to a significant change in its value. Care must be taken when interpreting PSD value as a stand-alone figure.

Therefore, the apparently more comprehensive risk stratification strategy that is based on the 5-year risk calculator can face several fundamental challenges. As discussed, the variability of IOP measurement and PSD value, even during baseline assessment, may add a considerable source of error to the risk calculation. Furthermore, due to the within-subject changes in risk factors' values during follow-up, the correlation between baseline and updated values may diminish with time [17]. One study has demonstrated that risk calculation is variable over time and that longitudinal changes in baseline variables correspond with changes in the risk estimation of glaucoma development [18]. In the study, the 5-year risk of POAG development was calculated by incorporating different measurements that assume the best-case scenario (baseline age, lowest PSD, highest CCT and lowest IOP) and the worst-case scenario (final age, highest PSD, lowest CCT and highest IOP). For the VCDR, a value of ±0.2 was applied to model interobserver and intraobserver variability (i.e. -0.2 in addition to the best-case scenario and + 0.2 in addition to the worst-case scenario). It was found that, within the same individual, the mean risk of POAG conversion could increase by almost 10-fold when comparing the worst- and best-case scenarios (5.0% vs. 45.7%, $P < 0.01$). Hence, risk stratification is dynamic, and risk estimations should be recalculated during follow-up visits as variables can fluctuate significantly within the same individual over time.

It is important to note that the VCDR data that derived the risk calculator was based on VCDR measurements on the optic disc stereophotography of the OHTS and EGPS cohorts. In the RCTs, the measurement and evaluation of the optic nerve head (ONH) were performed by highly trained, independent graders at designated optic disc centres that followed a strict protocol in a non-clinical setting [19]. In clinical practice, the assessment of ONH and the measurement of VCDR by individual ophthalmologists are susceptible to intraobserver and interobserver variability [20]. The precision and quality of the ONH evaluation is unlikely to match those in the RCTs.

Nowadays, imaging technologies such as confocal scanning laser ophthalmoscopy by Heidelberg retinal tomography (HRT) and optical coherence tomography (OCT) provide an objective and reproducible measurement of optic disc parameters. However, different techniques of evaluating ONH (hence the VCDR measurement) may not agree with each other. For instance, there is a poor agreement in the optic disc measurements obtained from HRT and OCT [21]. A study that compared VCDR measurement obtained with OCT, HRT and stereophotography in untreated OHT patients showed that there were poor agreement and lack of interchangeability between different techniques [22]. This is due to the differences between

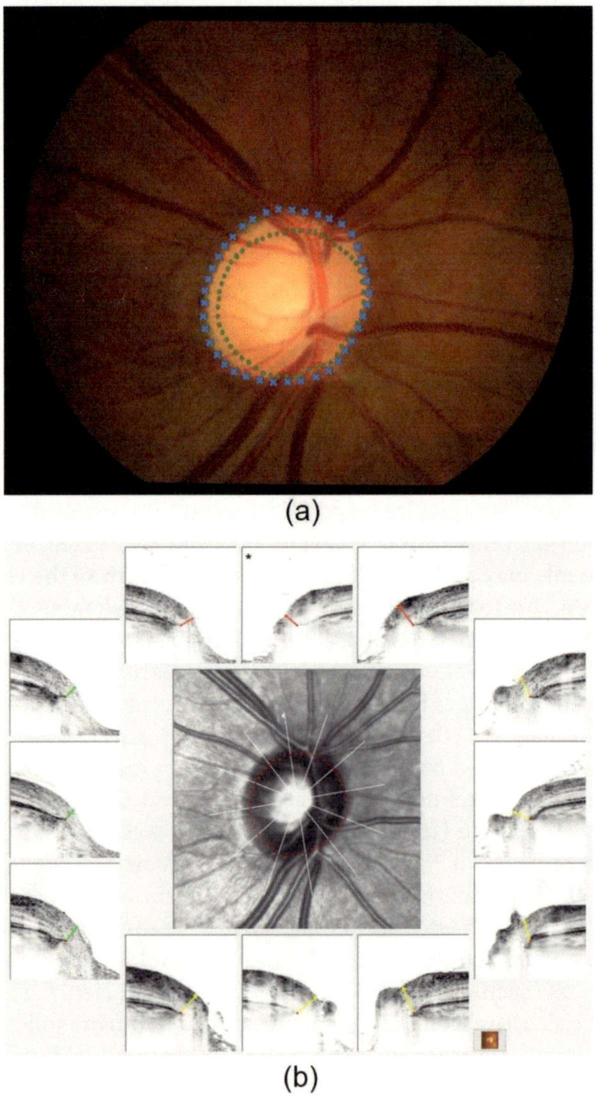

Figure 1.
Optic disc of a normal right eye (a) and corresponding spectral-domain optical coherence tomography (OCT, (b)) delineating the anatomical measurements of disc margin. The green dots on the fundus photo represent the Bruch's membrane opening (BMO) identified by spectral-domain optical coherence tomography (OCT). The blue crosses represent the disc margin that was identified by an examiner with stereophotography. Hence, the green dots and blue crosses represent the potential disc margins that could be identified by different examiners (adapted from Chauhan BC and Burgoyne CF 2013 [25]).

the techniques in defining optic disc margin and optic disc cup. The assessment of ONH in HRT and stereophotography relies on the examiners to define the disc margin, which can be variable. Spectral-domain OCT demonstrated that the 'perceived disc margin' of HRT and stereophotography rarely correlate with the Bruch's membrane opening (BMO) (**Figure 1**) [23, 24], which is considered to be the true outer border of the neural tissue because axons cannot pass through an intact Bruch's membrane to exit the eye [25]. The BMO is also unaltered under larger change of IOP [26]. Hence, it is a more reliable landmark, especially for eyes with OHT. Spectral-domain OCT is arguably more accurate in defining the ONH because it defines the BMO at every clock hour. It can also reliably identify the cup margin by measuring the minimum distance between the BMO and the internal limiting membrane in all meridians; the built-in software can then define the maximal vertical diameter to be the vertical cup diameter. In comparison, the definition of vertical cup diameter by stereoscopic photography and HRT are likely to be less accurate. Both are based on subjective judgement of examiners in defining the cup and disc margin. In some cases of small cups that do not pass through the midline of the optic disc, HRT has difficulties in calculating the VCDR because it obtains the vertical cup diameter along the vertical axis at the midline of the disc. Hence, the value of VCDR becomes '0' if the cup does not pass through the vertical midline.

The study that compared VCDR measured by OCT, HRT and stereophotography of the ONH in patients with untreated OHT also investigated how the degree of disagreement extended to their corresponding 5-year risk estimation when other risk factors were kept contant [22]. In the study, ONH images of 140 untreated OHT eyes (of 75 patients) were taken by fundus camera (stereoscopic images), OCT and HRT. ONH stereophotographs were evaluated with a stereo-viewer by two glaucoma specialists, and the VCDR was measured with the ImageJ software. VCDR measurements obtained with stereophotography, OCT and HRT were used to calculate the estimated 5-year risk. The study showed that there was disagreement in VCDR measurements between the three methods. This disagreement also extended to their corresponding 5-year risk estimation of POAG development [22]. When the comparison was made on the Bland–Altman plots, the range of discrepancies tended to widen with increasing mean risk, especially beyond the estimated

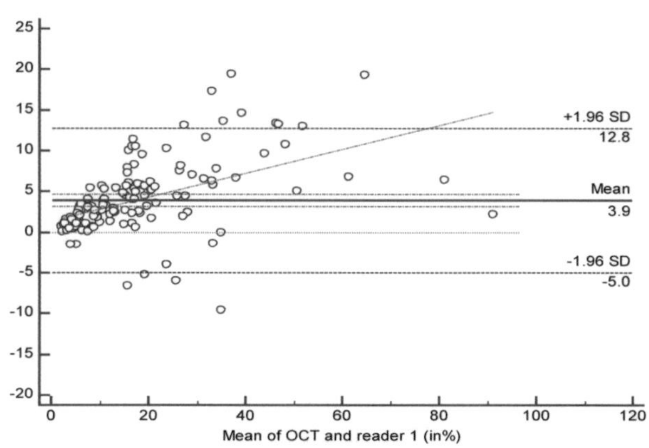

Figure 2.
Bland-Altman plot: comparison of 5-year risk estimations of POAG conversion that were calculated by vertical cup-to-disc ratio measured by different vertical cup-to-disc ratio measured by spectral-domain optical coherence tomography (OCT) and stereophotography performed by a glaucoma specialist. Notice that the range of discrepancies widen with increasing mean risk, especially beyond the estimated risk of >15%. OCT, optical coherence tomography; reader 1, stereophotography evaluation (adopted from Chan PP et al., 2019 [22]).

risk of >15% (**Figure 2**). We should be careful when using the 5-year risk of >15% as our treatment threshold when using VCDR values that are obtained from different measurement techniques. This can dramatically alter the management approach for any OHT subjects, especially if they have a relatively high baseline estimated risk and/or larger VCDR. In the cohort of untreated OHT eyes from this study, up to 72 eyes (51.2%) would require treatment if OCT was used for assessing the VCDR, according to the ≥15% 5-year risk cut-off. On the other hand, only 54 eyes (38.6%) would require treatment if the VCDR measurements were obtained from stereophotography by one of the glaucoma specialists. Therefore, one must be cautious when applying the risk estimation obtained from the other means of measuring VCDR.

4. Detection of retinal nerve fibre layer defect and early diagnosis of glaucoma

The diagnosis of glaucoma requires a confirmed glaucomatous VF defect that correlates with structural change. A glaucomatous visual field loss is defined as a cluster of ≥3 non-edged points in the PSD plot in a single hemifield with p value <5%, one of which must have a p value <1%; glaucoma hemifield test outside normal limits; and PSD with p value <5%. Any one of these criteria, if repeatable, was considered as sufficient evidence of a glaucomatous VF defect [27]. This has been considered as the gold standard of diagnosing glaucoma. OCT has gained popularity in the past decades and is now the standard for assessing structural damage of retinal nerve fibre layer (RNFL) and ONH for the detection of structural glaucomatous change. Indeed, RNFL and ONH measured by OCT were shown to be useful in differentiating normal eyes from even mild glaucoma [28]. Evidence suggests that RNFL thinning measured by OCT can detect glaucomatous damage several years before detectable functional deficits by VF testing [28–30]. The 10th World Glaucoma Association consensus meeting stated that 'detecting progressive glaucomatous RNFL thinning and neuroretinal rim narrowing is the best currently available gold standard for glaucoma diagnosis [31]'. This emphasised the importance of detecting RNFL abnormalities in terms of the diagnosis of glaucoma. Since OCT is becoming an invaluable tool for detecting early changes of ONH and RNFL thinning, especially because of its repeatability and objectiveness, it is logical to suggest that a risk scoring system for OHT patients should include OCT measurements.

On the contrary, the measurement of VCDR by stereoscopic photography or during clinical examination remains the only parameter in the risk calculator that reflects the structural status of the complex architecture of the ONH. During the slow and progressive process of glaucoma development, enlargement of VCDR could happen much later than the occurrence of RNFL thinning and other subtle structural glaucomatous damage. It is important to note that the powerful and carefully designed OHTS and EGPS were performed in the era when OCT was not widely used as an investigative tool. The two studies ruled out glaucoma patients from OHT mainly based on VF criteria and the absence of detectable structural damage on stereoscopic photography. Therefore, it might not be cavalier to suggest that a portion of these subjects might already have 'asymptomatic disease' (or preperimetric glaucoma) (**Figure 3**), and this damage was undetectable on stereoscopic photography, which was also suggested by Weinreb et al. [11]. The ever-evolving OCT technology and the concepts of ONH assessment can provide valuable data and new parameters for further refinement of the existing risk calculator, for instance, integrating other factors of OHN and RNFL based on OCT measurement [22]. The glaucoma risk model needs refinement that involves the advancing OCT technologies and concepts in measuring VCDR. Reliable risk estimation is

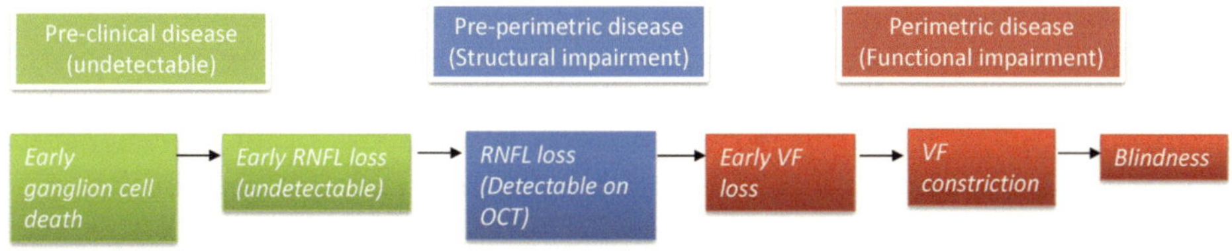

Figure 3.
Spectrum of disease in glaucoma. RNFL, retinal nerve fibre layer. OCT, optical coherence tomography. VF, visual field (adapted from Weinreb et al., 2004 [11]).

important as it may guide treatment decision, which in turn has consequences on both health economics and patients' quality of life.

5. The new trends of early detection of glaucoma and disease progression

5.1 Detecting of RNFL thinning and disease progression

Evidence shows that RNFL abnormalities can often be evident without detectable VF damage [32–35]. Therefore, measuring the change of RNFL is likely to be useful in detecting early disease progression. Spectral-domain OCT is now the invaluable investigation tool for glaucoma patients because it can measure RNFL thickness reliably [36] with high sensitivity and specificity to detect glaucoma [37, 38] and its progression [39]. Commercially available software event-based algorithm, such as the Guided Progression Analysis (GPA, Carl Zeiss Meditec), can detect progressive RNFL thinning using RNFL thickness maps. A study has demonstrated that GPA can detect and visualise different patterns of progressive RNFL thinning [39]. Trend-Based Progression Analysis (TPA) is another algorithm for detecting progressive RNFL thinning by measuring the rate of change in RNFL thickness for each superpixel of the RNFL thickness map (50 x 50 superpixels). A study that involved 139 POAG patients (240 eyes) followed up for ≥5 years showed that progressive RNFL thinning determined by GPA and TPA was predictive of detectable functional decline in glaucoma. The study showed that TPA outperformed GPA in detecting more eyes with progressive RNFL thinning at a similar level of specificity (84.2% vs. 81.7% for TPA and GPA, respectively) [40]. Furthermore, TPA also provides visualisation of the distribution of the rate of RNFL thinning. It was suggested that the detection of progressive RNFL loss can serve as a biomarker to reflect disease deterioration behaviour and hence guide glaucoma management [40]. However, TPA is not without its limitations. A minimum of four follow-up visits is required for the construction of the TPA, and performance can be undermined with fewer visits. In situations where there are abrupt RNFL changes or in eyes with large test-retest variability, the event-based analysis may be more useful [41]. The authors concluded that TPA enhances but may not replace GPA for topographic analysis of RNFL thinning.

5.2 The dynamic target IOP, disease progression and quality of life: The LiGHT trial

Clinical trials usually define a treatment IOP-lowering target. For instance, the OHT study aimed for an IOP lowering by 20% from baseline for patients in the treatment arm [3], whereas the Collaborative Normal Tension Glaucoma (CNTG) study targeted an IOP lowering by 30% from baseline [42]. The Laser in Glaucoma and Ocular Hypertension (LiGHT) trial is a multicentre RCT that compared eye drops versus selective laser trabeculoplasty as first-line treatment for POAG or OHT [43]. The study is unique with its well-constructed algorithm for detecting disease progression and guiding treatment escalation [44]. It has a novel approach to defining target IOP. Firstly, the target IOP is specific for each patient at baseline, based on disease severity and lifetime risk of loss of vision at recruitment (e.g. different target pressure and percentage IOP reduction according to the disease stratification suggested by Mills et al. [45]). Secondly, the IOP was adjustable based on IOP control and disease progression [44]. The disease progression (either glaucoma deterioration or conversion of OHT to POAG) was determined by a decision support software based on objective visual field and optic disc imaging criteria. Disease progression was defined as 'strong evidence', with the Humphrey GPA software showing 'likely progression' and/or HRT rim area > 1% per year (at $P < 0.001$), and 'less strong evidence' with GPA showing 'possible progression' and/or HRT rim area > 1% per year (at $P < 0.01$). 'Likely visual field progression' is the presence of three or more points on the GPA at <0.05 probability for change on three consecutive occasions, while 'possible visual field progression' is the same criterion but on only two consecutive occasions [44]. Optic disc progression was defined as the rate of neuroretinal rim loss exceeding 1% of baseline rim area/year on a minimum of five repeat HRT images, where this is equivalent to approximately twice the value of normal age-related rim area loss [22]. Following treatment escalation, there is a resetting of both the target IOP and visual field and optic disc baselines against which future assessments will be compared with.

Although the LiGHT trial is probably more complex in its target IOP setting algorithm compared with other glaucoma trials which defined treatment success based on the proportion of patients achieving a particular target percentage reduction of IOP, it resembled closer to our clinical practice. For instance, further IOP lowering beyond the 'target IOP' is probably required for patients with progressive disease. In some cases, patients might request to reduce medication use even when the target IOP is not achieved (e.g. OHT patients with IOP at 24 mmHg who do not want treatment and show no signs of POAG conversion). Furthermore, the LiGHT trial is also unique in that it included the evaluation of quality of life as an outcome measure. These are all novel features that might become important components for future glaucoma study design.

6. Conclusion

It is more cost-effective to selectively treat OHT subjects who have a higher risk of POAG conversion. However, risk assessment can be difficult due to the variabilities in the measurement of the baseline variables of the glaucoma risk calculator. In the era of advancing OCT technology and knowledge of glaucoma, there may be a need to refine our existing risk assessment methodology.

Conflict of interest

All authors have no financial/proprietary interest in the subject matters of the manuscript.

Author details

Claire Chow[1,2] and Poemen Pui-man Chan[1,2*]

1 Department of Ophthalmology and Visual Sciences, The Chinese University of Hong Kong, Hong Kong Eye Hospital, Kowloon, Hong Kong, The People's Republic of China

2 Hong Kong Eye Hospital, Hong Kong, SAR, The People's Republic of China

*Address all correspondence to: poemen@gmail.com

References

[1] Tham YC, Li X, Wong TY, Quigley HA, Aung T, Cheng CY. Global prevalence of glaucoma and projections of glaucoma burden through 2040: A systematic review and meta-analysis. Ophthalmology. 2014;**121**:2081-2090

[2] Gordon MO, Kass MA. The Ocular Hypertension Treatment Study: Design and baseline description of the participants. Archives of Ophthalmology. 1999;**117**:573-583

[3] Kass MA, Heuer DK, Higginbotham EJ, et al. The Ocular Hypertension Treatment Study: A randomized trial determines that topical ocular hypotensive medication delays or prevents the onset of primary open-angle glaucoma. Archives of Ophthalmology. 2002;**120**:701-713. discussion 829-30

[4] Stewart WC, Stewart JA, Nasser QJ, Mychaskiw MA. Cost-effectiveness of treating ocular hypertension. Ophthalmology. 2008;**115**:94-98

[5] Kymes SM, Kass MA, Anderson DR, Miller JP, Gordon MO, Ocular Hypertension Treatment Study Group. Management of ocular hypertension: A cost-effectiveness approach from the Ocular Hypertension Treatment Study. American Journal of Ophthalmology. 2006;**141**:997-1008

[6] National Institute for Clinical Excellence. Guide to the methods of technology appraisal. London: NICE; 2004. Available from: http://www.nice.org.uk

[7] van Gestel A, Webers CA, Beckers HJ, et al. The relationship between visual field loss in glaucoma and health-related quality-of-life. Eye (London, England). 2010;**24**:1759-1769

[8] Hodapp E, Parrish RK, Anderson DR. Clinical decisions in glaucoma. St Louis: Mosby; 1993

[9] NCCfAC (UK). Glaucoma: Diagnosis and Management of Chronic Open Angle Glaucoma and Ocular Hypertension. London: NCCfAC (UK); 2009

[10] Miglior S, Zeyen T, Pfeiffer N, et al. Results of the European glaucoma prevention Study. Ophthalmology. 2005;**112**:366-375

[11] Weinreb RN, Friedman DS, Fechtner RD, et al. Risk assessment in the management of patients with ocular hypertension. American Journal of Ophthalmology. 2004;**138**:458-467

[12] Chan PP, Leung CK, Chiu V, et al. Protocol-driven adjustment of ocular hypotensive medication in patients at low risk of conversion to glaucoma. The British Journal of Ophthalmology. 2015;**99**:1245-1250

[13] Ocular Hypertension Treatment Study G, European Glaucoma Prevention Study G, Gordon MO, et al. Validated prediction model for the development of primary open-angle glaucoma in individuals with ocular hypertension. Ophthalmology. 2007;**114**:10-19

[14] Leung DY, Iliev ME, Chan P, et al. Pressure–cornea–vascular index (PCVI) for predicting disease progression in normal tension glaucoma. British Journal of Ophthalmology. 2011;**95**:1106-1110

[15] Bhorade AM, Gordon MO, Wilson B, Weinreb RN, Kass MA, Ocular Hypertension Treatment Study G. Variability of intraocular pressure measurements in observation participants in the ocular hypertension treatment study. Ophthalmology. 2009;**116**:717-724

[16] Gardiner SK, Demirel S, Gordon MO, Kass MA, Ocular

Hypertension Treatment Study G. Seasonal changes in visual field sensitivity and intraocular pressure in the ocular hypertension treatment study. Ophthalmology. 2013;**120**:724-730

[17] Clarke R, Shipley M, Lewington S, et al. Underestimation of risk associations due to regression dilution in long-term follow-up of prospective studies. American Journal of Epidemiology. 1999;**150**:341-353

[18] Song C, De Moraes CG, Forchheimer I, Prata TS, Ritch R, Liebmann JM. Risk calculation variability over time in ocular hypertensive subjects. Journal of Glaucoma. 2014;**23**:1-4

[19] Feuer WJ, Parrish RK 2nd, Schiffman JC, et al. The Ocular Hypertension Treatment Study: Reproducibility of cup/disk ratio measurements over time at an optic disc reading center. American Journal of Ophthalmology. 2002;**133**:19-28

[20] Tielsch JM, Katz J, Quigley HA, Miller NR, Sommer A. Intraobserver and interobserver agreement in measurement of optic disc characteristics. Ophthalmology. 1988;**95**:350-356

[21] Yang B, Ye C, Yu M, Liu S, Lam DS, Leung CK. Optic disc imaging with spectral-domain optical coherence tomography: Variability and agreement study with Heidelberg retinal tomograph. Ophthalmology. 2012;**119**:1852-1857

[22] Chan PP, Chiu V, Wong MO. Variability of vertical cup to disc ratio measurement and the effects of glaucoma 5-year risk estimation in untreated ocular hypertensive eyes. The British Journal of Ophthalmology. 2019;**103**:361-368

[23] Reis AS, O'Leary N, Yang H, et al. Influence of clinically invisible, but optical coherence tomography detected, optic disc margin anatomy on neuroretinal rim evaluation. Investigative Ophthalmology & Visual Science. 2012;**53**:1852-1860

[24] Reis AS, Sharpe GP, Yang H, Nicolela MT, Burgoyne CF, Chauhan BC. Optic disc margin anatomy in patients with glaucoma and normal controls with spectral domain optical coherence tomography. Ophthalmology. 2012;**119**:738-747

[25] Chauhan BC, Burgoyne CF. From clinical examination of the optic disc to clinical assessment of the optic nerve head: A paradigm change. American Journal of Ophthalmology. 2013;**156**:218-227

[26] Reis AS, O'Leary N, Stanfield MJ, Shuba LM, Nicolela MT, Chauhan BC. Laminar displacement and prelaminar tissue thickness change after glaucoma surgery imaged with optical coherence tomography. Investigative Ophthalmology & Visual Science. 2012;**53**:5819-5826

[27] Anderson DR, Chauhan B, Johnson C, Katz J, Patella VM, Drance SM. Criteria for progression of glaucoma in clinical management and in outcome studies. American Journal of Ophthalmology. 2000;**130**:827-829

[28] Mwanza JC, Oakley JD, Budenz DL, Anderson DR, Cirrus Optical Coherence Tomography Normative Database Study Group. Ability of cirrus HD-OCT optic nerve head parameters to discriminate normal from glaucomatous eyes. Ophthalmology. 2011;**118**:241-248

[29] Bowd C, Weinreb RN, Williams JM, Zangwill LM. The retinal nerve fiber layer thickness in ocular hypertensive, normal, and glaucomatous eyes with optical coherence tomography. Archives of Ophthalmology. 2000;**118**:22-26

[30] Kuang TM, Zhang C, Zangwill LM, Weinreb RN, Medeiros FA. Estimating

Lead time gained by optical coherence tomography in detecting glaucoma before development of visual field defects. Ophthalmology. 2015;**122**:2002-2009

[31] 10th World Glaucoma Association Consensus: Diagnosis of Primary Open Angle Glaucoma. 22 April 2016. Available from: https://wga.one/wga/consensus-10-preliminary-report/

[32] Sehi M, Bhardwaj N, Chung YS, Greenfield DS, Advanced Imaging for Glaucoma Study G. Evaluation of baseline structural factors for predicting glaucomatous visual-field progression using optical coherence tomography, scanning laser polarimetry and confocal scanning laser ophthalmoscopy. Eye (London, England). 2012;**26**:1527-1535

[33] Wollstein G, Kagemann L, Bilonick RA, et al. Retinal nerve fibre layer and visual function loss in glaucoma: The tipping point. The British Journal of Ophthalmology. 2012;**96**:47-52

[34] Sung KR, Kim S, Lee Y, Yun SC, Na JH. Retinal nerve fiber layer normative classification by optical coherence tomography for prediction of future visual field loss. Investigative Ophthalmology & Visual Science. 2011;**52**:2634-2639

[35] Lalezary M, Medeiros FA, Weinreb RN, et al. Baseline optical coherence tomography predicts the development of glaucomatous change in glaucoma suspects. American Journal of Ophthalmology. 2006;**142**:576-582

[36] Leung CK, Cheung CY, Weinreb RN, et al. Retinal nerve fiber layer imaging with spectral-domain optical coherence tomography: A variability and diagnostic performance study. Ophthalmology. 2009;**116**:1257-1263

[37] Leung CK, Lam S, Weinreb RN, et al. Retinal nerve fiber layer imaging with spectral-domain optical coherence tomography: Analysis of the retinal nerve fiber layer map for glaucoma detection. Ophthalmology. 2010;**117**:1684-1691

[38] Leung CK, Chiu V, Weinreb RN, et al. Evaluation of retinal nerve fiber layer progression in glaucoma: A comparison between spectral-domain and time-domain optical coherence tomography. Ophthalmology. 2011;**118**:1558-1562

[39] Leung CK, Yu M, Weinreb RN, Lai G, Xu G, Lam DS. Retinal nerve fiber layer imaging with spectral-domain optical coherence tomography: Patterns of retinal nerve fiber layer progression. Ophthalmology. 2012;**119**:1858-1866

[40] Yu M, Lin C, Weinreb RN, Lai G, Chiu V, Leung CK. Risk of visual field progression in glaucoma patients with progressive retinal nerve fiber layer thinning: A 5-year prospective Study. Ophthalmology. 2016;**123**:1201-1210

[41] Yu M, Weinreb RN, Yiu C, et al. Computer simulation of progressive retinal nerve fiber layer loss in glaucoma: Performance of event and trend analyses. Investigative Ophthalmology & Visual Science. 2011;**52**:9674-9683

[42] Collaborative Normal-Tension Glaucoma Study Group. Comparison of glaucomatous progression between untreated patients with normal-tension glaucoma and patients with therapeutically reduced intraocular pressures. American Journal of Ophthalmology. 1998;**126**:487-497

[43] Gazzard G, Konstantakopoulou E, Garway-Heath D, et al. Selective laser trabeculoplasty versus eye drops for first-line treatment of ocular

hypertension and glaucoma (LiGHT): A multicentre randomised controlled trial. Lancet. 2019;**393**:1505-1516

[44] Gazzard G, Konstantakopoulou E, Garway-Heath D, et al. Laser in glaucoma and Ocular Hypertension (LiGHT) trial. A multicentre, randomised controlled trial: Design and methodology. The British Journal of Ophthalmology. 2018;**102**:593-598

[45] Mills RP, Budenz DL, Lee PP, et al. Categorizing the stage of glaucoma from pre-diagnosis to end-stage disease. American Journal of Ophthalmology. 2006;**141**:24-30

Section 3

Macular Degeneration and Diabetic Retinopathy: Visual Impairment, Pathophysiology, Clinical Features, Imaging/ Management and Treatment

Chapter 8

Introductory Chapter: Macular Degeneration: Mechanisms of Action

Giuseppe Lo Giudice

1. Introduction

Macular degeneration refers as a progressive condition in which patients are suffering of a disease that is a leading cause of blindness in the elderly worldwide. In particular age-related macular degeneration (AMD) is characterized by two forms, wet and dry, that are classified on the presence or absence of new blood vessels (CNV) [1]. However, there is emerging evidence that significantly overlap which exists in the underlying pathogenetic mechanisms of these clinical conditions. Clarification of the overlapping process that lead to wet and dry diseases will be crucial for the future development in the prevention and treatment of AMD.

By definition, early AMD is characterized by confluent regions of drusen, which are multicomponent, heterogeneous aggregates that lie both external and internal to the retinal pigment epithelium (RPE) cells [2–3]. They are located primarily at the macular region of the retina with relative sparing of the surrounding peripheral retina.

A slow growth of drusen occurs over years or decades with RPE cell death and synaptic dysfunction during the advanced stage of AMD, with the development of advanced AMD (CNV or geographic atrophy (GA)) [4]. All we know about pathogenetic mechanism underlying AMD is that it has the RPE as the fulcrum of AMD pathogenesis. However, whereas, the stepwise development of certain maladies is relatively well-defined, no such hallmarks of disease progression have been identified in AMD.

2. The RPE: at the core of AMD disease

The RPE is the fulcrum of AMD pathogenesis. In general, in spite of interindividual heterogeneity, RPE dysfunction and atrophy precedes the final stages of AMD [5–6]. The RPE cells integrate numerous stimuli to regulate its own health, while also receiving and broadcasting signals to and from the retinal microenvironment. There are several human AMD samples displaying significant interindividual variation in RPE transcript expression, which supports the concept that heterogenic stress responses underlie a categorical AMD phenotype. The effect of specific AMD-associated stresses and AMD in retinal molecular composition have been cataloged by mean genome-wide stress-response transcriptome and proteome assays on whole-genome RPE gene. Such studies reveal common protective and deleterious RPE gene responses that could clarify the key molecular basis of the disease. One of the most important evidences involved in the AMD pathology is the crosstalk of RPE with immune and vascular system. Indeed there are numerous overlapping proangiogenic mechanisms that underlie AMD, many of which involve

IntechOpen

the intersection of immune and vascular system. Whether this immunovascular axis modulates RPE cell is not clear. However in the presence of the AMD pathogenesis, the critical event from which there is not return is RPE dysfunction and damage, although perturbations in other tissues (e.g., choroid, Bruch's membrane, and photoreceptors) are important burdens [7–9].

3. RPE vascular response in neovascular AMD

Response to complement and oxidative stress represent the two major pathways by which the RPE secretes VEGF-A [10–12]. Oxidative stress is the oxidation of cellular macromolecules and complement system, if left unregulated, can directly damage host tissue and recruit immune cells to the vicinity of active complement activation. Also these stresses may act inducing complement-induced RPE secretion of VEGF-A and other vasculogenic molecules in response to oxidative stress and activated complement [13]. However, it is important to emphasize as RPE not be only source of proangiogenic factors, the latter ones could originate from various immune cells or other cell types but RPE is a central player in CNV developing by two important step: (1) the potential for multiple distinct stresses to converge to produce a common (proangiogenic) effect and (2) the diversity of response molecules produced by the RPE that could drive angiogenesis.

4. RPE and immune response in neovascular AMD

There are multiple pathways by which the RPE can regulate the retinal immune-landscape, which in turn can regulate neovascularization in AMD:

1. Macrophages. The macrophages might be the hallmark of CNV [14]. Whether macrophages are critical for CNV development is not clear. The most macrophage activity in CNV development seems to be linked to complex local macrophage-polarizing factors. The role of a complex local regulation of macrophage vascular-modifying activity might be related to the vascular modeling during neovascular process. Among the many factors that control macrophage chemotaxis, VEGF-A has a well-defined role in recruitment of proangiogenic macrophages. However, there are still several questions, the answer to which has important therapeutic implications; whether suppression of VEGF-A dramatically increased the number of retinal macrophages within human neovascular membranes also increasing the activity of proangiogenic macrophages by inflammatory cell recruitment and leukocyte-endothelial adhesion, can this finding does explain the tachyphylaxis that occurs with multiple anti-VEGF-A treatments? Microenvironmental influences in CNV remains an area of needed research [15–16].

2. Microglia. Microglia are another immune cell type that might modulate human CNV pathogenesis. However, while macrophages accumulate in human CNV, it is not known whether microglia do. In the largest histopathologic characterization of microglia in AMD, which observed microglia at various stages of AMD pathology, there was a change in microglia morphology, but not in number AMD compared to nondiseased retinas. Interestingly, one-third of all infiltrating cells (immune and nonimmune cells) in experimental CNV are not classified, and immune cells besides macrophages and microglia could modify CNV. Future work could provide a comprehensive assessment of the composition of cellular infiltrate in CNV specimens. Full understanding of the

immunopathology of CNV will require an assessment of all potential vascular-modifying immune cells and their subsets, in health, disease, and following therapeutic intervention [17].

5. Dry AMD

Toxic accumulations, either within the RPE cell or at the RPE-Bruch membrane interface, are the molecular hallmarks of dry AMD [18]. Dry AMD may be considered as a form of a metabolic storage disease; two approaches to preventing their formation or removing them after formation are attempts to prevent RPE damage. AMD and other neurodegenerative disorders occur when a particular cell or group of cells die. In this scenario, AMD might share some pathogenetic mechanisms with several common neurodegenerative diseases of aging, such as Alzheimer's disease, Parkinson's disease, amyotrophic lateral sclerosis, and Huntington's disease in which mitochondrial defects, DNA mutations, impaired structural integrity, and defective mitochondrial function. Other toxins accumulate in AMD; an excessive amount of "lipofuscin," which is non-degradable debris that accumulates in the RPE with age, is associated with AMD. In the presence of light, lipofuscin forms ROS and is toxic to RPE cells [19–20].

6. Autophagy and damage control

Cells are equipped with machinery to discard toxic accumulations with a self-cleansing process called macroautophagy. Autophagy of the mitochondria and other cellular debris could rejuvenate cells by disposing defunct organelles, a concept which has been reviewed for AMD. Autophagy may also regulate RPE health by reducing cytotoxicity that is secondary to a primary insult. Future work should address several basic questions about this cell survival mechanism in AMD [21–23].

7. Environmental risk factors

Smoking of cigarette confers the greatest numerical risk for AMD with two to three times likely than nonsmokers to develop AMD (smoking cessation reduces the risk of developing AMD) [24]. Several nutritional deficiencies are associated with AMD risk. In a recent epidemiologic study, omega-3 fatty acid (FA) intake was associated with a lower risk of AMD [25]. The protective effect of statins on AMD is not well established and would require long-term prospective interventional studies to confirm its relevance to AMD pathogenesis.

8. Genetics

One prevailing approach in AMD research was the genome-wide association studies (GWAS) that have been used in attempt to predict risk of disease, understand pathogenesis, and identify potential therapeutic target [26]. GWAS have indeed identified several genetic loci, which harbor genetic variants known as single nucleotide polymorphisms (SNPs) that are associated with an increased risk of AMD. Factor H (CFH) represents the complement gene variant conferring the greatest quantitative statistical AMD risk. CFH inhibits a key activation step in complement activation, thereby reducing complement-induced host cell damage and inflammation [27]. The predictive power of AMD risk assessment can be augmented greatly by considering genetic information from multiple loci in combination with epidemiologic and environmental risk factors. In contrast taking into consideration disease prevalence, the positive predictive value of genetic variation to assess AMD risk is inconclusive, even when multiple genetic loci are considered. Next-generation sequencing technologies combined with rigorous biological definition of mechanistic implications of the identified variants are likely to yield more valuable insights both into disease pathogenesis and rational development of novel diagnostics and therapeutics in the coming decade.

Author details

Giuseppe Lo Giudice
San Paolo Ophthalmic Center, San Antonio Hospital, Padua, Italy

*Address all correspondence to: giuseppe.logiudice@aulss6.veneto.it

References

[1] Bird AC. Therapeutic targets in age-related macular disease. The Journal of Clinical Investigation. 2010;**120**:3033-3041

[2] Klein R, Meuer SM, Knudtson MD, Iyengar SK, Klein BE. The epidemiology of retinal reticular drusen. American Journal of Ophthalmology. 2008;**145**:317-326

[3] Klein ML, Ferris FL 3rd, Francis PJ, Lindblad AS, Chew EY, Hamon SC, et al. Progression of geographic atrophy and genotype in age-related macular degeneration. Ophthalmology. 2010;**117**:1554-1559

[4] Zweifel SA, Imamura Y, Spaide TC, Fujiwara T, Spaide RF. Prevalence and significance of subretinal drusenoid deposits (reticular pseudodrusen) in age-related macular degeneration. Ophthalmology. 2010;**117**:1775-1781

[5] Booij JC, ten Brink JB, Swagemakers SM, Verkerk AJ, Essing AH, van der Spek PJ, et al. A new strategy to identify and annotate human RPE-specific gene expression. PLoS ONE. 2010;**5**:e9341

[6] Newman AM, Gallo NB, Hancox LS, Miller NJ, Radeke CM, Maloney MA, et al. Systems-level analysis of age-related macular degeneration reveals global biomarkers and phenotype-specific functional networks. Genome Medicine. 2012;**4**:16

[7] Kurji KH, Cui JZ, Lin T, Harriman D, Prasad SS, Kojic L, et al. Microarray analysis identifies changes in inflammatory gene expression in response to amyloid-beta stimulation of cultured human retinal pigment epithelial cells. Investigative Ophthalmology & Visual Science. 2010;**51**:1151-1163

[8] Cai H, Del Priore LV. Bruch membrane aging alters the gene expression profile of human retinal pigment epithelium. Current Eye Research. 2006;**31**:181-189

[9] Glenn JV, Mahaffy H, Dasari S, Oliver M, Chen M, Boulton ME, et al. Proteomic profiling of human retinal pigment epithelium exposed to an advanced glycation-modified substrate. Graefe's archive for clinical and experimental ophthalmology. Albrecht von Graefes Archiv für Klinische und Experimentelle Ophthalmologie. 2011;**32**:1407-1416

[10] Rohrer B, Long Q, Coughlin B, Wilson RB, Huang Y, Qiao F, et al. A targeted inhibitor of the alternative complement pathway reduces angiogenesis in a mouse model of age-related macular degeneration. Investigative Ophthalmology & Visual Science. 2009;**50**:3056-3064

[11] Thurman JM, Renner B, Kunchithapautham K, Ferreira VP, Pangburn MK, Ablonczy Z, et al. Oxidative stress renders retinal pigment epithelial cells susceptible to complement mediated injury. The Journal of Biological Chemistry. 2009;**284**:16939-16947

[12] Fukuoka Y, Strainic M, Medof ME. Differential cytokine expression of human retinal pigment epithelial cells in response to stimulation by C5a. Clinical and Experimental Immunology. 2003;**131**:248-253

[13] Bhutto IA, McLeod DS, Hasegawa T, Kim SY, Merges C, Tong P, et al. Pigment epithelium-derived factor (PEDF) and vascular endothelial growth factor (VEGF) in aged human choroid and eyes with age related macular degeneration. Experimental Eye Research. 2006;**82**:99-110

[14] Cherepanoff S, McMenamin P, Gillies MC, Kettle E, Sarks SH. Bruch's

membrane and choroidal macrophages in early and advanced age-related macular degeneration. The British Journal of Ophthalmology. 2010;**94**:918-925

[15] Wang Y, Wang VM, Chan CC. The role of anti-inflammatory agents in age-related macular degeneration (AMD) treatment. Eye (London, England). 2011;**25**:127-139

[16] Cursiefen C, Chen L, Borges LP, Jackson D, Cao J, Radziejewski C, et al. VEGF-A stimulates lymphangiogenesis and hemangiogenesis in inflammatory neovascularization via macrophage recruitment. The Journal of Clinical Investigation. 2004;**113**:1040-1050

[17] Espinosa-Heidmann DG, Reinoso MA, Pina Y, Csaky KG, Caicedo A, Cousins SW. Quantitative enumeration of vascular smooth muscle cells and endothelial cells derived from bone marrow precursors in experimental choroidal neovascularization. Experimental Eye Research. 2005;**80**:369-378

[18] Lin MT, Beal MF. Mitochondrial dysfunction and oxidative stress in neurodegenerative diseases. Nature. 2006;**443**:787-795

[19] Schmitz-Valckenberg S, Fleckenstein M, Scholl HP, Holz FG. Fundus autofluorescence and progression of age-related macular degeneration. Survey of Ophthalmology. 2009;**54**:96-117

[20] Winkler BS, Boulton ME, Gottsch JD, Sternberg P. Oxidative damage and age-related macular degeneration. Molecular Vision. 1999;**5**:32

[21] Klionsky DJ. Autophagy: From phenomenology to molecular understanding in less than a decade. Nature Reviews. Molecular Cell Biology. 2007;**8**:931-937

[22] Zhou J, Jang YP, Kim SR, Sparrow JR. Complement activation by photooxidation products of A2E, a lipofuscin constituent of the retinal pigment epithelium. Proceedings of the National Academy of Sciences of the United States of America. 2006;**103**:16182-16187

[23] Zhou R, Yazdi AS, Menu P, Tschopp J. A role for mitochondria in NLRP3 inflammasome activation. Nature. 2011;**469**:221-225

[24] Chen Y, Zeng J, Zhao C, Wang K, Trood E, Buehler J, et al. Assessing susceptibility to age-related macular degeneration with genetic markers and environmental factors. Archives of Ophthalmology. 2011;**129**:344-351

[25] Christen WG, Schaumberg DA, Glynn RJ, Buring JE. Dietary u-3 fatty acid and fish intake and incident age-related macular degeneration in women. Archives of Ophthalmology. 2011;**129**:921-929

[26] Patel N, Adewoyin T, Chong NV. Age-related macular degeneration: A perspective on genetic studies. Eye (London, England). 2008;**22**:768-776

[27] Jakobsdottir J, Gorin MB, Conley YP, Ferrell RE, Weeks DE. Interpretation of genetic association studies: Markers with replicated highly significant odds ratios may be poor classifiers. PLoS Genetics. 2009;**5**:e1000337

Chapter 9

Prologue: My Experience with Photoreceptors - The Peroxidation of Lipids

Angel Catala

1. Introduction

In this chapter, I described several studies on the lipid peroxidation of membrane phospholipids in retina. Particular emphasis is placed on the molecular modifications of very long chain polyunsaturated fatty acids associated with protein changes during peroxidation of photoreceptor membranes. Retina possesses membranes with high content of polyunsaturated fatty acids. Reactive oxygen species begins chain reactions of lipid peroxidation which damage the retina, especially the membranes that play important roles in visual function. Furthermore, biomolecules such as proteins or amino lipids can be covalently modified by lipid decomposition products. In retinal membranes, peroxidation of lipids is also usually accompanied by oxidation of membrane proteins. In consequence, lipid peroxidation may alter the arrangement of proteins in bilayers and by that it interferes with their physiological role on the membrane function.

2. Brief description of photoreceptor

The photoreceptors are the only cells that can convert incoming light into an electrical signal that can be carried to the brain (via the optic nerve) to generate conscious vision. Photoreceptors (rods and cones) are highly polarized and specialized neurons with distinct compartments: cell body, inner segment (IS), and outer segment (OS). Although both rods and cones share a similar overall arrangement of the different compartments, they are diverse in their shape, size, and light-detecting capacities. Rods are highly sensitive to light (only active in starlight vision at night) and show long cylindrical structures with the ciliary OS membrane including many membranous discs, which are loaded with the photopigment rhodopsin and other proteins that participate in the phototransduction cascade.

3. Photoreceptor cell damage

Retina is very rich in membranes containing polyunsaturated fatty acids. Reactive oxygen species initiates chain reactions of lipid peroxidation which injure the retina, especially the membranes that play important roles in visual function. Furthermore, biomolecules such as proteins or amino lipids can be covalently modified by lipid decomposition products. In retinal membranes, peroxidation of lipids is also usually accompanied by oxidation of membrane proteins. In consequence,

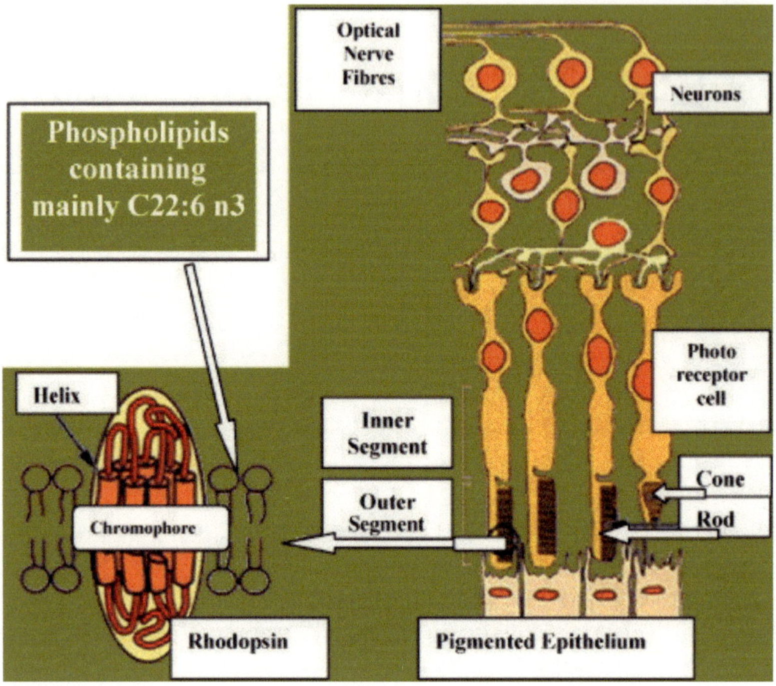

Figure 1.
Schematic diagram of rhodopsin in the membrane of the photoreceptor cell. Taken from: The International Journal of Biochemistry & Cell Biology. 2006; 38(9):1482-95.

lipid peroxidation may alter the arrangement of proteins in bilayers and by that it interferes with their physiological role on the membrane function. Here, we review several studies on the lipid peroxidation of membrane phospholipids in retina. Particular emphasis is placed on the molecular changes of very long chain polyunsaturated fatty acids associated with protein modifications during peroxidation of photoreceptor membranes **Figure 1**.

4. My participation in studies with photoreceptor

I started researching lipids almost six decades ago. My main interest was focused on the study of fatty acids. From 1990 up to now, our laboratory has been interested in the lipid peroxidation of biological membranes from various tissues and different species as well as liposomes prepared with phospholipids rich in PUFAs, as a consequence and considering that the retina is a tissue with enormous amounts of polyunsaturated fatty acids, our studies focused on the lipid peroxidation of photoreceptor membranes. In our first study, it was investigated if soluble-binding proteins for fatty acids (FABPs) present in neural retina show protection from in vitro lipoperoxidation of rod outer segment membranes (ROS). [1] Also we studied the effect of alpha-tocopherol, all-trans retinol, and retinyl palmitate on the nonenzymatic lipid peroxidation of rod outer segments [2].

Retina is highly susceptible to oxidative damage due to its high content of polyunsaturated fatty acids (PUFAs), mainly docosahexaenoic acid (22:6 n3). Lipid peroxidation process is thought to be involved in many physiological and pathological events. Many model membranes can be used to learn more about issues that cannot be studied in biological membranes. Sonicated liposomes (SL) and non-sonicated liposomes (NSL) prepared with lipids isolated from bovine retina and characterized by dynamic light-scattering were submitted to lipid peroxidation, under air atmosphere at 22°C, with Fe(2+) or Fe(3+) as initiator, in different aqueous media. We verified that peroxidation of liposomes made of retinal lipids is affected not only by type of initiator but also by aqueous media. This model constitutes a useful system to study formation of lipid peroxidation intermediaries and products in an aqueous environment [3]. Furthermore, using rod outer segments and/or liposomes made of retinal lipids, we have analyzed the effect of alpha-tocopherol, all-trans retinol, and retinyl palmitate on the nonenzymatic lipid peroxidation of rod outer segments [2]; the selective inhibition of the nonenzymatic lipid peroxidation of phosphatidylserine in rod outer segments by alpha-tocopherol [4]. We have studied also how retinal fatty acid binding protein reduces lipid peroxidation stimulated by long chain fatty acid hydroperoxides on rod outer segments [5], the protective effect of indoleamines on in vitro ascorbate-Fe2+-dependent lipid peroxidation of rod outer segment membranes of bovine retina [6], and lipid-protein modifications during ascorbate-Fe2+ peroxidation of photoreceptor membranes—protective effect of melatonin [7]. In addition, we have determined that melatonin and structural analogues do not possess antioxidant properties on Fe (2+)-initiated peroxidation of sonicated liposomes made of retinal lipids [8]; for reviews, see [9, 10].

5. General remarks, conclusions, and perspectives

It has been attractive to follow the field of photoreceptor cell damage research during almost three decades. Quantitative proteomics and lipidomics analysis are now accessible for measurement of the main components of the photoreceptor cell. From my experience, it is impossible to predict which aspects of photoreceptor cell damage research will dominate in the future.

Acknowledgements

Studies in the author laboratory were supported by PIP 2008-0157 and PIP 4097, granted to AC National Research Council (CONICET) and Secretaría de Ciencia y Técnica, Universidad Nacional de La Plata. Agencia Nacional de Promoción Científica y Tecnológica (ANPCyT) PICT-13399 and bilateral Grant HU/PA03-BI/008.

Author details

Angel Catala
Instituto de Investigaciones Fisicoquímicas Teóricas y Aplicadas, (INIFTA-CCT La Plata-CONICET), Facultad de Ciencias Exactas, Universidad Nacional de La Plata, Argentina

*Address all correspondence to: catala@inifta.unlp.edu.ar

References

[1] Terrasa A, Guajardo M, Catalá A. Lipoperoxidation of rod outer segments of bovine retina is inhibited by soluble binding proteins for fatty acids. Molecular and Cellular Biochemistry. 1998;**178**:181-186

[2] Guajardo M, Terrasa A, Catalá A. The effect of alpha tocopherol, all-trans retinol and retinyl palmitate on the non enzymatic lipid peroxidation of rod outer segments. Molecular and Cellular Biochemistry. 1999;**197**:173-178

[3] Fagali N, Catalá A. Fe2+ and Fe3+ initiated peroxidation of sonicated and non-sonicated liposomes made of retinal lipids in different aqueous media. Chemistry and Physics of Lipids. 2009;**159**:88-94

[4] Terrasa A, Guajardo M, Catalá A. Selective inhibition of the non-enzymatic lipid peroxidation of phosphatidylserine in rod outer segments by alpha-tocopherol. Molecular and Cellular Biochemistry. 2000;**211**:39-45

[5] Guajardo MH, Terrasa AM, Catalá A. Retinal fatty acid binding protein reduce lipid peroxidation stimulated by long-chain fatty acid hydroperoxides on rod outer segments. Biochimica et Biophysica Acta. 2002;**1581**:65-74

[6] Guajardo MH, Terrasa AM, Catalá A. Protective effect of indoleamines on in vitro ascorbate-Fe2+ dependent lipid peroxidation of rod outer segment membranes of bovine retina. Journal of Pineal Research. 2003;**35**:276-282

[7] Guajardo MH, Terrasa AM, Catalá A. Lipid-protein modifications during ascorbate-Fe2+ peroxidation of photoreceptor membranes: Protective effect of melatonin. Journal of Pineal Research. 2006;**41**:201-210

[8] Fagali N, Catalá A. Melatonin and structural analogues do not possess antioxidant properties on Fe(2+)-initiated peroxidation of sonicated liposomes made of retinal lipids. Chemistry and Physics of Lipids. 2011;**164**:688-695

[9] Catalá A. A synopsis of the process of lipid peroxidation since the discovery of the essential fatty acids. Biochemical and Biophysical Research Communications. 2010;**399**:318-323

[10] Catala A. Lipid peroxidation of membrane phospholipids in the vertebrate retina. Frontiers in Bioscience (Scholar Edition). 2011;**3**:52-60

Chapter 10

Zebrafish Photoreceptor Degeneration and Regeneration Research to Understand Hereditary Human Blindness

Maria Iribarne

Abstract

Humans with mutations in photoreceptor-related genes develop forms of retinal degeneration, such as retinitis pigmentosa, cone dystrophy, or Leber congenital amaurosis. Similarly, numerous photoreceptor mutant animal models present phenotypes that resemble retinal degeneration. Zebrafish retina manifests anatomical organization and development remarkably conserved in humans, making these fish a good model to study photoreceptor development and disease. Zebrafish are ideal for forward genetic screens to isolate mutants with visual defects. More recently, CRISPR/Cas system-mediated genome editing has enabled establishment of specific zebrafish photoreceptor mutants. Here, I review zebrafish models of inherited retinal diseases, focusing on rod versus cone photoreceptor mutants. Because zebrafish possess robust regeneration capacity to replace the lost photoreceptors, here I review the current understanding of molecular mechanisms underlying this response.

Keywords: photoreceptor, degeneration, genetic mutant, regeneration, Müller glia, genome editing, CRISPR/Cas9 system, zebrafish

1. Introduction

Photoreceptor degeneration includes a heterogeneous group of diseases characterized by death of photoreceptors and progressive loss of vision. Photoreceptor degeneration is a major cause of blindness in developed countries, for which there is currently no effective treatment [1]. Zebrafish are a good model to study photoreceptor development and disease, because the anatomical organization and development of the retina are remarkably conserved among vertebrates. In contrast to the mammalian retina, which is rod-rich, zebrafish have cone- and rod-rich retinas, facilitating the study of cones. Cone visual acuity can be evaluated by simple optokinetic response (OKR), even at very early stages of development. In this review, I discuss why the zebrafish model is useful to unravel mechanisms of photoreceptor loss. In addition, unlike mammals, zebrafish have the capacity to fully regenerate dead photoreceptors, raising the hope of future treatments for this disorder. Here I summarize our current understanding of this regeneration response.

IntechOpen

1.1 Photoreceptors in the zebrafish retina

Zebrafish neural retina, like those of other vertebrates, comprises three nuclear layers, separated by two synaptic layers (**Figure 1**). The outer nuclear layer (ONL) comprises rod and cone photoreceptors, the light-sensing neurons. The inner nuclear layer (INL) consists of bipolar, horizontal, and amacrine neurons, the second-order neurons. The ganglion cell layer is formed by ganglion cells, axons of which exit the retina, forming the optic nerve, which connects with the tectum. These neurons interconnect by synapses in the plexiform layers. The neural retina is located adjacent to the retinal pigment epithelium (RPE), which supports general homeostasis of photoreceptors, such as recycling 11-cis retinal for visual pigment regeneration [2, 3].

Photoreceptors are polarized neurons with characteristic morphology. They display very specialized cell regions, including outer segments (OSs), connecting cilia, cell bodies, and terminal synapses. OS structure is important for phototransduction. The cell bodies possess the machinery to support all cell functions, and their synaptic termini transduce signals to bipolar neurons. OSs are formed by hundreds of cell membrane discs stacked horizontally and associated with a high concentration of proteins for phototransduction. These proteins are synthetized in cell bodies, and then are transported to the OS through connecting cilia.

Photoreceptors are sensory neurons that produce electrical responses when stimulated by light. In the OS, photons are captured by photopigment molecules to initiate phototransduction cascades [4]. Phototransduction is a complex signaling process that results in closing of voltage-gated ion channels, producing a change in membrane potential. Then, this electrical signal is amplified by other cell types in the inner retina and conducted to the brain. Although this signaling pathway is common to both rods and cones, signaling proteins are mostly encoded by distinct sets of rod- and cone-specific genes. Cone and rod photoreceptors have different sensitivity to light. Rods are extremely sensitive to low-intensity light, while cones function at higher light intensity, and enable color discrimination. In zebrafish, four different subtypes of cones are organized in a precise mosaic pattern. Cones are

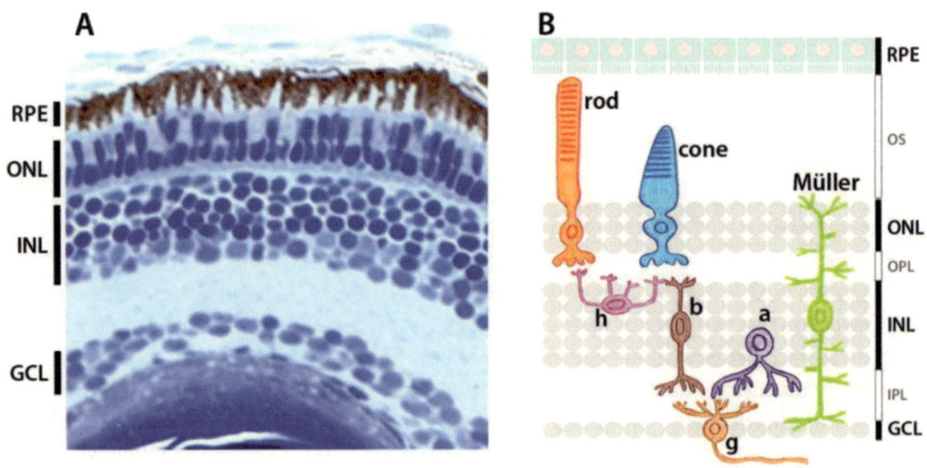

Figure 1.
Zebrafish retinal organization. (A) Semi-thin section of a zebrafish retina at 7 days post-fertilization (dpf). The neural retina is organized into 3 layers. The ONL is formed of cone and rod photoreceptors. (B) Schematic representation of all components of the retina. ONL: outer nuclear layer; INL: inner nuclear layer; GCL: ganglion cell layer; RPE: retinal pigmentary epithelium; h: horizontal; b: bipolar; a: amacrine; g: ganglion neuron.

abundant throughout the zebrafish retina, unlike that of humans, in which cones are at high density in the fovea. Like humans, zebrafish are diurnal.

1.2 Zebrafish as a model to study hereditary eye diseases in humans

Hereditary diseases of the retina involve heterogeneous mutations that result in progressive photoreceptor death, leading to blindness. Mutations in over 200 genes are currently known to be associated with retinal disorders [Retinal Information Network (RetNet): https://sph.uth.edu/retnet]. Retinal degeneration includes multifactorial diseases such as retinitis pigmentosa, Leber congenital amaurosis (LCA), cone-rod dystrophy, and age-related macular degeneration (AMD). In many cases, these diseases are similar in morphological pathogenicity, whereas their genetic origins may be due to mutations affecting different proteins, such as opsins, proteins of the transduction cascade, ciliary protein, or metabolic proteins.

Retinal degeneration can affect rods, cones, or both. Retinitis pigmentosa is a remarkable disease, caused by a mutation in rod photoreceptors that progresses to affect wild-type cone photoreceptors. It is characterized by progression from night blindness due to rod photoreceptor death, to dysfunction and degeneration of cones concentrated in the fovea at the center of the retina [5]. Retinitis pigmentosa is the most common inherited retinal dystrophy (IRD), affecting approximately 1 in 4000 people [6]. AMD is a multi-factorial disease that affects RPE, and leads to the loss of central vision, sustained by cone photoreceptors. AMD is the leading cause of blindness in industrialized countries [7]. Age and a positive family history of AMD are the two strongest risk factors for AMD. This disease is characterized by pigmentation changes at the level of the RPE and deposition of extracellular deposits called drusen, between the basal surface of the RPE and Bruch's membrane in the macula [8].

Leber congenital amaurosis is a group of monogenic, inherited, retinal degenerative disorders that typically show early onset and severe visual dysfunction, with progressive degeneration [9]. At least 25 genes involved in the retinoid cycle and phototransduction, photoreceptor morphogenesis, and protein trafficking in the connecting cilia are associated with LCA. Cone and cone-rod dystrophies are a clinically and genetically heterogeneous group of inherited retinal diseases, involving as many as 30 genes. Initially cone photoreceptors degenerate, followed by rod photoreceptor loss. These disorders typically present progressive loss of central vision, color vision disturbances, and photophobia [10].

Why use zebrafish to research inherited retinal dystrophy? Zebrafish are small tropical fish that are easy to maintain, and that produce many eggs. They have transparent embryos that develop very rapidly, with a 3–4-month generation time. Zebrafish are also easy to modify genetically [11]. The visual system is highly conserved. It is already functional just 5 days post-fertilization (dpf), and it can be assessed by OKR [12]. The fish retina is cone-rich. Because several genes have extra paralogs caused by gene duplication in teleost fish, several genes are cone and rod-specific, making them suitable to study both types of photoreceptors independently [13]. The pioneering work of Streisinger, which produced mutants using UV-irradiated sperm, hydrostatic pressure, heat shock, or gamma irradiation, proved that genetics could be studied using the zebrafish [14, 15]. Soon after that, wide-ranging mutant collections that develop retinal degeneration were isolated, propelling zebrafish into ophthalmologic research.

1.2.1 Forward genetic screens to isolate mutants with visual defects

A special issue of *Development* in 1996 published 37 papers coming mainly from Nüsslein-Volhard's lab in Tübingen and Wolfgang Driever's lab in Boston. These groups performed large-scale mutagenesis screens from founder fish chemically mutagenized with N-ethyl-N-nitrosourea (ENU) [16–18] to provide researchers with thousands of mutants (**Figure 2**). This special issue described roughly 1500 mutations in more than 400 genes involved in processes that govern development and organogenesis [19]. These initial screens were based on evaluations of phenotype by stereomicroscope, without staining or complex microscopy. Additionally, behavioral screens to isolate visual mutants were carried out [12, 20–23]. In these cases, OKR and optomotor responses (OMR) of mutagenized larvae were measured during a three-generation screen for recessive mutations (**Figure 2**). Other screening used F1 generation fish (8–10 months old) derived by ENU mutagenesis, and evaluated their escape responses to a threatening object in order to isolate dominant mutants [24, 25].

The zebrafish genome has been sequenced, providing targets for reverse genetics through use of morpholinos [26]. The use mutants identified from screening in combination with morpholino knock-down has been a widely employed strategy to understand mechanisms underlying many biological processes, including vision. Morpholinos are antisense oligonucleotides designed to temporarily downregulate gene function by blocking translation or splicing [27]. However, morpholinos limit

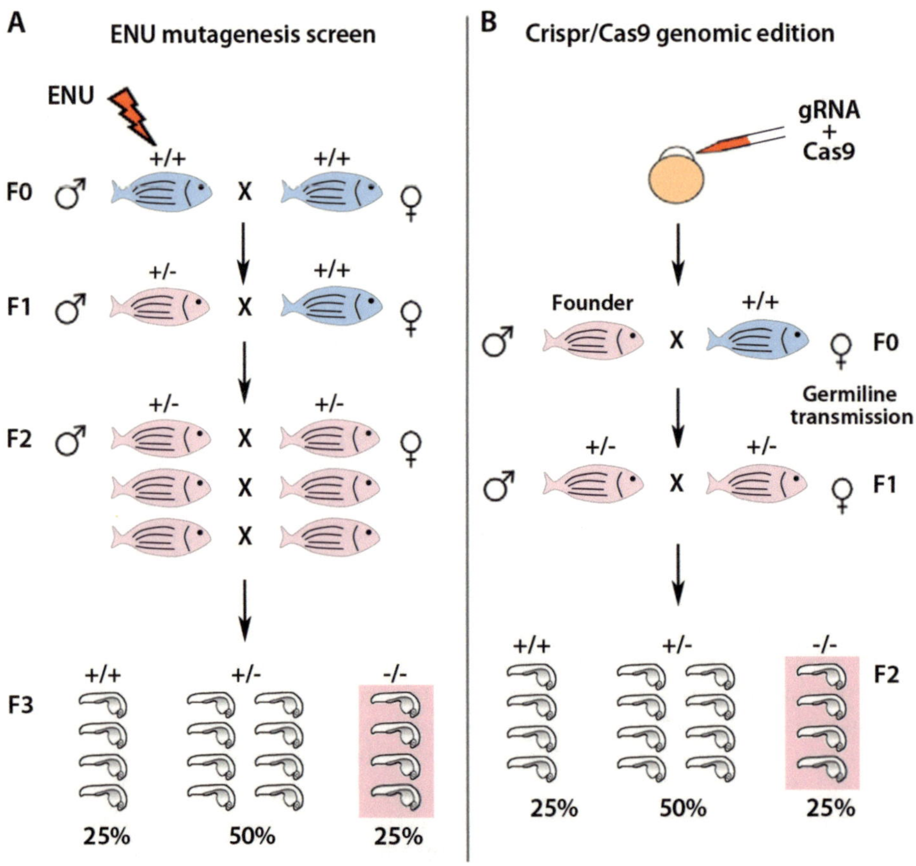

Figure 2.
Genetic strategies to isolate zebrafish visual mutants. (A) Three-generation forward screening. Male zebrafish are treated with the mutagenic drug, ENU, followed by 3 generations of crossing to isolate homozygous recessive mutants. Larvae are usually screened using visual behavior tests. (B) Reverse genetic screening based on Crispr/Cas9 technology. 1–4 cell eggs are microinjected with gRNA and Cas9 mix to target a specific gene of interest. Founders need to be screened in the next generation according to the inheritance of the mutation. Homozygous recessive mutants are evaluated to find abnormal phenotypes.

embryonic development. Usually 1 to 4-cell embryos are injected and effects can be studied up to 4–5 dpf. Mutagenic screening of zebrafish revealed conserved functions of numerous genes across vertebrate lineages and identified zebrafish orthologs for 82% of known human retinal disease genes.

1.2.2 Discerning specific signaling pathways between cone or rod photoreceptors

Genetic screens in zebrafish have shed light on the molecular bases of photoreceptor functions by isolation of visual mutants. Photoreceptor mutants have been isolated, characterized, and mapped. Cone function can be evaluated by OKR and OMR under normal light in 5–7-dpf larvae. A breakthrough discovery in retinal dystrophy was the identification of mutants of phosphodiesterase 6c (pde6c), a novel cone-specific phototransduction gene [12, 28]. *Pde6c*$^{-/-}$ was identified as a blind zebrafish mutant with rapid degeneration of cone photoreceptors having secondary, but transitory degeneration of rod photoreceptors. These two achromatopsia zebrafish mutants were the first visual disorders linked to cone-specific degeneration, and helped to identify human PDE6c mutations in patients [29, 30]. These findings indicated that like zebrafish pde6c mutants, cone-specific degeneration also occurs in humans.

The maturation and functional integrity of PDE6 depends on aryl hydrocarbon receptor-interacting protein-like 1 (AIPL1) [31]. We reported an *aipl1* mutant that was blind and developed cone photoreceptor degeneration accompanied by rod degeneration only at an early stage of development [32]. Retinal phenotypes of *aipl1* mutants are very similar to those of zebrafish hypomorphic *pde6c* mutants. Such results were not surprising, given the role of aipl1 in supporting pde6c functions. We confirm the absence of pd6c protein in the *aipl1* mutant. Unexpectedly, the level of guanylate cyclase-3 (gc-3), another important cone-specific phototransduction molecule, was also affected. At the moment, the molecular mechanism underlying the coupling of Pde6 and Gc3 maintenance in photoreceptors remains unknown. *gc3* mutants have been isolated by OKR and OMR screening and they present abnormal visual behavior, although their retinal morphology is normal during larval stages [22]. It would be interesting to study *gc3* mutants to elucidate the relationship between pde6c and gc3.

Though mutants isolated through OKR or OMR behavioral screening evaluate cone function, several mutants exhibited rod degeneration as well. Since rod and cone photoreceptor OSs are continually phagocytosed by the covering RPE, they need to be renewed actively by transport of molecules from the cell body to the OS through connecting cilia. This is called Intraflagellar Transport (IFT) [33]. Several genes have been identified as components of the IFT, such as ift52, ift57, ift80, ift88, and ift172 [23, 34]. In *ift88* zebrafish mutants, cilia are generated, but not maintained, causing an absence of photoreceptor OSs [35]. *ift57* mutant zebrafish had short OSs whereas *ift172* mutants lack OSs completely at 5 dpf [23, 36]. Degeneration of mutant photoreceptors is partly caused by ectopic accumulation of opsins. These results illustrate the unique mechanism of IFT, which is very different from cytosolic transport, and is important for OS formation and maintenance.

Intracellular vesicular transport is important for cytosolic distribution and recycling of molecules. *β-SNAP* cooperates with N-ethylmaleimide-sensitive factor (NSF) to recycle the SNAP receptor (SNARE) by disassembling the cis-SNARE complex generated during the vesicular fusion process. *β-SNAP*$^{-/-}$ presents photoreceptors degeneration, in which photoreceptors undergo apoptosis in a BH3- only, protein BNip1-dependent mechanism due to failure to disassemble the SNARE. *β-SNAP* mutant was the first zebrafish mutant to link photoreceptor degeneration to vesicular transport defects [37].

Unlike photopic cone-mediated vision mutants, which can easily be isolated by behavioral tests from genetic screens, rod mutant screens are much more laborious and time consuming. Scotopic vision needs to be evaluated under dim light, and rod maturation takes up to 3 weeks post-fertilization (wpf). The escape response has been used to screen adult male F1-generation zebrafish treated with ENU, looking for dominant inherited retinal mutants [24, 25, 38, 39]. When a fish is swimming in a circular container and is threatened, it reacts by turning away from the threat. Individuals that failed to show the escape response under dim light illumination were isolated, and named *night blindness a-g*. A spectrum of retinal phenotypes was observed, from photoreceptor degeneration in a patchy array (*nba*$^{+}/^{-}$; *nbe*$^{+/-}$), thinner OSs or degenerated OSs (*nbc*$^{+/-}$; *nbd*$^{+}/^{-}$; *nbg*$^{+}/^{-}$), to absence of photoreceptor degeneration (*nbb*$^{+}/^{-}$). Homozygous mutant embryos of the F3 generation in most cases died after several days of development, indicating that these mutations are not photoreceptor-specific.

1.2.3 CRISPR/Cas editing genome technology to produce photoreceptor mutants

Forward genetic screens have proven very powerful for isolating mutants. However, they do not allow specific genes or pathways to be investigated. Programmable nucleases have revolutionized genetics by allowing precise targeted genome modifications to produce mutants. There are several types of tools for genome editing, such as zinc finger nucleases (ZFNs), transcription activator-like effector nucleases (TALENs), and clustered regularly interspaced short palindromic repeat (CRISPR) systems. These tools have facilitated widespread DNA editing in various organisms, including zebrafish. High specificity and efficiency, flexible design and simple methodology are the most relevant features. CRISPR/Cas enzyme stands out for its extremely utility based on RNA–DNA interaction, while ZFNs and TALENs recognize specific DNA sequences through protein–DNA interactions. Any researcher with basic skill in molecular biology can easily implement CRISPR technology. CRISPR/Cas can target virtually any gene of interest with a customizable short RNA guide to produce knock-out of individual genes [40, 41]. CRISPR requires two key components, a nuclease, most commonly Cas9, and sgRNA (single-guide RNA) which targets the nuclease to a specific DNA location (**Figure 2**) [42]. By simply designing the sgRNA, CRISPR can be targeted to different genome locations. By expressing several sgRNAs, the system also enables multiplex genome editing with high efficiency [43].

1.2.4 Zebrafish photoreceptor-specific genes edited to model human retinal pathologies

Genome editing technologies have been employed in zebrafish for retinal studies. While it is quite easy to produce knock-outs, creating knock-in zebrafish remains challenging. Several photoreceptor knock-out mutants have been recovered in zebrafish that showed the involvement of several genes in photoreceptor development and survival. Mutations in over 50 genes, such as RP2, have been identified as causes of retinitis pigmentosa. RP2 is a GTPase activator protein for ARL3 and participates in trafficking of ciliary proteins. Fei Liu et al. generated an *RP2* knock-out zebrafish line using TALEN technology to understand the RP2 degeneration mechanism [44]. *RP2* knock-out zebrafish display progressive retinal degeneration, with a degeneration of rod OSs, followed by degeneration of cone OSs. RP2 knock-down by morpholinos resulted in abnormal retinal localization of GRK1 and rod transducin subunits, GNAT1 and GNB1. Furthermore, distribution of farnesylated proteins in zebrafish retina was also affected by

RP2 ablation. The same lab also produced *cerkl* knock-out zebrafish, a model for a rod-cone dystrophy [45]. Progressive degeneration of rods and cones, with an accumulation of shed OSs in the interphotoreceptor matrix was observed, suggesting that cerkl may regulate phagocytosis of OSs by the RPE. In addition, the phagocytosis-associated protein, MERTK, was significantly reduced in *cerkl* mutants. Despite a number of genes that have been implicated in retinitis pigmentosa pathogenesis, the mechanism of the disease remains unknown. Zebrafish have proven useful for modeling these ocular diseases.

Photoreceptor genesis requires precise regulation of progenitor cell competence, cell cycle exit, and differentiation. Several transcription factors that control photoreceptor-specific gene expression have been identified. The basic helix–loop–helix transcription factor NeuroD governs photoreceptor genesis, but the signaling pathway through which it functions is unknown. NeuroD was knocked-down with morpholinos, and knocked-out with CRISPR/Cas9 [46]. NeuroD induces cell cycle exit and photoreceptor maturation through cell–cell signaling. NeuroD knockdown resulted in failure to exit the cell cycle, but did not affect expression of photoreceptor lineage markers, Nr2e3 and Crx. NeuroD increased Notch gene expression. Notch inhibition rescued the cell cycle exit, but not photoreceptor maturation. The nuclear receptor transcription factor, Nr2e3, is expressed in photoreceptors. It forms a complex with Crx, which enhances expression of rod-specific genes and represses expression of cone-specific genes in rods [47]. CRISPR-edited *Nr2e3* knock-out animals displayed rod precursors undergoing terminal mitoses, but failed to differentiate into rods. They did not express rod-specific genes and the OS fails to develop. Cone differentiation was normal; however, later, progressive degeneration of OS of double cones began, with a reduction of phototransduction proteins. Nr2e3 acts synergistically with Crx and Nrl to enhance rhodopsin gene expression, without affecting cone opsin expression [47].

A large number of genetic defects can disrupt OS morphology to impair photoreceptor function and viability. Kinesin family members and IFT motors are important for trafficking proteins to photoreceptor OSs [33]. Edited-knock-out *osm-3/kif17* and *cos2/kif7* mutants have comparable OS developmental delays, although via different mechanisms [48]. *Cos2/kif7* mutant dysfunction depends on Hedgehog signaling, which leads to generalized, non-photoreceptor-specific delay of retinal neurogenesis, while *osm-3/kif17* OS morphogenesis delays are associated with initial disc morphogenesis of photoreceptors. The ciliary protein C2orf71a/pcare1 is almost exclusively expressed in photoreceptors, and modulates the ciliary membrane through recruitment of an actin assembly module. Embryos and adult retinas of *C2orf71a/pcare1*$^{-/-}$ zebrafish display disorganization of photoreceptor OSs [49]. This mutant shows visual impairment assessed by OKR and OMR in larvae. Lack of *pcare1* in zebrafish causes similar retinal phenotype to that in humans and indicates that the function of the pcare gene is conserved across species. When mutated, Eye shut homolog (EYS), another ciliary protein, causes retinitis pigmentosa and cone-rod dystrophy. Since eys is absent from several rodent genomes, including mice, zebrafish hold promise as a model for EYS-deficient patients. Several groups established an *eys* knock-out zebrafish model using CRISPR/Cas9 and TALEN technology [50–52]. Embryos and adult retinas showed disorganization of photoreceptor OSs. *eys*$^{-/-}$ zebrafish presented mislocalization of several OS proteins, such as rhodopsin, opn1lw, opn1sw1, GNB3 and PRPH2, and disruption of actin filaments in photoreceptors [50–52]. All these new zebrafish mutants present phenotypes that mimic clinical manifestations of patients, suggesting the utility of these animal models for studying the etiology of these retinopathies.

Gene target editing technologies enable production of rod-specific photoreceptor mutants, which were challenging to isolate using behavioral screening.

Mutations in rhodopsin are the most common cause of retinitis pigmentosa in humans [53]. The human rhodopsin mutation Q344X was expressed in zebrafish to study photoreceptor degeneration. Early mislocalization of hRho Q334X led to rod apoptosis, without affecting cone survival. Activation of phototransduction signaling through transduction and adenylyl cyclase increased photoreceptor loss [54]. Recently, CRISPR/Cas9-induced mutations were used to target the major zebrafish Rho locus, rh1–1, and several mutants were recovered [55]. These mutants were characterized by rapid degeneration of rod photoreceptors, but not of cones. These novel lines will provide badly needed *in vivo* models to study pathology of retinitis pigmentosa.

All these examples of mutants recovered by reverse genetic approaches have been used to identify key molecular pathways required for photoreceptor development and function. Nonetheless, they are generally limited in terms of the number of targets that can be evaluated. Reverse genetic screening techniques have been used with invertebrate animal models and cell culture systems to identify genes and pathways involved in various biological processes; however, their use with *in vivo* vertebrate model systems has been challenging [56]. Recently, several zebrafish labs have shown the feasibility of CRISPR/Cas-based mutagenesis assays to isolate high numbers of mutants focused on synapsis [56], thyroid morphogenesis and function [57], and the Fanconi Anemia pathway, which is involved in genomic instability syndrome, resulting in aplastic anemia [58]. One study screened 54 ciliary genes and isolated 8 mutants that were required for retinal development [59].

In summary, these descriptions of zebrafish phenotypic models isolated from forward mutagenesis screens and reverse genetic approaches targeting genes important in retinal biology have shown how it is possible to advance studies of retinal degeneration through zebrafish research. There still remain several unknown genes associated with retinal degeneration. Their eventual exploration will provide a deeper understanding of molecular mechanisms underlying photoreceptor degeneration and death.

1.3 Therapeutic treatments for retinal degeneration in humans

Several photoreceptor diseases such as retinitis pigmentosa, Leber congenital amaurosis, and macular degeneration produce photoreceptor cell death which leads to blindness. Current treatments of such diseases are ineffective; thus, several different strategies to treat them are being pursued. Neuroprotective approaches with drugs have been evaluated with different degrees of success. These include cGMP analogue treatment [60], calcium-channel blockers [61], and rod-derived cone viability factor [62]. These strategies aim to treat patients during early stages of retinal degeneration, since the disease cannot be reversed. On the other hand, neuroprotective strategies do not depend on any specific mutation and may provide a longer time window for other treatments [63]. Gene therapy has been applied to improve vision in patients with LCA caused by mutations in RPE65. In 2008, three groups reported success in delivering a healthy RPE65 gene using an AAV2 vector to the retina of three LCA patients [64–66], but the improvement may not persist [67]. External devices have been used to electrically stimulate neurons in the inner part of the retina. High visual acuity cannot be achieved, but face and object recognition, and orientation in unknown environments are possible [63].

The most promising therapies are cell transplantation and regeneration based on Müller cells. Using induced-pluripotent stem cells (iPSCs) it is possible to produce eyecup-like structures [68]. These eyecups present a layered structure similar to a retina, with photoreceptor-like cells that contain outer segments, express phototransduction proteins, and some light response [69]. When photoreceptors are transplanted, they need to integrate into and establish synaptic connections with the remaining retina. Animal experiments showed that few photoreceptors integrate to produce functional recovery of vision [70, 71]. Unexpectedly, recently research demonstrated that the improvement in vision is due to exchange of cytoplasmic material (RNA and/or proteins) between donor cells and the host retina, and not to integration of transplanted photoreceptors [70, 72, 73], making it unclear through which mechanism restoration of vision is achieved. The goal of regeneration is to replace photoreceptors through induction of endogenous progenitor cells. Unfortunately, neurons in the mammalian central nervous systems cannot be replaced. In contrast, lower vertebrates such as reptiles, amphibians, and fish, have the capacity to regenerate lost neurons in brain, spinal cord, and sensory organs, such as the retina and ear [74]. Defining mechanisms of zebrafish retinal repair may offer a key to regenerative medicine.

1.3.1 Müller cell response to retinal injury

In response to injury, mammalian Müller cells exhibit signs of reactive gliotic, featuring cell hypertrophy and upregulation of glial fibrillary acidic protein (GFAP) [75, 76]. Initially this reactive gliosis is neuroprotective, but eventually leads to loss of retinal neurons and causes scarring. Unlike mammals, zebrafish retina responds to neuronal damage by proliferation of Müller glia, which can replace all neuron types, including photoreceptors. Müller glia are the major glial cell type in the retina and contribute to retinal structure and homeostasis [77]. Nuclei are located in the inner nuclear layer, and these cells present apical and basal projections that extend all through the retina (**Figure 1**). Apical feet form the outer limiting membrane. Müller glia are located so that they can monitor the entire retina and contribute to retinal structure and function.

When loss of neurons occurs, Müller glia respond by dedifferentiating, re-entering the cell cycle and producing neuronal progenitor cells (**Figure 3**). These progenitors amplify their numbers, and then migrate to the injured region. Then neuronal progenitor cells exit the cell cycle and differentiate into replacement neurons. All types of retinal neurons can be produced and replaced in injured zebrafish retina to achieve morphological and functional recovery of the retina [78–81]. Identifying molecular signals and pathways that drive this regeneration response is the focus of regenerative medicine.

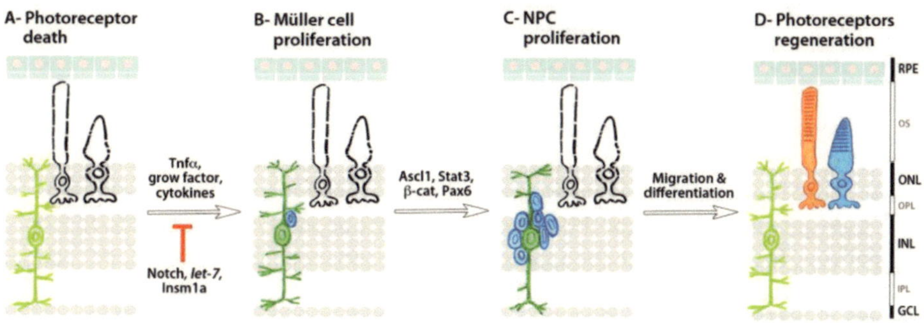

Figure 3.
Photoreceptor degeneration induces a regenerative response based on Müller cell activity. (A) Photoreceptor loss and/or other cells produce stress signals such as TNFα, growth factors, etc. to induce cell Müller activation. (B) Müller cells dedifferentiate to stem cells, and divide asymmetrically to produce one NPC and one Müller glial cell. Müller cells express Ascl1 and Stat3. (C) NPCs proliferate to increase the number of progenitor cells. (D) NPCs exit the cell cycle and differentiate into photoreceptor lineage cells to reverse loss of these neurons. NPC: neuronal proliferative cells.

1.3.2 Positive and negative signaling to modulate Müller cell proliferation in the regenerative response

Understanding mechanisms by which zebrafish can regenerate injured retina may provide strategies for stimulating retinal regeneration in mammals. Given the similarity of anatomy, cell types, and gene conservation between teleost fish and mammals, the regenerative approach offers hope for clinical treatment. Both species present Müller cells that are the primary cell type responsible for regeneration.

Acute injury models have been useful for dissecting many signaling pathways, and great progress has been achieved. Several secreted signaling molecules that participate in Müller glia dedifferentiation and proliferation have been identified. These include TNFα [82], HB-EFG [83], Wnt [84], TFGb [85], insulin, and Fgf2 [86] (**Figure 3**). In addition, Müller cells activate different transcription factors, and initiate signaling essential to differentiation and/or proliferation, such as Ascl1b [87], Stat3 [88, 89], Pax6 [90, 91], PCNA [90], Lin-28 [87]. Interestingly, it still has not been confirmed that these transcription factors and signaling molecules are also expressed and activated in genetic mutants with slow degeneration.

When a regeneration response occurs, around 50% of Müller cells dedifferentiate and proliferate in the injured region, while the other Müller cells remain as differentiated glia. Let-7, Notch and Insm1a [87, 92, 93] are involved in this quiescent Müller cell population. It may be important that some Müller cells remain quiescent to avoid an excessive neurogenesis and remodeling of the retina, as well to maintain homeostasis of healthy neurons.

Important results have come from uninjured retinas in relation to the external delivery of activation signals or transcription factors that are able to generate a regenerative response. For example, Tnfα intravitreal injection into adult fish induced a moderate proliferative response [82]. Tnfα combined with repressing Notch (γ-secretase inhibitor) via intravitreal injection produced a much stronger proliferative response [92]. These results suggest that identifying key molecules for the regenerative response, and modulating them can induce a proliferative response by Müller cells.

Recently, some exciting results came from studies in adult mice [94]. NMDA-damaged retinas, with injury to the inner part of the retina, were treated with a histone deacetylase inhibitor and overexpressed Ascl1. Under these conditions, Müller glia were induced to produce functional neurons via a trans differentiation mechanism. $Gnat1^{rd17}Gnat2^{cpfl3}$ double mutant mice, a model of congenital blindness, were treated by gene transfer of β-catenin, and subsequent gene transfer of transcription factors essential for rod cell fate specification and determination. Müller glia-derived rods restored visual responses [95].

1.3.3 Genetic mutant models to investigate regeneration mechanisms

Most current studies use acute approaches to injure adult retinas, like light damage [79, 96], retinal puncture [80], chemical injection [81], or loss of specific cell populations due to activation of a toxic transgene (nitroreductase: NTR) [97, 98]. Light damage and toxic transgene NTR induce photoreceptor death, while retinal puncture kills specific neurons. These animal models use powerful, rapid damage that resembles traumatic injury in human patients. To model inherited photoreceptor degeneration diseases, better models need to be used.

Only a few studies have employed zebrafish photoreceptor genetic mutants [32]. Iribarne et al. used cone- or rod-specific mutants with a very rapid loss of photoreceptors, and observed that regeneration started as early as 1 wpf. Cone-specific mutant regeneration relied on Müller cell proliferation, while rod photoreceptor-specific mutant regeneration was based on rod progenitor proliferation [99]. Another cone mutant, *Aipl1*$^{-/-}$, which developed a slower and progressive degeneration, surprisingly did not show an increase in Müller cell or rod progenitor proliferation, even though cell death was detected [32]. Both studies used larval animals (1 and 2 wpf) and lacked the information of later stages and the adult regenerative response. Further investigation during development and adulthood should be performed to gain a better understanding of the response of Müller cells to damage.

Interestingly, all these injury models elicited a Müller cell response that was similar overall. However, some molecules revealed injury-dependent induction. Hbegf was necessary for retinal regeneration following a mechanical injury, but it was not necessary for regeneration following photoreceptor damage by light [82, 83]. These adult acute models have proven to be powerful in revealing many of the molecular signals that drive the regenerative response. However, for modeling human photoreceptor genetic diseases, which usually proceed from embryogenesis or childhood to adulthood to completely degenerate, a more specific model needs to be used.

1.3.4 CRISPR/Cas system screening to isolate defective regenerative retinal processes

The high efficiency and multiplexing capabilities of CRISPR enable high-throughput, forward screening of "genotype to phenotype" functions in various model systems [43]. So far, several zebrafish labs have utilized CRISPR/Cas system screening (check Section 2.2.4 in this chapter). However, few screening studies have focused on regeneration. A screening method for hair cell regeneration identified 7 genes involved in this response [100]. To evaluate genes important for retinal regeneration, large-scale, reverse genetic screening has been established by applying a multiplexed gene disruption strategy [101]. This screening used an automated reporter quantification-based assay to identify cellular regeneration-deficient phenotypes in transgenic fish. Over 300 regeneration genes were targeted, and so far, data have been obtained from 120 targeted genomic sites. This screening is ongoing, and regeneration-defective mutants still have not been published. It will be interesting to see what types of new genes are associated with the regeneration response.

2. Conclusions

Inherited retinal degenerative diseases are characterized by photoreceptor death that leads to blindness. The underlying genetic causes of these disorders are numerous and diverse, and most involve photoreceptor-specific genes. Zebrafish are amenable to large-scale genetic manipulation and genome editing technology, which as I have illustrated, can generate a great mutant collection. These mutants are helping to uncover molecular mechanisms underlying retinal degeneration disorders. Currently, there are no effective treatments for these diseases in humans to reduce or impede the progression of degeneration; thus, different approaches have been investigated to develop medical interventions for the patients. Zebrafish exhibit extraordinary neuronal regeneration, including retinal photoreceptors, making them an excellent model to develop regenerative therapies to treat photoreceptor degeneration.

Acknowledgements

I thank Steven D. Aird for editing this chapter.

Conflict of interest

The author has no competing interests.

Author details

Maria Iribarne
University of Notre Dame, Notre Dame, United States

*Address all correspondence to: miribarn@nd.edu

References

[1] Angueyra JM, Kindt KS. Leveraging zebrafish to study retinal degenerations. Frontiers in Cell and Development Biology. 2018;**6**:110

[2] Fan J, Rohrer B, Frederick JM, Baehr W, Crouch RK. Rpe65−/− and Lrat−/− mice: Comparable models of leber congenital amaurosis. Investigative Ophthalmology & Visual Science. 2008;**49**(6):2384-2389

[3] Iribarne M, Canto-Soler MV, Torbidoni V, Suburo AM. Controlling retinal pigment epithelium injury after experimental detachment of the retina. Investigative Ophthalmology & Visual Science. 2007;**48**(3):1348-1354

[4] Iribarne M, Masai I. Do cGMP levels drive the speed of photoreceptor degeneration? Advances in Experimental Medicine and Biology. 2018;**1074**:327-333

[5] Narayan DS, Wood JP, Chidlow G, Casson RJ. A review of the mechanisms of cone degeneration in retinitis pigmentosa. Acta Ophthalmologica. 2016;**94**(8):748-754

[6] Verbakel SK, van Huet RAC, Boon CJF, den Hollander AI, Collin RWJ, Klaver CCW, et al. Non-syndromic retinitis pigmentosa. Progress in Retinal and Eye Research. 2018;**66**:157-186

[7] Jonasson F, Arnarsson A, Eiriksdottir G, Harris TB, Launer LJ, Meuer SM, et al. Prevalence of age-related macular degeneration in old persons: Age, gene/environment susceptibility Reykjavik study. Ophthalmology. 2011;**118**(5):825-830

[8] Lynch AM, Mandava N, Patnaik JL, Frazer-Abel AA, Wagner BD, Palestine AG, et al. Systemic activation of the complement system in patients with advanced age-related macular degeneration. European Journal of Ophthalmology. 2019. DOI: 10.1177/1120672119857896

[9] Cideciyan AV, Jacobson SG. Leber congenital amaurosis (LCA): Potential for improvement of vision. Investigative Ophthalmology & Visual Science. 2019;**60**(5):1680-1695

[10] Gill JS, Georgiou M, Kalitzeos A, Moore AT, Michaelides M. Progressive cone and cone-rod dystrophies: Clinical features, molecular genetics and prospects for therapy. British Journal of Ophthalmology. 2019;**103**(5):711

[11] Westerfield M. The Zebrafish Book: A Guide for the Laboratory Use of Zebrafish (*Brachydanio rerio*). M. Westerfield: Eugene, OR; 1993

[12] Nishiwaki Y, Komori A, Sagara H, Suzuki E, Manabe T, Hosoya T, et al. Mutation of cGMP phosphodiesterase 6alpha'-subunit gene causes progressive degeneration of cone photoreceptors in zebrafish. Mechanisms of Development. 2008;**125**(11-12):932-946

[13] Iribarne M, Masai I. Neurotoxicity of cGMP in the vertebrate retina: From the initial research on rd mutant mice to zebrafish genetic approaches. Journal of Neurogenetics. Sep 2017;**31**(3):59-60

[14] Streisinger G, Walker C, Dower N, Knauber D, Singer F. Production of clones of homozygous diploid zebra fish (*Brachydanio rerio*). Nature. 1981;**291**(5813):293-296

[15] Walker C, Streisinger G. Induction of mutations by gamma-rays in pregonial germ cells of zebrafish embryos. Genetics. 1983;**103**(1):125-136

[16] Solnica-Krezel L, Schier AF, Driever W. Efficient recovery of ENU-induced mutations from the zebrafish germline. Genetics. 1994;**136**(4):1401-1420

[17] Mullins MC, Hammerschmidt M, Haffter P, Nusslein-Volhard C. Large-scale mutagenesis in the zebrafish: In search of genes controlling development in a vertebrate. Current Biology. 1994;**4**(3):189-202

[18] Haffter P, Granato M, Brand M, Mullins MC, Hammerschmidt M, Kane DA, et al. The identification of genes with unique and essential functions in the development of the zebrafish, Danio rerio. Development. 1996;**123**:1-36

[19] Nusslein-Volhard C. The zebrafish issue of development. Development. 2012;**139**(22):4099-4103

[20] Brockerhoff SE, Hurley JB, Janssen-Bienhold U, Neuhauss SC, Driever W, Dowling JE. A behavioral screen for isolating zebrafish mutants with visual system defects. Proceedings of the National Academy of Sciences of the United States of America. 1995;**92**(23):10545-10549

[21] Neuhauss SC, Biehlmaier O, Seeliger MW, Das T, Kohler K, Harris WA, et al. Genetic disorders of vision revealed by a behavioral screen of 400 essential loci in zebrafish. The Journal of Neuroscience. 1999;**19**(19):8603-8615

[22] Muto A, Orger MB, Wehman AM, Smear MC, Kay JN, Page-McCaw PS, et al. Forward genetic analysis of visual behavior in zebrafish. PLoS Genetics. 2005;**1**(5):e66

[23] Gross JM, Perkins BD, Amsterdam A, Egana A, Darland T, Matsui JI, et al. Identification of zebrafish insertional mutants with defects in visual system development and function. Genetics. 2005;**170**(1):245-261

[24] Li L, Dowling JE. A dominant form of inherited retinal degeneration caused by a non-photoreceptor cell-specific mutation. Proceedings of the National Academy of Sciences of the United States of America. 1997;**94**(21):11645-11650

[25] Maaswinkel H, Riesbeck LE, Riley ME, Carr AL, Mullin JP, Nakamoto AT, et al. Behavioral screening for nightblindness mutants in zebrafish reveals three new loci that cause dominant photoreceptor cell degeneration. Mechanisms of Ageing and Development. 2005;**126**(10):1079-1089

[26] Phillips JB, Westerfield M. Zebrafish models in translational research: Tipping the scales toward advancements in human health. Disease Models & Mechanisms. 2014;**7**(7):739-743

[27] Nasevicius A, Ekker SC. Effective targeted gene 'knockdown' in zebrafish. Nature Genetics. 2000;**26**(2):216-220

[28] Stearns G, Evangelista M, Fadool JM, Brockerhoff SE. A mutation in the cone-specific pde6 gene causes rapid cone photoreceptor degeneration in zebrafish. The Journal of Neuroscience. 2007;**27**(50):13866-13874

[29] Chang B, Grau T, Dangel S, Hurd R, Jurklies B, Sener EC, et al. A homologous genetic basis of the murine cpfl1 mutant and human achromatopsia linked to mutations in the PDE6C gene. Proceedings of the National Academy of Sciences of the United States of America. 2009;**106**(46):19581-19586

[30] Thiadens AA, den Hollander AI, Roosing S, Nabuurs SB, Zekveld-Vroon RC, Collin RW, et al. Homozygosity mapping reveals PDE6C mutations in patients with early-onset cone photoreceptor disorders. American Journal of Human Genetics. 2009;**85**(2):240-247

[31] Christiansen JR, Kolandaivelu S, Bergo MO, Ramamurthy V. RAS-converting enzyme 1-mediated

endoproteolysis is required for trafficking of rod phosphodiesterase 6 to photoreceptor outer segments. Proceedings of the National Academy of Sciences of the United States of America. 2011;**108**(21):8862-8866

[32] Iribarne M, Nishiwaki Y, Nakamura S, Araragi M, Oguri E, Masai I. Aipl1 is required for cone photoreceptor function and survival through the stability of Pde6c and Gc3 in zebrafish. Scientific Reports. 2017;7:45962

[33] Malicki J, Besharse JC. Kinesin-2 family motors in the unusual photoreceptor cilium. Vision Research. 2012;**75**:33-36

[34] Malicki J, Avidor-Reiss T. From the cytoplasm into the cilium: Bon voyage. Organogenesis. 2014;**10**(1):138-157

[35] Tsujikawa M, Malicki J. Intraflagellar transport genes are essential for differentiation and survival of vertebrate sensory neurons. Neuron. 2004;**42**(5):703-716

[36] Sukumaran S, Perkins BD. Early defects in photoreceptor outer segment morphogenesis in zebrafish ift57, ift88 and ift172 intraflagellar transport mutants. Vision Research. 2009;**49**(4):479-489

[37] Nishiwaki Y, Yoshizawa A, Kojima Y, Oguri E, Nakamura S, Suzuki S, et al. The BH3-only SNARE BNip1 mediates photoreceptor apoptosis in response to vesicular fusion defects. Developmental Cell. 2013;**25**(4):374-387

[38] Li L, Dowling JE. Disruption of the olfactoretinal centrifugal pathway may relate to the visual system defect in night blindness b mutant zebrafish. The Journal of Neuroscience. 2000;**20**(5):1883-1892

[39] Maaswinkel H, Ren JQ, Li L. Slow-progressing photoreceptor cell degeneration in night blindness c mutant zebrafish. Journal of Neurocytology. 2003;**32**(9):1107-1116

[40] Campbell LJ, Hyde DR. Opportunities for CRISPR/Cas9 gene editing in retinal regeneration research. Frontiers in Cell and Development Biology. 2017;**5**:99

[41] Jao LE, Wente SR, Chen W. Efficient multiplex biallelic zebrafish genome editing using a CRISPR nuclease system. Proceedings of the National Academy of Sciences of the United States of America. 2013;**110**(34):13904-13909

[42] Jinek M, Chylinski K, Fonfara I, Hauer M, Doudna JA, Charpentier E. A programmable dual-RNA-guided DNA endonuclease in adaptive bacterial immunity. Science. 2012;**337**(6096):816-821

[43] Varshney GK, Carrington B, Pei W, Bishop K, Chen Z, Fan C, et al. A high-throughput functional genomics workflow based on CRISPR/Cas9-mediated targeted mutagenesis in zebrafish. Nature Protocols. 2016;**11**(12):2357-2375

[44] Liu F, Chen J, Yu S, Raghupathy RK, Liu X, Qin Y, et al. Knockout of RP2 decreases GRK1 and rod transducin subunits and leads to photoreceptor degeneration in zebrafish. Human Molecular Genetics. 2015;**24**(16):4648-4659

[45] Yu S, Li C, Biswas L, Hu X, Liu F, Reilly J, et al. CERKL gene knockout disturbs photoreceptor outer segment phagocytosis and causes rod-cone dystrophy in zebrafish. Human Molecular Genetics. 2017;**26**(12):2335-2345

[46] Taylor SM, Alvarez-Delfin K, Saade CJ, Thomas JL, Thummel R, Fadool JM, et al. The bHLH transcription factor neurod governs photoreceptor genesis and regeneration

through delta-notch signaling. Investigative Ophthalmology & Visual Science. 2015;**56**(12):7496-7515

[47] Xie S, Han S, Qu Z, Liu F, Li J, Yu S, et al. Knockout of Nr2e3 prevents rod photoreceptor differentiation and leads to selective L−/M-cone photoreceptor degeneration in zebrafish. Biochimica et Biophysica Acta - Molecular Basis of Disease. 2019;**1865**(6):1273-1283

[48] Lewis TR, Kundinger SR, Pavlovich AL, Bostrom JR, Link BA, Besharse JC. Cos2/Kif7 and Osm-3/Kif17 regulate onset of outer segment development in zebrafish photoreceptors through distinct mechanisms. Developmental Biology. 2017;**425**(2):176-190

[49] Corral-Serrano JC, Messchaert M, Dona M, Peters TA, Kamminga LM, van Wijk E, et al. C2orf71a/pcare1 is important for photoreceptor outer segment morphogenesis and visual function in zebrafish. Scientific Reports. 2018;**8**(1):9675

[50] Lu Z, Hu X, Liu F, Soares DC, Liu X, Yu S, et al. Ablation of EYS in zebrafish causes mislocalisation of outer segment proteins, F-actin disruption and cone-rod dystrophy. Scientific Reports. 2017;**7**:46098

[51] Yu M, Liu Y, Li J, Natale BN, Cao S, Wang D, et al. Eyes shut homolog is required for maintaining the ciliary pocket and survival of photoreceptors in zebrafish. Biology Open. 2016;**5**(11):1662-1673

[52] Messchaert M, Dona M, Broekman S, Peters TA, Corral-Serrano JC, Slijkerman RWN, et al. Eyes shut homolog is important for the maintenance of photoreceptor morphology and visual function in zebrafish. PLoS One. 2018;**13**(7):e0200789

[53] al-Maghtheh M, Gregory C, Inglehearn C, Hardcastle A, Bhattacharya S. Rhodopsin mutations in autosomal dominant retinitis pigmentosa. Human Mutation. 1993;**2**(4):249-255

[54] Nakao T, Tsujikawa M, Notomi S, Ikeda Y, Nishida K. The role of mislocalized phototransduction in photoreceptor cell death of retinitis pigmentosa. PLoS One. 2012;**7**(4):e32472

[55] Zelinka CP, Sotolongo-Lopez M, Fadool JM. Targeted disruption of the endogenous zebrafish rhodopsin locus as models of rapid rod photoreceptor degeneration. Molecular Vision. 2018;**24**:587-602

[56] Shah AN, Davey CF, Whitebirch AC, Miller AC, Moens CB. Rapid reverse genetic screening using CRISPR in zebrafish. Nature Methods. 2015;**12**(6):535-540

[57] Trubiroha A, Gillotay P, Giusti N, Gacquer D, Libert F, Lefort A, et al. A rapid CRISPR/Cas-based mutagenesis assay in zebrafish for identification of genes involved in thyroid morphogenesis and function. Scientific Reports. 2018;**8**(1):5647

[58] Ramanagoudr-Bhojappa R, Carrington B, Ramaswami M, Bishop K, Robbins GM, Jones M, et al. Multiplexed CRISPR/Cas9-mediated knockout of 19 Fanconi anemia pathway genes in zebrafish revealed their roles in growth, sexual development and fertility. PLoS Genetics. 2018;**14**(12):e1007821

[59] Hu R, Huang W, Liu J, Jin M, Wu Y, Li J, et al. Mutagenesis of putative ciliary genes with the CRISPR/Cas9 system in zebrafish identifies genes required for retinal development. FASEB Journal: Official Publication of the Federation of American Societies for Experimental Biology. 2019;**33**(4):5248-5256

[60] Vighi E, Trifunovic D, Veiga-Crespo P, Rentsch A, Hoffmann D, Sahaboglu A, et al. Combination of cGMP analogue and drug delivery system provides functional protection in hereditary retinal degeneration. Proceedings of the National Academy of Sciences of the United States of America. 2018;**15**(13):E2997-E3006

[61] Frasson M, Sahel JA, Fabre M, Simonutti M, Dreyfus H, Picaud S. Retinitis pigmentosa: Rod photoreceptor rescue by a calcium-channel blocker in the rd mouse. Nature Medicine. 1999;**5**(10):1183-1187

[62] Ait-Ali N, Fridlich R, Millet-Puel G, Clerin E, Delalande F, Jaillard C, et al. Rod-derived cone viability factor promotes cone survival by stimulating aerobic glycolysis. Cell. 2015;**161**(4):817-832

[63] Scholl HP, Strauss RW, Singh MS, Dalkara D, Roska B, Picaud S, et al. Emerging therapies for inherited retinal degeneration. Science Translational Medicine. 2016;**8**(368):368rv6

[64] Bainbridge JW, Smith AJ, Barker SS, Robbie S, Henderson R, Balaggan K, et al. Effect of gene therapy on visual function in Leber's congenital amaurosis. The New England Journal of Medicine. 2008;**358**(21):2231-2239

[65] Cideciyan AV, Aleman TS, Boye SL, Schwartz SB, Kaushal S, Roman AJ, et al. Human gene therapy for RPE65 isomerase deficiency activates the retinoid cycle of vision but with slow rod kinetics. Proceedings of the National Academy of Sciences of the United States of America. 2008;**105**(39):15112-15117

[66] Maguire AM, Simonelli F, Pierce EA, Pugh EN Jr, Mingozzi F, Bennicelli J, et al. Safety and efficacy of gene transfer for Leber's congenital amaurosis. The New England Journal of Medicine. 2008;**358**(21):2240-2248

[67] Jacobson SG, Cideciyan AV, Roman AJ, Sumaroka A, Schwartz SB, Heon E, et al. Improvement and decline in vision with gene therapy in childhood blindness. The New England Journal of Medicine. 2015;**372**(20):1920-1926

[68] Eiraku M, Takata N, Ishibashi H, Kawada M, Sakakura E, Okuda S, et al. Self-organizing optic-cup morphogenesis in three-dimensional culture. Nature. 2011;**472**(7341):51-56

[69] Zhong X, Gutierrez C, Xue T, Hampton C, Vergara MN, Cao LH, et al. Generation of three-dimensional retinal tissue with functional photoreceptors from human iPSCs. Nature Communications. 2014;**5**:4047

[70] Pearson RA, Gonzalez-Cordero A, West EL, Ribeiro JR, Aghaizu N, Goh D, et al. Donor and host photoreceptors engage in material transfer following transplantation of post-mitotic photoreceptor precursors. Nature Communications. 2016;**7**:13029

[71] Leveillard T, Klipfel L. Mechanisms underlying the visual benefit of cell transplantation for the treatment of retinal degenerations. International Journal of Molecular Sciences. 2019;**20**(3):E557

[72] Santos-Ferreira T, Llonch S, Borsch O, Postel K, Haas J, Ader M. Retinal transplantation of photoreceptors results in donor-host cytoplasmic exchange. Nature Communications. 2016;**7**:13028

[73] Singh MS, Balmer J, Barnard AR, Aslam SA, Moralli D, Green CM, et al. Transplanted photoreceptor precursors transfer proteins to host photoreceptors by a mechanism of cytoplasmic fusion. Nature Communications. 2016;**7**:13537

[74] Lahne M, Hyde DR. Live-cell imaging: New avenues to investigate retinal regeneration.

Neural Regeneration Research. 2017;**12**(8):1210-1219

[75] Bringmann A, Wiedemann P. Muller glial cells in retinal disease. Ophthalmologica. 2012;**227**(1):1-19

[76] Iribarne M, Ogawa L, Torbidoni V, Dodds CM, Dodds RA, Suburo AM. Blockade of endothelinergic receptors prevents development of proliferative vitreoretinopathy in mice. The American Journal of Pathology. 2008;**172**(4):1030-1042

[77] Reichenbach A, Bringmann A. New functions of Muller cells. Glia. 2013;**61**(5):651-678

[78] Yurco P, Cameron DA. Responses of Muller glia to retinal injury in adult zebrafish. Vision Research. 2005;**45**(8):991-1002

[79] Bernardos RL, Barthel LK, Meyers JR, Raymond PA. Late-stage neuronal progenitors in the retina are radial Muller glia that function as retinal stem cells. The Journal of Neuroscience. 2007;**27**(26):7028-7040

[80] Fausett BV, Goldman D. A role for alpha1 tubulin-expressing Muller glia in regeneration of the injured zebrafish retina. The Journal of Neuroscience. 2006;**26**(23):6303-6313

[81] Fimbel SM, Montgomery JE, Burket CT, Hyde DR. Regeneration of inner retinal neurons after intravitreal injection of ouabain in zebrafish. The Journal of Neuroscience. 2007;**27**(7):1712-1724

[82] Nelson CM, Ackerman KM, O'Hayer P, Bailey TJ, Gorsuch RA, Hyde DR. Tumor necrosis factor-alpha is produced by dying retinal neurons and is required for Muller glia proliferation during zebrafish retinal regeneration. The Journal of Neuroscience. 2013;**33**(15):6524-6539

[83] Wan J, Ramachandran R, Goldman D. HB-EGF is necessary and sufficient for Muller glia dedifferentiation and retina regeneration. Developmental Cell. 2012;**22**(2):334-347

[84] Ramachandran R, Zhao XF, Goldman D. Ascl1a/Dkk/beta-catenin signaling pathway is necessary and glycogen synthase kinase-3beta inhibition is sufficient for zebrafish retina regeneration. Proceedings of the National Academy of Sciences of the United States of America. 2011;**108**(38):15858-15863

[85] Lenkowski JR, Qin Z, Sifuentes CJ, Thummel R, Soto CM, Moens CB, et al. Retinal regeneration in adult zebrafish requires regulation of TGFbeta signaling. Glia. 2013;**61**(10):1687-1697

[86] Wan J, Zhao XF, Vojtek A, Goldman D. Retinal injury, growth factors, and cytokines converge on beta-catenin and pStat3 signaling to stimulate retina regeneration. Cell Reports. 2014;**9**(1):285-297

[87] Ramachandran R, Fausett BV, Goldman D. Ascl1a regulates Muller glia dedifferentiation and retinal regeneration through a Lin-28-dependent, let-7 microRNA signalling pathway. Nature Cell Biology. 2010;**12**(11):1101-1107

[88] Kassen SC, Ramanan V, Montgomery JE. C TB, Liu CG, Vihtelic TS, et al. Time course analysis of gene expression during light-induced photoreceptor cell death and regeneration in albino zebrafish. Developmental Neurobiology. 2007;**67**(8):1009-1031

[89] Nelson CM, Gorsuch RA, Bailey TJ, Ackerman KM, Kassen SC, Hyde DR. Stat3 defines three populations of Muller glia and is required for initiating maximal muller glia proliferation in the regenerating zebrafish retina. The

Journal of Comparative Neurology. 2012;**520**(18):4294-4311

[90] Raymond PA, Barthel LK, Bernardos RL, Perkowski JJ. Molecular characterization of retinal stem cells and their niches in adult zebrafish. BMC Developmental Biology. 2006;**6**:36

[91] Thummel R, Enright JM, Kassen SC, Montgomery JE, Bailey TJ, Hyde DR. Pax6a and Pax6b are required at different points in neuronal progenitor cell proliferation during zebrafish photoreceptor regeneration. Experimental Eye Research. 2010;**90**(5):572-582

[92] Conner C, Ackerman KM, Lahne M, Hobgood JS, Hyde DR. Repressing notch signaling and expressing TNFalpha are sufficient to mimic retinal regeneration by inducing Muller glial proliferation to generate committed progenitor cells. The Journal of Neuroscience. 2014;**34**(43):14403-14419

[93] Ramachandran R, Zhao XF, Goldman D. Insm1a-mediated gene repression is essential for the formation and differentiation of Muller glia-derived progenitors in the injured retina. Nature Cell Biology. 2012;**14**(10):1013-1023

[94] Jorstad NL, Wilken MS, Grimes WN, Wohl SG, VandenBosch LS, Yoshimatsu T, et al. Stimulation of functional neuronal regeneration from Muller glia in adult mice. Nature. 2017;**548**(7665):103-107

[95] Yao K, Qiu S, Wang YV, Park SJH, Mohns EJ, Mehta B, et al. Restoration of vision after de novo genesis of rod photoreceptors in mammalian retinas. Nature. 2018;**560**(7719):484-488

[96] Vihtelic TS, Hyde DR. Light-induced rod and cone cell death and regeneration in the adult albino zebrafish (Danio rerio) retina. Journal of Neurobiology. 2000;**44**(3):289-307

[97] Montgomery JE, Parsons MJ, Hyde DR. A novel model of retinal ablation demonstrates that the extent of rod cell death regulates the origin of the regenerated zebrafish rod photoreceptors. The Journal of Comparative Neurology. 2010;**518**(6):800-814

[98] Hagerman GF, Noel NC, Cao SY, DuVal MG, Oel AP, Allison WT. Rapid recovery of visual function associated with blue cone ablation in zebrafish. PLoS One. 2016;**11**(11):e0166932

[99] Morris AC, Scholz TL, Brockerhoff SE, Fadool JM. Genetic dissection reveals two separate pathways for rod and cone regeneration in the teleost retina. Developmental Neurobiology. 2008;**68**(5):605-619

[100] Pei W, Xu L, Huang SC, Pettie K, Idol J, Rissone A, et al. Guided genetic screen to identify genes essential in the regeneration of hair cells and other tissues. NPJ Regenerative Medicine. 2018;**3**:11

[101] Unal Eroglu A, Mulligan TS, Zhang L, White DT, Sengupta S, Nie C, et al. Multiplexed CRISPR/Cas9 targeting of genes implicated in retinal regeneration and degeneration. Frontiers in Cell and Development Biology. 2018;**6**:88

Chapter 11

Mechanistic Dissection of Macular Degeneration Using the Phosphorylation Interactome

Weilue He, Srinivas R. Sripathi, Madu Joshua, Ruonan Zhang, Fabunmi Tosin, Patrick Ambrose, Diana R. Gutsaeva and Wan Jin Jahng

Abstract

In the current study, we suggest that phosphorylation reactions of specific proteins in mitochondria and the nucleus are a key step in the progression of age-related macular degeneration (AMD). To determine the molecular mechanism of AMD, we examined proteomic changes under oxidative stress to establish the protein interaction map using *in vitro* and *in vivo* models that mimic the complex and progressive characteristics of AMD. We postulated that apoptosis can be initiated by phosphorylation reactions under chronic oxidative stress in a region-specific and tissue-specific manner. The analysis of AMD interactome and oxidative biomarker network demonstrated that the presence of tissue- and region-dependent post-translational mechanisms may contribute toward AMD progression through the mitochondrial-nuclear communication. The AMD interactome suggests that new therapeutic targets, including prohibitin, erythropoietin, vitronectin, crystalline, nitric oxide synthase, ubiquitin, and complement inhibition may exist as a proteome network. Further, immunocytochemistry demonstrated that mitochondria could enter the nucleus in the retinal pigment epithelium (RPE) under oxidative stress. The current interactome map implies that a positive correlation may exist between oxidative stress-mediated phosphorylation and AMD progression. The unbiased proteome network provides a basis for understanding oxidative stress-induced mitochondrial dysfunction in AMD and exploring effective therapeutic approaches to treat age-related neurodegeneration.

Keywords: protein interactome, mitochondria, phosphoproteomics, prohibitin, retrograde signaling, AMD target

1. Introduction

Age-related macular degeneration (AMD) is the leading cause of legal blindness in developed countries [1, 2]. Although the vision loss directly results from dysfunction and cell death of photoreceptors in the central retina, it has been demonstrated that the early stage of AMD involves the pathological changes in retinal pigment epithelium (RPE), the cell layer that plays pivotal roles in supporting photoreceptors. Due to the inevitable roles of RPE in supporting retinal function, it is critical to understand the physiological and pathological events in the RPE to prevent the development of AMD.

AMD symptoms include RPE atrophy, drusen accumulation, pigmentary changes, and choroidal neovascularization [1, 2]. Progressive cell death of post-mitotic RPE can lead to rod and cone apoptosis, resulting in AMD eventually. As AMD is a complex and multifactorial disease, AMD mechanisms could be discussed under environmental and genetic factors, including oxidative stress (smoking, light exposure, and hypoxia), RPE dysfunction (retinoid recycling, phagocytosis, aging, and apoptosis), accumulation of visual cycle waste, chronic inflammation (involving CFH, CFB/C2, C3, CF1, C5, and C9), drusen formation (lipid metabolism involving APOE, LIPC, and CETP), geographic atrophy, and choroidal neovascularization (VEGF signaling) [3–8].

Recently, mitochondrial alterations have drawn great deal of attention in understanding AMD [3]. Mitochondrion is the main cell compartment for cell respiration and cell signaling. Many studies have shown that RPE mitochondria undergo severe structural and functional changes during aging and AMD [3, 4]. The mitochondrial dysfunction causes the excessive generation and leaking of reactive oxidative species (ROS) from the respiration chain and RPE is one of the most susceptible cells to ROS. RPE is also responsible for phagocytosis of rod outer segments, where polyunsaturated fatty acids abound. Phagocytosis and oxidation of unsaturated fatty acids generate additional ROS. Further, RPE cells are exposed to chronic oxidative stress, including constant exposure to intense light and oxidants from mitochondria due to high levels of oxygen demand and consumption. The increased oxidative stress in RPE may in turn deteriorates mitochondria and causes RPE cell death. Our data suggested that mitochondrial morphology and functional integrity are closely related to apoptosis and cellular aging [9–11]. Insufficient bioenergetic processes may lead to drusen accumulation. A number of apoptotic regulators reside in mitochondria and various retrograde signaling mechanisms are also dependent on mitochondria.

Oxidative stress facilitates the formation of toxic lipids and protein peroxidation, resulting in drusen deposition. There are excessive generation and leaking of oxidants from the respiratory chain under oxidative stress. This explains why AMD is associated with the accumulation of advanced lipid peroxidation end products, leading to apoptosis of photoreceptors and RPE cells. In addition, phosphorylation of crystalline and vimentin may participate in the pathogenesis of AMD by forming soft drusen with longer chain of phosphatidylcholine and cholesteryl esters. With aging, lipids and cholesterol accumulate underneath the RPE and contribute toward drusen formation. The excessive drusen deposition may damage the RPE and lead to degeneration of collagen or elastin in Brook's membrane, the outer retina, and the choroid vasculature.

We have studied the mechanism of RPE cell death under various stress conditions [9–20]. Our data demonstrated that mitochondrial morphological changes and mitochondrial-nuclear shuttling of prohibitin are significant responses in the RPE under oxidative stress [9, 10, 18]. Herein, we discuss AMD mechanisms based on four distinctive subnetworks of protein interactome, including complement activation, transcriptional regulation, mitochondrial signaling, and apoptosis. We propose that altered retrograde mitochondrial-nuclear crosstalk may initiate the pathological reactions observed in aging and oxidative stress-mediated RPE cell death that can contribute to the pathogenesis of AMD.

2. Materials and methods

2.1 *In vivo* experimental design

All the animal procedures were performed in compliance with the Association for Research in Vision and Ophthalmology Statement for the humane use of laboratory animals. Human *postmortem* donor eye tissues were used following the tenets of the Declaration of Helsinki. Diabetic retinopathy (DR) human retinal tissues (n = 9, biological triplicate × technical triplicate) were obtained from the Georgia Eye Bank (Atlanta, GA). AMD retina (8 mm macular and peripheral punches), RPE (8 mm central and peripheral punches), and age-matched control eyes (n = 9, biological triplicate × technical triplicate) were provided by the Lions Eye Bank (Moran Eye Center, University of Utah). Phosphoproteomes of macula (I), peripheral retina (II), central RPE (III), and peripheral RPE (IV) were compared to age-matched control donor eyes to determine region-specific, senescence-associated molecular mechanisms during AMD progression. Phosphoproteins were enriched by charge-based spin column chromatography and resolved by 2D gel electrophoresis as previously reported [11, 16]. Trypsin-digested phosphopeptides from whole lysates were enriched using Ga^{3+}/TiO_2 immobilized metal ion chromatography. Eluted phosphopeptides were analyzed using MALDI-TOF-TOF and ESI MS/MS. Serine, threonine, and tyrosine phosphorylations were confirmed by phospho-Western blotting analysis.

2.2 ARPE-19 and HRP cells

For *in vitro* experiments, retinal pigment epithelial cells (ARPE-19) were purchased from ATCC (Manassas, VA) and retinal progenitor cells (HRP) were kindly donated by Dr. Harold J. Sheeldo at the University of North Texas Health Science Center. ARPE-19 and HRP cells were cultured in a 5% CO_2 incubator at 37°C in 100-mm dishes (Nalge Nunc International, Naperville, IL) using Dulbecco's modified Eagle's medium (DMEM) with fetal bovine serum (10%) and penicillin/streptomycin (1%). Confluent cells were trypsinized (5–7 min at 37°C) using a trypsin-EDTA buffer (0.1%, Sigma-Aldrich, St. Louis, MO), followed by centrifugation (300 × *g*, 7 min). Cells (eight to nine passages) were grown to confluence for 2–4 days and then were treated with H_2O_2 (200 μM), intense light (7000–10,000 lux, 1–24 h) or constant light (700 lux, 48 h). Then, cells were rinsed (Modified Dulbecco's PBS) and lysed using IP lysis buffer containing Tris (25 mM), NaCl (150 mM), EDTA (1 mM), NP-40 (1%), glycerol (5%), and protease inhibitor cocktail at pH 7.4 by incubating on ice for 5 min with periodic sonication (3 × 5 min), followed by centrifugation (13,000 × *g*, 10 min). Proteins (1 mg/ml, 200–400 μl) were loaded for immunoprecipitation and nonspecific bindings were avoided using control agarose resin cross-linked by 4% bead agarose. Amino-linked protein-A beads were used to immobilize antiprohibitin antibody with a coupling buffer (1 mM sodium phosphate, 150 mM NaCl, pH 7.2), followed by incubation (room temperature, 2 h) with sodium cyanoborohydride (3 μl, 5 M). Columns were washed using a washing buffer (1 M NaCl), and protein lysate was incubated in the protein A-antibody column with gentle rocking overnight at 4°C. The unbound proteins were spun down as flow-through, and the columns were washed three times using washing buffer to remove nonspecific binding proteins. The interacting proteins were eluted by incubating with elution buffer for 5 min at RT. The eluted proteins were equilibrated with Laemmli sample buffer (5X, 5% β-mercaptoethanol). Eluted proteins were separated using SDS-PAGE and stained using Coomassie blue (Pierce, IL) or silver staining kit (Bio-Rad, Hercules, CA). Immunoprecipitated proteins were reported previously [10] and were used to establish interactome in the current study.

2.3 *In vivo* oxidative stress

Constant light experiment was conducted as previously reported [21]. Female C3HeB/FeJ mice (12 weeks of age) were purchased from the Jackson Laboratory (Bar Harbor, ME) and housed under a 12-h light/12-h dark cyclic lighting condition

(250–300 lux of full spectra fluorescent room light) for 2 weeks. The first group of mice (light/dark group) was housed in the 12-h light/12-h dark condition and the second group (constant light group) was housed in constant room light (250–300 lux) for 7 days. After euthanasia, eyes were rapidly removed from animals and retinas were isolated by microscopic dissection. Retinas were then washed with a solution of 250 mM sucrose, 10 mM Tris–HCl, at pH 7.0 to remove contaminants before lysis in 30 mM Tris–HCl, 2 M thiourea, 7 M urea, 4% CHAPS, and protease inhibitors. Samples were then sonicated intermittently until cells were lysed. The crude lysate was centrifuged at 20817× *g* for 30 min at 4°C. Two-dimensional polyacrylamide gel electrophoresis (2D-PAGE) was performed using Ettan IPGphor system with 11 cm of immobilized pH gradient (IPG) strips (pH 5–8, ReadyStrip, Biorad) and 8–16% gradient Precast Gel (Criterion Precast Gel, Biorad). About 200 μg of retinal proteins were diluted to 200-μl solution with rehydration buffer (4% CHAPS, 8 M urea, 1% pharmalytes 3–10, 10 mM DTT). The mixture (200 μl) was incubated with IPG strip at room temperature for 30 min. IPG strips were rehydrated for 14 h at 30 V, followed by isoelectric focusing (IEF) performed at 500 V for 1 h, 500–8000 V for 6 h, and 8000 V for 1 h. After IEF, IPG strips were equilibrated for 15 min in 10-ml equilibration buffer containing 50 mM Tris–HCl (1.5 M, pH 8.8), 6 M urea, 30% glycerol (v/v), 2% SDS (w/v), trace amount of Bromophenol Blue, and 0.05 g DTT, and then re-equilibrated for another 15 min in the same buffer containing 0.45 g of iodoacetamide. Equilibrated strips were then placed on top of precast gradient gels and embedded in 0.5% agarose. Proteins were electrophoresed at 100 volts for about 2 h until the dye had reached the bottom of the gel. After electrophoresis, separated proteins were visualized using Coomassie blue staining. The Commassie blue-stained gels were scanned with a transmission scanner and differential protein expression was analyzed. Differentially expressed protein spots were excised from gels and analyzed by MALDI-TOF and the selected proteins were further analyzed by MALDI-TOF-TOF mass spectrometry. All experiments were repeated in triplicate.

2.4 Protein identification by MALDI-TOF and TOF-TOF mass spectrometry

Protein spots, manually excised from the gel, were de-stained with 100 mM NH_4HCO_3/50% acetonitrile (MeCN) at 37°C for 45 min twice. Gel slices were then incubated with 100% MeCN at room temperature for 5 min. After dehydration and drying, gel slices were incubated with 250 ng of trypsin (20 μg/20 μl, Promega) in 40 mM NH_4HCO_3/10% MeCN at 37°C overnight. Trypsin/digestion buffer (50 μl) was added so that the gel slices were completely covered. After trypsin treatment, peptides were collected and gel slices were washed for 1 h with extraction buffer (50% MeCN, 0.1% Trifluoroacetic acid (TFA)) with gentle agitation. Peptides were combined and concentrated in a speed vacuum. Ziptip has been used to purify peptides. About 0.6 μl of purified peptides were mixed with 0.6 μl of alpha-Cyano-4-hydroxy-cinnamic acid matrix solution saturated in 50% MeCN/0.1% TFA solution (1:1 vol/vol) onto a MALDI 100-well target plate. It was analyzed through matrix-assisted laser/desorption ionization time of flight mass spectrometry (Bruker Ultraflex MALDI-TOF-TOF Mass spectrometer) in a reflector mode. Mass spectra and tandem mass spectra were acquired manually with laser intensity at 2400 and 200 shots per spectrum in MS mode and laser intensity at 3800 and 400 shots in MS/MS mode. The spectra were analyzed using Flex analysis 2.0 and Biotools 2.2 software. Peptide mass was calibrated internally using two trypsin auto digest ions (m/z 842.509, m/z 2211.104). Protein identification was performed using Mascot software (www.matrixscience.com) to search the National Center for Biotechnology Information (NCBI) database with mouse taxonomy. A missed trypsin cleavage was not allowed and 100 ppm of mass tolerance was applied for the search for the matching peptide.

For MALDI-TOF and peptide fingerprinting, the probability-based Mowse score is used −10*Log (P), where P is the probability that the observed peptide match is a random event. Protein scores greater than 55 are considered significant ($p < 0.05$).

2.5 Immunocytochemical analysis

Cells were grown on sterile glass cover slips using DMEM/F12 medium with 10% FBS and 1% penicillin/streptomycin (Hyclone) in 5% CO_2 incubator at 37°C. Cells were treated under oxidative stress or intense light as previously reported [9–11, 18–20]. Cells were washed with PBS and incubated with MitoTracker Orange CMTMRos (100 nM, Molecular Probes, Carlsbad, CA) in serum-free culture medium (30 min, 37°C), followed by washing (PBS) and fixing (10% formaldehyde, 30 min, room temperature). Next, cells were treated using Triton X-100 (0.2%, Sigma-Aldrich, St. Louis, MO) in PBS (30 min) for permeabilization and blocked using complete medium (10% FBS, 0.05% Tween-20, 1 h). To stain cells, anti-actin, anti-tubulin, anti-vimentin antibody (1:100; Santa Cruz), and anti-prohibitin antibody (1:500, Genemed Synthesis Inc., San Antonio, TX, overnight, 4°C) were used; then, the cells were washed with PBS, followed by incubation with Alexa Fluor 488-conjugated anti-rabbit IgG secondary antibody (1:700; Molecular Probes, Carlsbad, CA, 1 h, room temperature). VECTASHIELD medium with DAPI (4,6-diamidino-2-phenylindole, the nucleus) was applied to mount the samples which were visualized using a Zeiss AxioVert fluorescent microscope (200 M Apo Tome, 63× magnification). Images were analyzed using ImageJ software (NIH).

2.6 AMD interactome map

Oxidative biomarker and AMD interactome were established using protein-protein interaction map software and databases, including STRING 10.0 (http://string-db.org/), MIPS (http://mips.helmholtz-muenchen.de/proj/ppi/), and iHOP (http://www.ihop-net.org/UniPub/iHOP/). Proteins found in AMD or oxidative stress conditions were added to establish the AMD interactome. Protein interactions were presented using eight categories, including neighborhood (green), gene fusion (red), co-occurrence (dark blue), co-expression (black), binding experiments (purple), databases (blue), text mining (lime), and homology (cyan). Protein interactions were determined and confirmed by genomic context, high-throughput experiments, co-expression, and previous publications in Pubmed. Protein database analysis showed the region-specific phosphorylation of specific proteins in AMD eyes. The AMD interactome was compared to the retina/RPE proteome under stress conditions.

3. Results

First, we determined the phosphorylation reactions in AMD samples to understand mitochondrial signaling, immune response, energy metabolism, and apoptosis under oxidative stress. The molecular network of altered phosphorylation is essential for determining molecular targets to treat AMD in the early stage. We built a comprehensive interaction map by combining several independent sets of *in vivo* and *in vitro* data including immunoprecipitation, co-expression, and protein domain information. The analysis of a large-scale phosphorylation reaction demonstrated that multiple phosphorylation motifs were implicated in the progression of AMD. A combination of phosphopeptide enrichment, high-performance liquid chromatography, and electrospray (ES)/time-of-flight (TOF) tandem mass spectrometry, followed by database search, provided an integrated phosphoproteome showing that the apoptotic pathway, energy metabolism, inflammation, cytoskeletal rearrangement, and mitochondrial dysfunction were involved in AMD mechanism (**Figure 1**).

The AMD interactome was connected together using phosphoproteomics data from AMD tissues, *in vivo* murine model, and *in vitro* data from ARPE-19 cells. STRING 10.0 software was used to establish the protein interaction map to analyze the molecular mechanisms involved in AMD progression in terms of oxidative stress, inflammation switch, energy metabolism, and transcriptional regulation. The interactome map demonstrated that four distinguished subnetworks may exist in AMD: (A) complement activation by SERPING1, transferrin, albumin, and HFE, which are connected to vimentin/vitronectin/plasminogen/matrix metallopeptidase 2 (MMP2); (B) transcriptional regulation by hypoxia signaling, which is connected to angiogenesis, vascularization switch as well as apoptosis involving ubiquitin downstream; (C) mitochondrial signaling through ATP synthase, PPA1, VDAC2, PRDX2, mitofilin (IMMT), and prohibitin; and (D) apoptosis/mitotic spindle checkpoint/NOTCH signaling by caspase, MAD, BUB 1/3, NOTCH/ZWINT, and cyclin-dependent kinases (CDC).

The AMD interactome with oxidative biomarkers demonstrated that several proteins that were previously characterized as unrelated to AMD, including ubiquitin, peroxiredoxin, MAP kinase, BUB 1/3, vimentin, and crystalline, were involved

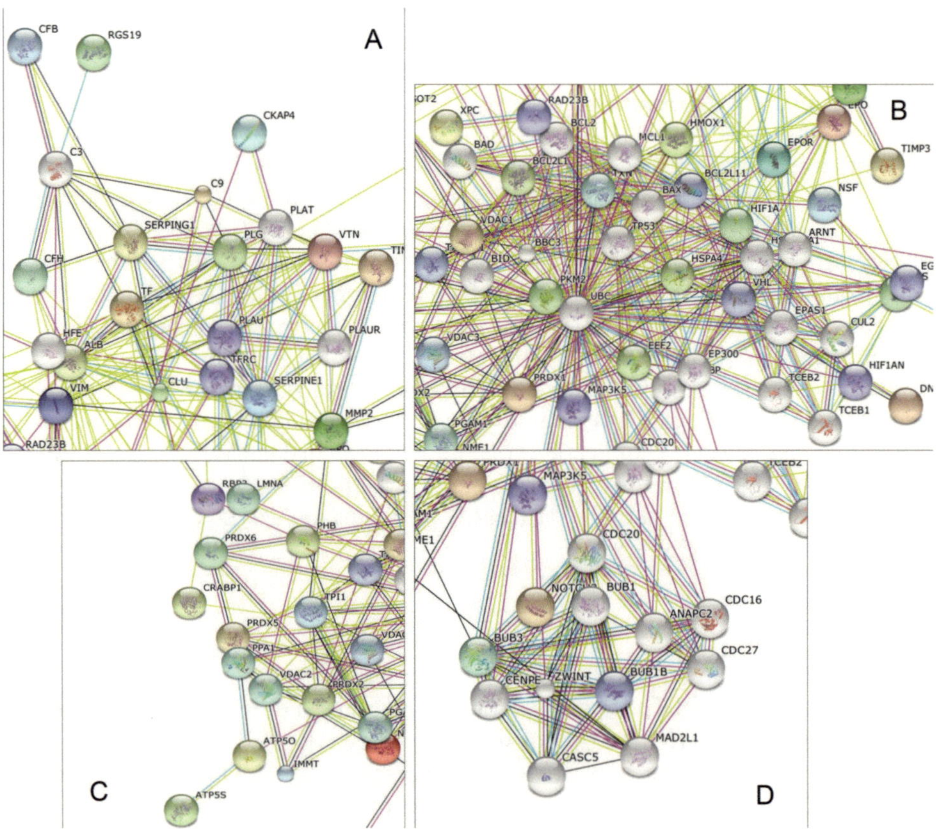

Figure 1.
Mechanistic dissection of AMD using the AMD biomarker interactome from proteomics data. AMD biomarkers from in vivo experiments using postmortem AMD eyes are connected using STRING software, followed by adding proteomics data from murine model in vivo and ARPE19 cells in vitro. The whole map was divided into four subnetworks presenting complement activation (A); transcriptional regulation including angiogenesis, vascularization, apoptosis (B); mitochondrial network (C); and apoptosis/mitotic spindle checkpoint/NOTCH signaling (D).

in AMD progression. Our interactome map suggests that mitochondrial protein trafficking, crystalline aggregation, and protein degradation may contribute to AMD pathway. To confirm oxidative stress biomarkers, specific cytoskeletal protein changes were determined *in vivo* using an animal model under constant light (C_3H female mice, 7 weeks old, 7 days of light). Results from mass spectrometry analysis showed that neurofilament, vimentin, and β-tubulin were up-regulated under 24 h of constant light compared to 12-h dark/12-h light condition (**Figure 2**).

Based on our proteomics data showing altered signaling of apoptosis in the retina and RPE, new targets for anti-apoptotic and anti-angiogenic therapy can be determined. The current interactome suggests the new biomarkers and targets in AMD including: (1) mitochondrial dysfunction in the peripheral RPE (depleted prohibitin, increased ATP synthase); (2) oxidative stress including intense and constant light (peroxiredoxin, thioredoxin, glutathione S-transferase); (3) cytoskeletal/mitochondrial remodeling by microtubule, actin filament, and intermediate filament (tubulin, actin, vimentin); (4) high concentration of nitric oxide (nitric oxide synthase); (5) hypoxia responses (HIF1, erythropoietin, VEGF); (6) disrupted circadian clock (melatonin); (7) apoptotic downstream (pJAK2, pSTAT3, Bclxl, caspases); (8) altered lipid concentrations (cardiolipin, cholesterol); (9) altered visual cycle (CRABP, CRALBP, RPE65); (10) altered energy metabolism (S/T vs. Y kinases, carnitine, pyruvate, ATP synthase); (11) aggregation of heat shock proteins and crystallins; and (12) inflammation switch (CFH, C3, collagen, vitronectin).

Next, we examined light-induced protein regulation to determine oxidative stress biomarkers *in vivo*. Unbiased proteomic approaches, including 2D electrophoresis and mass spectrometry analysis were used. Upregulated tubulin beta4/5 and vimentin were found under constant light (24 light) compared to 12-h light/12-h dark *in vivo*. Their up-regulation in constant light-exposed retina is possibly due to hyperphosphorylation of tubulin/vimentin and increased apoptosis. Melatonin mediated downregulation of PP2A, which may stabilize vimentin and negatively regulated apoptosis to protect retina from light-induced damages (data not shown).

To determine the interdependence of mitochondrial trafficking versus oxidative stress, we examined β-tubulin and vimentin dynamics under stress conditions (**Figure 3A**). Constant or intense light accelerated β-tubulin aggregation as well as nuclear localization. Mitochondrial trafficking was colocalized with tubulin polymerization, whereas vimentin was more likely to determine mitochondrial morphology in the dark. Intense light also led to actin filament aggregation in cytosol in

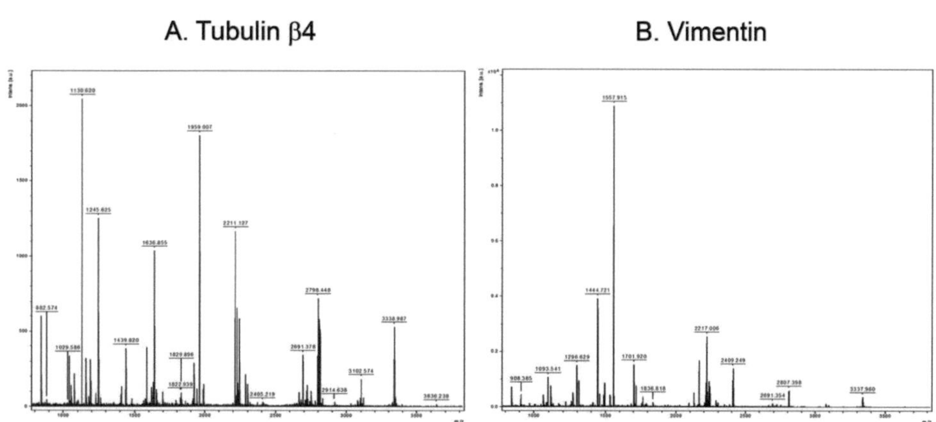

Figure 2.
Identification of β-tubulin (A) and vimentin (B) by MALDI-TOF-TOF spectrometry analysis. Proteins were separated from mouse retina using 2D electrophoresis under constant light (24 light) group compared to control group (12 h light/12 h dark). β-tubulin and vimentin were up-regulated under constant light in vivo.

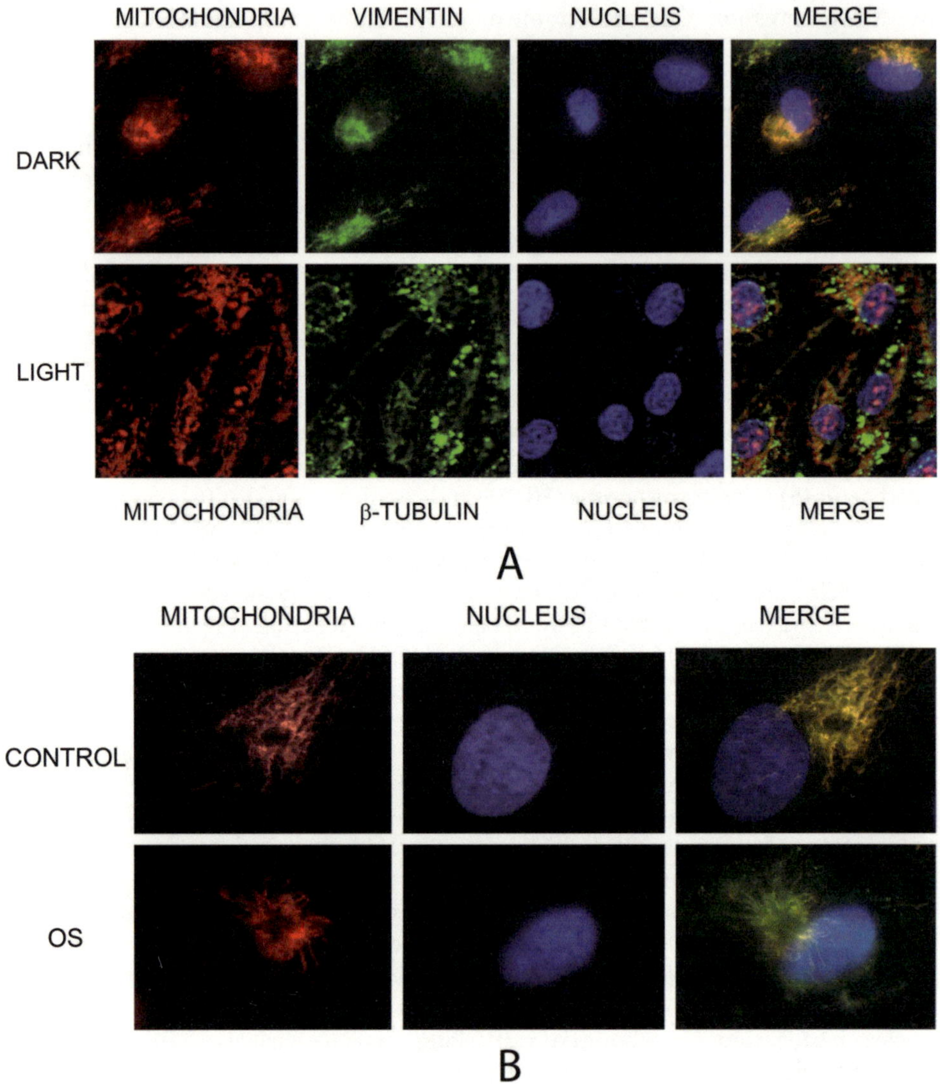

Figure 3.
Immunocytochemistry of mitochondrial trafficking using tubulin, vimentin, and prohibitin. β-tubulin and vimentin dynamics under stress conditions were analyzed (panel A). Constant or intense light accelerated β-tubulin aggregation as well as nuclear localization. Mitochondrial trafficking was colocalized with tubulin polymerization, whereas vimentin determines mitochondrial morphology in the dark. Vimentin was shown as an extended filamentous structure in control; however, it was aggregated around the nucleus under intense light (7000 lux). Mitochondrial prohibitin moved into the nucleus under intense light or oxidative stress (panel B).

the RPE. Cytosolic β-actin in the dark entered the nucleus under stress conditions. Immunocytochemistry of tubulin and actin demonstrated oxidative stress-mediated mitochondrial aggregation and size changes along with mitochondrial decay. Vimentin was shown as an extended filamentous structure in control; however, it was aggregated around the nucleus under stress conditions, that is oxidative stress and intense light (7000 lux). Mitochondrial proteins and cytoskeletal proteins, including prohibitin, actin, tubulin, and vimentin moved toward the nucleus under oxidative stresses (**Figure 3B**).

Translocalization of prohibitin might be related to post-transcriptional regulation and mitochondrial membrane depolarization. Down- or up-regulation of prohibitin in specific concentrations of H_2O_2 may imply one of several anti-apoptotic or pro-apoptotic responses depending on the intensity and temporal pattern of the stress. In our previous experiment, NF-κB was translocated into the nucleus in oxidative stress as a survival factor. It is important to note that prohibitin and NF-κB moved in parallel or opposite directions between the nucleus and mitochondria under various conditions. This coordinated translocalization may determine cell viability and apoptotic population in the retina and RPE.

We also examined the nuclear function of prohibitin by immunoprecipitation. Prohibitin binds with many transcription factors and nucleotide-binding proteins, including TFIIIB, DNA mismatch repair protein, ski2-type helicase, Cyclin-D-binding Myb-like transcription factor 1, DNA ligase, elongation factor, and BRCA1-A complex subunit RAP80. Additional interacting proteins have been reported such as E2F, retinoblastoma-associated protein, cellular tumor antigen p53, Heatshock 70: Stress-70 protein, and histone deacetylase (HDAC1). We confirmed transcriptional regulation of prohibitin by immunoprecipitation and protein-nucleotide binding assay.

Next, we established the signaling network of AMD using the interactome results. Based on our proteomics and interactome data, the potential AMD mechanisms were integrated as shown in **Figure 4**, suggesting altered energy metabolism, mitochondrial dysfunction, retinoid metabolism, circadian clock, inflammation, angiogenesis, lipid metabolism, and apoptosis.

Previous data demonstrated that Hsp70 (c-Jun N-terminal kinase), crystallins (Akt), and the increased expression of VDAC might be involved in AMD progression [22–26]. Altered phosphorylations of mitochondrial heat shock protein mtHsp70, αA/aB crystalline, vimentin, and ATP synthase were observed in RPE cell death under oxidative stress [9, 22, 27–29]. Retinoid-binding proteins, including CRABP, RPE65, and RLBP1, could be involved in the advanced stages of AMD [30–32]. It was reported that accumulation of all-*trans*-retinal (atRAL), an important intermediate of the visual cycle, led to NADPH (reduced nicotinamide adenine dinucleotide phosphate) activation, resulting in ROS production and apoptosis of RPE cells [33–37]. Therefore, atRAL can play an important role in AMD pathogenesis, and its action can be underlined by oxidative stress, which can be potentiated by mitochondrial impairment; however, it is elusive whether dysfunctions in atRAL clearance belong to the initiation or consequence of AMD [35–37].

We observed altered lipid compositions that include increased carbon number of fatty acids, double bond saturation, higher cholesterol, and phosphatidylcholine, whereas cardiolipin levels decreased in RPE apoptosis [9, 10, 18]. Changes in lipid concentrations seem to diminish the membrane fluidity and accelerate protein aggregation in the RPE [38–44].

In vivo data demonstrated that PP2A and vimentin are modulated by constant light and are key elements involved in cytoskeletal signaling in rd1 mutation model [19, 45, 46]. The expression levels of vimentin and PP2A are significantly increased when C_3HeB/FeJ mice (rd1 allele; 12 weeks; photoreceptors degenerated) are exposed under continuous light for 7 days compared to a condition of 12-h light/dark cycling exposure. When melatonin is administered to animals while they are exposed to continuous light, the increased levels of vimentin and PP2A return to a normal level. Further, vimentin has been shown to be a target of PP2A that directly binds vimentin and dephosphorylates it. Vimentin is present in all mesenchymal cells, and often used as a differentiation marker. Like other intermediate filaments, vimentin acts to maintain cellular integrity; however, vimentin phosphorylation level determines RPE survival by the polymerization/depolymerization mechanism.

A positive correlation between the levels of PP2A and vimentin under light-induced stress suggests that cytoskeletal dynamics are regulated by vimentin phosphorylation. We postulate that light may induce post-translational modifications of vimentin. Stabilized vimentin may act as an anti-apoptotic agent when cells are under stress.

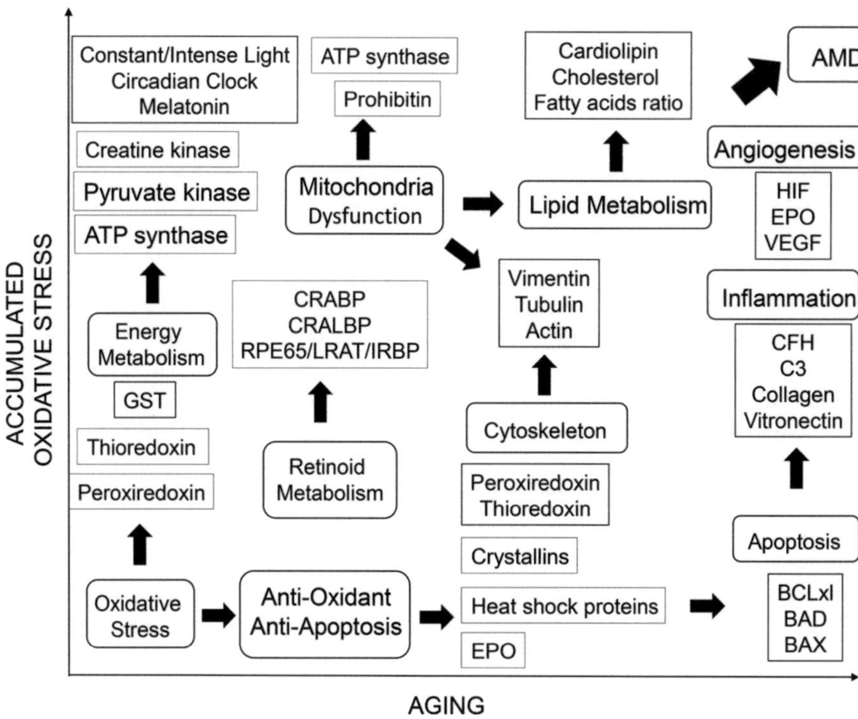

Figure 4.
AMD interactome and mechanistic dissection of AMD interpreted by phosphorylation reactions. Phosphoproteome alterations in the retina and RPE may lead to the pathological pathway which would be suited as targets for anti-apoptotic and anti-angiogenic therapy in AMD: (1) mitochondrial dysfunction in the peripheral RPE; (2) oxidative stress including intense and constant light; (3) cytoskeletal remodeling by actin, tubulin, and vimentin; (4) high concentration of nitric oxide; (5) hypoxia; (6) disrupted circadian clock; (7) apoptotic pathway through pJAK2, pSTAT3, Bclxl; (8) altered lipid concentrations; (9) altered visual cycle; (10) altered energy metabolism (ATP synthase, carnitine kinase, pyruvate kinases); (11) aggregation of heat shock proteins and crystallins, and inflammation (CFH, C3, collagen, vitronectin). Based on our proteomics data, we tested the following anti-apoptotic or anti-angiogenic molecules: (1) prohibitin (anti-apoptotic mitochondrial-nuclear shuttle); (2) erythropoietin as an anti-apoptotic protein via JAK2/STAT3 pathway; (3) melatonin as an anti-apoptotic and anti-angiogenic molecule protecting cytoskeletal reorganization through PP2A/vimentin pathway; (4) okadaic acid, arginine, and SNAP to control nitric oxide concentration; (5) cardiolipin and cholesterol; (6) anthocyanin (anti-angiogenic via VEGFR2 pathway); (7) phospholipids, fatty acids, cyclodextrin to control lipids and cholesterol concentration.

The current interactome suggests that altered phosphoproteome interactions, including pyruvate kinase, tyrosine kinase, and vimentin, exist in the retina and RPE in AMD. Phospho-Western blotting analysis revealed that phosphorylations of intermediate filament vimentin (Ser38, Ser55) and mitochondrial heat shock protein mtHsp70 were modulated in the RPE *in vitro* [9, 19, 22, 28, 47]. Changes of vimentin phosphorylation are directed to reorganization of the intermediate filament network and altered function of RPE cells.

4. Discussion

We used bioinformatics approaches to integrate molecular events associated with the progression of AMD. Proteomics data obtained using the oxidative stress animal model as well as the *in vitro* model were combined with previous AMD interactome results. We highlighted the importance of mitochondrial and cytoskeletal proteins in the oxidative stress responses in AMD models, including prohibitin, tubulin, and vimentin. In addition, we used immunocytochemistry analysis to validate the AMD interactome data, showing that mitochondria moved to the nucleus under intense light or oxidative stress conditions possibly through the tubulin/vimentin filament reorganization mechanism.

The current interactome mapping also suggests that changes in phosphoprotein levels in response to oxidative stress may induce complement activation, transcriptional regulation, mitochondrial dysfunction, and apoptosis. The phosphorylation signaling may explain why AMD is induced by oxidative stress and how the downstream of phosphorylations are associated with the changes of mitochondrial protein expressions, cytoskeleton reorganization, membrane remodeling, and lipid oxidation. For example, previous observations of vimentin derived from human choroidal neovascular membranes in AMD, as well as in drusen and melanolipofuscin, support the positive correlation between the biomarkers we characterized in RPE cells under stress and the AMD proteomics.

The AMD interactome map also elucidates the regulatory mechanism of apoptotic cell death governed by phosphorylation. Changes in the global phosphoproteome could be one of indications of early signaling events, including an increase of longer chain fatty acids, especially phosphatidylcholine and cholesteryl esters. The phosphoprotein interactome also provides a connection between oxidative stress-induced mitochondrial trafficking changes and AMD.

We also emphasize that mitochondria play a significant role in stress response in RPE cells, and this in turn influences the progression of AMD. The number of RPE mitochondria decreases with aging [48]. Through the observation by scanning electron microscope, mitochondrial shape becomes more oval in normal aged samples, while it is more bacillus-like in young eyes. The number of cristae decreases and cristae structure is less organized in aged tissue. In addition, mitochondrial matrix shows less electron density along with aging. In AMD samples, loss of cristae structure and matrix density is more obvious. Bleb formation on mitochondrial membrane and loss of mitochondrial membrane integrity were also observed in AMD [32, 49, 50].

Previously, quantitative analysis of mitochondrial morphology reveals that mitochondrial structure and functionality are closely associated with aging and AMD [9, 22, 32, 51–57]. In both aging and AMD samples, mitochondrion number per cell, cristae per mitochondrion, and mean area of mitochondrion per cell are declined. A similar trend was also observed in oxidative stressed ARPE-19, where mitochondrial distribution also changed. It is important to note that a mitochondrion is a highly dynamic organelle in response to different environmental factors, and those responses may determine the cell fate. RPE mitochondria undergo loss of structural integrity under oxidative stress and aging, indicating that mitochondrial signaling could be interrupted in AMD.

The retrograde communication from mitochondria to the nucleus has been demonstrated by our previous data by tracking the chaperon protein prohibitin using fluorescent microscopy techniques [10, 18, 58]. Mitochondrial components may also determine cell signaling in the nucleus, including change of mitochondrial membrane potential, mitochondrial DNA (mtDNA), and mitochondrial protein expressions. When cumulative damages hit the threshold where mitochondria cannot maintain their structural integrity, there is a decrease of mitochondrial membrane potential, along with a number of mitochondrial components released into the cytosol, including cardiolipin, cytochrome c, and Ca^{2+}. Release of cytochrome c initiates the caspase-dependent apoptosis and triggers more Ca^{2+} release from endoplasmic reticulum, whereas elevation of cytosolic Ca^{2+} level can cause more cytochrome c release and activation of caspase-9.

Mitochondrial DNA (mtDNA) is susceptible to oxidative stress damage. Compared to nuclear DNA (nDNA), mtDNA is located in mitochondrial matrix in close proximity to the ROS source in the cell. MtDNA is lack of histones and contains no introns that also increases its susceptibility to oxidative damage. Meanwhile, mtDNA mainly encodes electron transport chain proteins, including ATP synthase, cytochrome b, cytochrome c oxidase, and NADH dehydrogenase. Damaged mtDNA will lead to impaired electron transport chain proteins, further deteriorating cell energy production, generating more ROS, and inducing extra damages to mtDNA. Previous studies have revealed that abnormal mtDNA leads to reduced energy production and initiation of apoptosis [59–62]. Loss of mtDNA in ARPE-19 cells led to the change of nuclear gene expression, especially the up-regulation of genes related to glycolysis [63–65].

The mitochondrial-nuclear crosstalk could be a mechanism that the RPE cell uses to compensate the insufficient energy productions due to the mitochondrial dysfunction. Other changes in nuclear gene expressions caused by loss of mtDNA include up-regulation of proteins related to uptake of ROS and drusen, extracellular matrix and matrix enzymes, lipid transport-related proteins, and inflammation-related regulators. Therefore, damaged mtDNA has been considered as an important biomarker of oxidative stressed RPE and progression of AMD [50, 66, 67]. Fragments of mtDNA have been found to migrate to the nucleus and be inserted into the nuclear genome [68–71]. The entrance of mitochondria into the nucleus has been reported to promote both the attack of mitochondria by nuclear protein and the attack of nuclear DNA and protein by protein of the mitochondrial intermembrane space [65, 68–74]. Mitochondria move to the nucleus under stress to fulfill energy demand of the nucleus. Therefore, our observation that mitochondria entering the nucleus could be one of the mechanisms to explain mitochondrial diseases and the aging process.

Our AMD interactome map implies that a positive correlation exists between AMD mechanism and early oxidative stress biomarkers, as well as inflammation switch, apoptosis, transcriptional regulation, and mitochondrial dysfunction [26, 32, 52, 75–77]. The mechanistic dissection of our AMD interactome map is the initial delineation of the underlying physiology of oxidative stress-mediated phosphorylation signaling in RPE apoptosis which can lead to AMD progression. In addition, the phosphoprotein interactome provides a stimulus for understanding oxidative stress-induced mitochondrial changes and the mechanism of aggregate formation induced by protein phosphorylations. As a consequence, an effective therapeutic approach to treat AMD based on the modulation of phosphorylation reactions is expected to result.

Author details

Weilue He[1], Srinivas R. Sripathi[2], Madu Joshua[3], Ruonan Zhang[4], Fabunmi Tosin[3], Patrick Ambrose[3], Diana R. Gutsaeva[5] and Wan Jin Jahng[3]*

1 Department of Biomedical Engineering, Michigan Technological University, Houghton, MI, USA

2 Department of Ophthalmology, Wilmer Eye Institute, The Johns Hopkins University School of Medicine, Baltimore, MD, USA

3 Retina Proteomics Laboratory, Department of Petroleum Chemistry, American University of Nigeria, Yola, Adamawa, Nigeria

4 Department of Ophthalmology, University of South Carolina, Columbia, SC, USA

5 Department of Ophthalmology, Augusta University, Augusta, GA, USA

*Address all correspondence to: wan.jahng@aun.edu.ng

References

[1] Zarbin MA. Current concepts in the pathogenesis of age-related macular degeneration. Archives of Ophthalmology (Chicago, IL, 1960). 2004;**122**:598-614. DOI: 10.1001/archopht.122.4.598

[2] Kanagasingam Y, Bhuiyan A, Abràmoff MD, Smith RT, Goldschmidt L, Wong TY. Progress on retinal image analysis for age related macular degeneration. Progress in Retinal and Eye Research. 2014;**38**:20-42. DOI: 10.1016/j.preteyeres.2013.10.002

[3] Edwards AO, Ritter R, Abel KJ, Manning A, Panhuysen C, Farrer LA. Complement factor H polymorphism and age-related macular degeneration. Science. 2005;**308**:421-424. DOI: 10.1126/science.1110189

[4] Wu Z, Lauer TW, Sick A, Hackett SF, Campochiaro PA. Oxidative stress modulates complement factor H expression in retinal pigmented epithelial cells by acetylation of FOXO3. The Journal of Biological Chemistry. 2007;**282**:22414-22425. DOI: 10.1074/jbc.M702321200

[5] Jiang M, Esteve-Rudd J, Lopes VS, Diemer T, Lillo C, Rump A, et al. Microtubule motors transport phagosomes in the RPE, and lack of KLC1 leads to AMD-like pathogenesis. The Journal of Cell Biology. 2015;**210**:jcb.201410112. DOI: 10.1083/jcb.201410112

[6] Alcazar O, Hawkridge AM, Collier TS, Cousins SW, Bhattacharya SK, Muddiman DC, et al. Proteomics characterization of cell membrane blebs in human retinal pigment epithelium cells. Molecular & Cellular Proteomics. 2009;**8**:2201-2211. DOI: 10.1074/mcp.M900203-MCP200

[7] Spencer KL, Olson LM, Anderson BM, Schnetz-Boutaud N, Scott WK, Gallins P, et al. C3 R102G polymorphism increases risk of age-related macular degeneration. Human Molecular Genetics. 2008;**17**:1821-1824. DOI: 10.1093/hmg/ddn075

[8] Grimm C, Wenzel A, Hafezi F, Yu S, Redmond TM, Remé CE. Protection of Rpe65-deficient mice identifies rhodopsin as a mediator of light-induced retinal degeneration. Nature Genetics. 2000;**25**:63-66. DOI: 10.1038/75614

[9] Sripathi SR, He W, Sylvester OD, Neksumi M, Um JY, Dluya T, et al. Altered cytoskeleton as a mitochondrial decay signature in the retinal pigment epithelium. The Protein Journal. 2016;**35**:179-192. DOI: 10.1007/s10930-016-9659-9

[10] Sripathi SR, Sylvester O, He W, Moser T, Um J-Y, Lamoke F, et al. Prohibitin as the molecular binding switch in the retinal pigment epithelium. The Protein Journal. 2016;**35**:1-16. DOI: 10.1007/s10930-015-9641-y

[11] Sripathi S, He W, Prigge CL, Sylvester O, Um J-Y, Powell FL, et al. Interactome mapping guided by tissue-specific phosphorylation in age-related macular degeneration. International Journal of Scientific and Engineering Research. 2017;**8**:680-698. DOI: 10.14299/ijser.2017.02.010

[12] Xue L, Gollapalli DR, Maiti P, Jahng WJ, Rando RR. A palmitoylation switch mechanism in the regulation of the visual cycle. Cell. 2004;**117**:761-771. DOI: 10.1016/j.cell.2004.05.016

[13] Jahng WJ. New Biomarkers in the Retina and RPE Under Oxidative Stress. Ocular Diseases, Adedayo Adio. Rijeka, Croatia: InTechOpen; 2012. DOI: 10.5772/1678

[14] Chung H, Lee H, Lamoke F, Hrushesky WJM, Wood PA,

Jahng WJ. Neuroprotective role of erythropoietin by antiapoptosis in the retina. Journal of Neuroscience Research. 2009;**87**:2365-2374. DOI: 10.1002/jnr.22046

[15] Lee H, Chung H, Arnouk H, Lamoke F, Hunt RC, Hrushesky WJM, et al. Cleavage of the retinal pigment epithelium-specific protein RPE65 under oxidative stress. International Journal of Biological Macromolecules. 2010;**47**:104-108. DOI: 10.1016/j.ijbiomac.2010.05.014

[16] Lee H, Chung H, Lee SH, Jahng WJ. Light-induced phosphorylation of crystallins in the retinal pigment epithelium. International Journal of Biological Macromolecules. 2011;**48**:194-201. DOI: 10.1016/j.ijbiomac.2010.11.006

[17] Arnouk H, Lee H, Zhang R, Chung H, Hunt RC, Jahng WJ. Early biosignature of oxidative stress in the retinal pigment epithelium. Journal of Proteomics. 2011;**74**:254-261. DOI: 10.1016/j.jprot.2010.11.004

[18] Sripathi SR, He W, Atkinson CL, Smith JJ, Liu Z, Elledge BM, et al. Mitochondrial-nuclear communication by prohibitin shuttling under oxidative stress. Biochemistry. 2011;**50**:8342-8351. DOI: 10.1021/bi2008933

[19] Sripathi SR, He W, Um JY, Moser T. Nitric oxide leads to cytoskeletal reorganization in the retinal pigment epithelium under oxidative stress. Advances in Bioscience and Biotechnology. 2012;**03**:1167-1178. DOI: 10.4236/abb.2012.38143

[20] Sripathi SR, Prigge CL, Elledge B, He W, Offor J, Gutsaeva DR, et al. Melatonin modulates prohibitin and cytoskeleton in the retinal pigment epithelium. International Journal of Scientific and Engineering Research. 2017;**8**:502-506. DOI: 10.14299/ijser.2017.07.001

[21] Zhang R, Hrushesky WJM, Wood PA, Lee SH, Hunt RC, Jahng WJ. Melatonin reprogrammes proteomic profile in light-exposed retina in vivo. International Journal of Biological Macromolecules. 2010;**47**:255-260. DOI: 10.1016/j.ijbiomac.2010.04.013

[22] Nordgaard CL, Karunadharma PP, Feng X, Olsen TW, Ferrington DA. Mitochondrial proteomics of the retinal pigment epithelium at progressive stages of age-related macular degeneration. Investigative Ophthalmology & Visual Science. 2008;**49**:2848-2855. DOI: 10.1167/iovs.07-1352

[23] Nakata K, Crabb JW, Hollyfield JG. Crystallin distribution in Bruch's membrane-choroid complex from AMD and age-matched donor eyes. Experimental Eye Research. 2005;**80**: 821-826. DOI: 10.1016/j.exer.2004.12.011

[24] Crabb JW, Miyagi M, Gu X, Shadrach K, West KA, Sakaguchi H, et al. Drusen proteome analysis: An approach to the etiology of age-related macular degeneration. Proceedings of the National Academy of Sciences of the United States of America. 2002;**99**:14682-14687. DOI: 10.1073/pnas.222551899

[25] Umeda S, Suzuki MT, Okamoto H, Ono F, Mizota A, Terao K, et al. Molecular composition of drusen and possible involvement of anti-retinal autoimmunity in two different forms of macular degeneration in cynomolgus monkey (Macaca fascicularis). The FASEB Journal. 2005;**19**:1683-1685. DOI: 10.1096/fj.04-3525fje

[26] Nita M, Grzybowski A, Ascaso FJ, Huerva V. Age-related macular degeneration in the aspect of chronic low-grade inflammation (pathophysiological parainflammation). Mediators of Inflammation. 2014;**2014**:930671. DOI: 10.1155/2014/930671

[27] Aoki H, Hara A, Nakagawa S, Motohashi T, Hirano M, Takahashi Y, et al. Embryonic stem cells that differentiate into RPE cell precursors in vitro develop into RPE cell monolayers in vivo. Experimental Eye Research. 2006;**82**:265-274. DOI: 10.1016/j.exer.2005.06.021

[28] Kaempf S, Walter P, Salz AK, Thumann G. Novel organotypic culture model of adult mammalian neurosensory retina in co-culture with retinal pigment epithelium. Journal of Neuroscience Methods. 2008;**173**:47-58. DOI: 10.1016/j.jneumeth.2008.05.018

[29] Huang H, Li F, Alvarez RA, Ash JD, Anderson RE. Downregulation of ATP synthase subunit-6, cytochrome c oxidase-III, and NADH dehydrogenase-3 by bright cyclic light in the rat retina. Investigative Ophthalmology & Visual Science. 2004;**45**:2489-2496. DOI: 10.1167/iovs.03-1081

[30] Lakkaraju A, Finnemann SC, Rodriguez-Boulan E. The lipofuscin fluorophore A2E perturbs cholesterol metabolism in retinal pigment epithelial cells. Proceedings of the National Academy of Sciences of the United States of America. 2007;**104**:11026-11031. DOI: 10.1073/pnas.0702504104

[31] Yuan X, Gu X, Crabb JSW, Yue X, Shadrach K, Hollyfield JG, et al. Quantitative proteomics: Comparison of the macular Bruch membrane/choroid complex from age-related macular degeneration and normal eyes. Molecular & Cellular Proteomics. 2010;**9**:1031-1046. DOI: 10.1074/mcp.M900523-MCP200

[32] Suter M, Remé C, Grimm C, Wenzel A, Jäättela M, Esser P, et al. Age-related macular degeneration: The lipofuscin component N-retinyl-N-retinylidene ethanolamine detaches proapoptotic proteins from mitochondria and induces apoptosis in mammalian retinal pigment epithelial cells. The Journal of Biological Chemistry. 2000;**275**:39625-39630. DOI: 10.1074/jbc.M007049200

[33] Zhu X, Wang K, Zhang K, Zhou F, Zhu L. Induction of oxidative and nitrosative stresses in human retinal pigment epithelial cells by all-trans-retinal. Experimental Cell Research. 2016;**348**:87-94. DOI: 10.1016/j.yexcr.2016.09.002

[34] Wang H, Wittchen ES, Hartnett ME. Breaking barriers: Insight into the pathogenesis of neovascular age-related macular degeneration. Eye Brain. 2011;**3**:19-28. DOI: 10.2147/EB.S24951

[35] Mata NL, Tzekov RT, Liu X, Weng J, Birch DG, Travis GH. Delayed dark-adaptation and lipofuscin accumulation in abcr+/– mice: Implications for involvement of ABCR in age-related macular degeneration. Investigative Ophthalmology and Visual Science. 2001;**42**:1685-1690

[36] Ueda K, Zhao J, Kim HJ, Sparrow JR. Photodegradation of retinal bisretinoids in mouse models and implications for macular degeneration. Proceedings of the National Academy of Sciences, United States of America. 2016;**113**:6904-6909. DOI: 10.1073/pnas.1524774113

[37] Zhang J, Kiser PD, Badiee M, Palczewska G, Dong Z, Golczak M, et al. Molecular pharmacodynamics of emixustat in protection against retinal degeneration. The Journal of Clinical Investigation. 2015;**125**:2781-2794. DOI: 10.1172/JCI80950

[38] Wang L, Clark ME, Crossman DK, Kojima K, Messinger JD, a Mobley J, et al. Abundant lipid and protein components of drusen. PLoS One. 2010;**5**:e10329. DOI: 10.1371/journal.pone.0010329

[39] Nikolaeva O, Moiseyev G, Rodgers KK, Ma J-X. Binding to lipid membrane induces conformational changes in RPE65: Implications for

its isomerohydrolase activity. The Biochemical Journal. 2011;**436**:591-597. DOI: 10.1042/BJ20110091

[40] Bretillon L, Thuret G, Grégoire S, Acar N, Joffre C, Bron AM, et al. Lipid and fatty acid profile of the retina, retinal pigment epithelium/choroid, and the lacrimal gland, and associations with adipose tissue fatty acids in human subjects. Experimental Eye Research. 2008;**87**:521-528. DOI: 10.1016/j.exer.2008.08.010

[41] Yuan Q, Kaylor JJ, Miu A, Bassilian S, Whitelegge JP, Travis GH. Rpe65 isomerase associates with membranes through an electrostatic interaction with acidic phospholipid headgroups. The Journal of Biological Chemistry. 2010;**285**:988-999. DOI: 10.1074/jbc.M109.025643

[42] Trudel E, Beaufils S, Renault A, Breton R, Salesse C. Binding of RPE65 fragments to lipid monolayers and identification of its partners by glutathione S-transferase pull-down assays. Biochemistry. 2006;**45**:3337-3347. DOI: 10.1021/bi0519405

[43] Golczak M, Kiser PD, Lodowski DT, Maeda A, Palczewski K. Importance of membrane structural integrity for RPE65 retinoid isomerization activity. The Journal of Biological Chemistry. 2010;**285**:9667-9682. DOI: 10.1074/jbc.M109.063941

[44] Kopitz J, Holz FG, Kaemmerer E, Schutt F. Lipids and lipid peroxidation products in the pathogenesis of age-related macular degeneration. Biochimie. 2004;**86**:825-831. DOI: 10.1016/j.biochi.2004.09.029

[45] Turowski P, Myles T, a Hemmings B, a Fernandez NJ. Lamb, Vimentin dephosphorylation by protein phosphatase 2A is modulated by the targeting subunit B55. Molecular Biology of the Cell. 1999;**10**:1997-2015. Available from: http://www.pubmedcentral.nih.gov/articlerender.fcgi?artid=25403&tool=pmcentrez&rendertype=abstract

[46] Eriksson JE, He T, Trejo-Skalli AV, Härmälä-Braskén A-S, Hellman J, Chou Y-H, et al. Specific in vivo phosphorylation sites determine the assembly dynamics of vimentin intermediate filaments. Journal of Cell Science. 2004;**117**:919-932. DOI: 10.1242/jcs.00906

[47] Guidry C, Medeiros NE, Curcio CA. Phenotypic variation of retinal pigment epithelium in age-related macular degeneration. Investigative Ophthalmology & Visual Science. 2002;**43**:267-273. Available from: http://www.ncbi.nlm.nih.gov/pubmed/11773041

[48] He Y, Ge J, Burke JM, Myers RL, Dong ZZ, Tombran-Tink J. Mitochondria impairment correlates with increased sensitivity of aging RPE cells to oxidative stress. Journal of Ocular Biology, Diseases, and Informatics. 2010;**3**:92-108. DOI: 10.1007/s12177-011-9061-y

[49] Feher J, Kovacs I, Artico M, Cavallotti C, Papale A, Balacco Gabrieli C. Mitochondrial alterations of retinal pigment epithelium in age-related macular degeneration. Neurobiology of Aging. 2006;**27**:983-993. DOI: 10.1016/j.neurobiolaging.2005.05.012

[50] Liang F-QQ, Godley BF. Oxidative stress-induced mitochondrial DNA damage in human retinal pigment epithelial cells: A possible mechanism for RPE aging and age-related macular degeneration. Experimental Eye Research. 2003;**76**:397-403. DOI: 10.1016/S0014-4835(03)00023-X

[51] Markovets AM, Fursova AZ, Kolosova NG. Therapeutic action of the mitochondria-targeted antioxidant SkQ1 on retinopathy in OXYS rats linked

with improvement of VEGF and PEDF gene expression. PLoS One. 2011;**6**:1-8. DOI: 10.1371/journal.pone.0021682

[52] Terluk MR, Kapphahn RJ, Soukup LM, Gong H, Gallardo C, Montezuma SR, et al. Investigating mitochondria as a target for treating age-related macular degeneration. The Journal of Neuroscience. 2015;**35**:7304-7311. DOI: 10.1523/JNEUROSCI.0190-15.2015

[53] Karunadharma PP, Nordgaard CL, Olsen TW, a Ferrington D. Mitochondrial DNA damage as a potential mechanism for age-related macular degeneration. Investigative Ophthalmology & Visual Science. 2010;**51**:5470-5479. DOI: 10.1167/iovs.10-5429

[54] a Voloboueva L, Killilea DW, Atamna H, Ames BN. N-tert-butyl hydroxylamine, a mitochondrial antioxidant, protects human retinal pigment epithelial cells from iron overload: Relevance to macular degeneration. The FASEB Journal. 2007;**21**:4077-4086. DOI: 10.1096/fj.07-8396com

[55] Paraoan L, Ratnayaka A, Spiller DG, Hiscott P, White MRH, Grierson I. Unexpected intracellular localization of the AMD-associated cystatin C variant. Traffic. 2004;**5**:884-895. DOI: 10.1111/j.1600-0854.2004.00230.x

[56] Finley LWS, Haigis MC. The coordination of nuclear and mitochondrial communication during aging and calorie restriction. Ageing Research Reviews. 2009;**8**:173-188. DOI: 10.1016/j.arr.2009.03.003

[57] Hoye AT, Davoren JE, Wipf P, Fink MP, Kagan VE. Targeting mitochondria. Accounts of Chemical Research. 2008;**41**:87-97. DOI: 10.1021/ar700135m

[58] Lee H, Arnouk H, Sripathi S, Chen P, Zhang R, Bartoli M, et al. Prohibitin as an oxidative stress biomarker in the eye. International Journal of Biological Macromolecules. 2010;**47**:685-690. DOI: 10.1016/j.ijbiomac.2010.08.018

[59] Tuppen HAL, Blakely EL, Turnbull DM, Taylor RW. Mitochondrial DNA mutations and human disease. Biochimica et Biophysica Acta. 2010;**1797**:113-128. DOI: 10.1016/j.bbabio.2009.09.005

[60] Rudel T, Kepp O, Kozjak-Pavlovic V, Santhanam S, Venkatraman A, Ramakrishna BS, et al. Mitochondrial dysfunction and insulin resistance: An update. Journal of Pediatric Gastroenterology and Nutrition. 2014;**4**:1172-1184. DOI: 10.1007/s00535-009-0119-6

[61] Kenney MC, Atilano SR, Boyer D, Chwa M, Chak G, Chinichian S, et al. Characterization of retinal and blood mitochondrial DNA from age-related macular degeneration patients. Investigative Ophthalmology and Visual Science. 2010;**51**:4289-4297. DOI: 10.1167/iovs.09-4778

[62] Hill BG, Benavides GA, Lancaster JJR, Ballinger S, Dell'Italia L, Zhang J, et al. Integration of cellular bioenergetics with mitochondrial quality control and autophagy. Biological Chemistry. 2012;**393**:1485-1512. DOI: 10.1515/hsz-2012-0198

[63] Gramajo AL, Zacharias LC, Neekhra A, Luthra S, Atilano SR, Chwa M, et al. Mitochondrial DNA damage induced by 7-ketocholesterol in human retinal pigment epithelial cells in vitro. Investigative Ophthalmology & Visual Science. 2010;**51**:1164-1170. DOI: 10.1167/iovs.09-3443

[64] Liang F-Q, Green L, Wang C, Alssadi R, Godley BF. Melatonin protects human retinal pigment epithelial (RPE) cells against oxidative stress. Experimental Eye Research. 2004;**78**:1069-1075. DOI: 10.1016/j.exer.2004.02.003

[65] Spinazzola A, Zeviani M. Disorders of nuclear-mitochondrial intergenomic

signaling. Gene. 2005;**354**:162-168. DOI: 10.1016/j.gene.2005.03.025

[66] SanGiovanni JP, Arking DE, Iyengar SK, Elashoff M, Clemons TE, Reed GF, et al. Mitochondrial DNA variants of respiratory complex I that uniquely characterize haplogroup T2 are associated with increased risk of age-related macular degeneration. PLoS One. 2009;**4**:e5508. DOI: 10.1371/journal.pone.0005508

[67] Wang AL, Lukas TJ, Yuan M, Du N, Tso MO, Neufeld AH. Autophagy and exosomes in the aged retinal pigment epithelium: Possible relevance to drusen formation and age-related macular degeneration. PLoS One. 2009;**4**:e4160. DOI: 10.1371/journal.pone.0004160

[68] Bakeeva LE, Skulachev VP, Sudarikova YV, Tsyplenkova VG. Mitochondria enter the nucleus (one further problem in chronic alcoholism). Biochemistry Biokhimiia. 2001;**66**:1335-1341. DOI: 10.1023/A:1013374410540

[69] Delsite R, Kachhap S, Anbazhagan R, Gabrielson E, Singh KK. Nuclear genes involved in mitochondria-to-nucleus communication in breast cancer cells. Molecular Cancer. 2002;**1**:6. Available from: http://www.pubmedcentral.nih.gov/articlerender.fcgi?artid=149409&tool=pmcentrez&rendertype=abstract

[70] Amuthan G, Biswas G, Zhang SY, Klein-Szanto A, Vijayasarathy C, Avadhani NG. Mitochondria-to-nucleus stress signaling induces phenotypic changes, tumor progression and cell invasion. The EMBO Journal. 2001;**20**:1910-1920. DOI: 10.1093/emboj/20.8.1910

[71] Park SY, Lee S, Park KS, Lee HK, Lee W. Proteomic analysis of cellular change involved in mitochondria-to-nucleus communication in L6 GLUT4myc myocytes. Proteomics. 2006;**6**:1210-1222. DOI: 10.1002/pmic.200500284

[72] Woo DK, Phang TL, Trawick JD, Poyton RO. Multiple pathways of mitochondrial-nuclear communication in yeast: Intergenomic signaling involves ABF1 and affects a different set of genes than retrograde regulation. Biochimica et Biophysica Acta. 2009;**1789**:135-145. DOI: 10.1016/j.bbagrm.2008.09.008

[73] Yakes FM, Van Houten B. Mitochondrial DNA damage is more extensive and persists longer than nuclear DNA damage in human cells following oxidative stress. Proceedings of the National Academy of Sciences of the United States of America. 1997;**94**:514-519. DOI: 10.1073/pnas.94.2.514

[74] Blasiak J, Glowacki S, Kauppinen A, Kaarniranta K. Mitochondrial and nuclear DNA damage and repair in age-related macular degeneration. International Journal of Molecular Sciences. 2013;**14**:2996-3010. DOI: 10.3390/ijms14022996

[75] Abu-Asab MS, Salazar J, Tuo J, Chan C-C. Systems biology profiling of AMD on the basis of gene expression. Journal of Ophthalmology. 2013;**2013**:453934. DOI: 10.1155/2013/453934

[76] Sreekumar PG, Ishikawa K, Spee C, Mehta HH, Wan J, Yen K, et al. The mitochondrial-derived peptide humanin protects RPE cells from oxidative stress, senescence, and mitochondrial dysfunction. Investigative Ophthalmology & Visual Science. 2016;**57**:1238-1253. DOI: 10.1167/iovs.15-17053

[77] Biasutto L, Chiechi A, Couch R, Liotta VE. Retinal pigment epithelium (RPE) exosomes contain signaling phosphoproteins affected by oxidative stress. Experimental Cell Research. 2013;**319**:2113-2123. DOI: 10.1016/j.yexcr.2013.05.005

Chapter 12

The Role of Imaging in Age-Related Macular Degeneration

Andi Arus Victor

Abstract

Age-related macular degeneration (ARMD) is the leading cause of blindness affecting adults. The disease alters the macula, center of the retina, responsible for the keenest vision. Although ARMD is part of the aging process, the exact pathophysiology is still unknown. The evidence suggests that oxidative stress, lipofuscin accumulation, drusen accumulation, chronic inflammation, choroidal neovascularization, and mutations of the complement contribute to the development of ARMD. Early recognition and prompt treatment halt the progression of the disease. The advanced technology in imaging modalities provides comprehensive and complete management at the earliest stage of ARMD.

Keywords: macular degeneration, age-related macular degeneration, imaging, fundus photography, fundus autofluorescence, fundus fluorescence angiography, indocyanine green angiography, optical coherence tomography, optical coherence tomography angiography

1. Introduction

Macular degeneration or age-related macular degeneration (ARMD) is the leading cause of blindness affecting elder individuals. In 2004, it was estimated that 1.75 million people over 40 years old in the USA develop ARMD, and the number is expected to increase twice the number in the next decades [1]. The prevalence of ARMD varies among ethnicity group. A study by Wong et al. gathered the pooled prevalence (age ranges from 45 to 85 years) was 8.69%, with the highest prevalence found in European decent 11.9% and the lowest among Asian decent 6.81% [2]. The progression of the disease is worsening with age, a systematic review of European studies found increasing trend of early ARMD prevalence from 3.5% in age group 55–59 years to 17.6% in age group >85 years old and from 0.1% in those aged 55–59 years to 9.8% in those aged >85 years old for late ARMD [3]. Thus, aging is the pivotal factors behind ARMD development and progression.

Age at diagnosis of ARMD is the key element to halt ARMD progression [4]. Advancement in technology of imaging modalities provides a comprehensive and complete examination of the ocular condition at the earliest stage of ARMD. Imaging modalities include fundus photography, fundus fluorescence angiography, indocyanine green angiography (ICGA), fundus autofluorescence, optical coherence tomography (OCT), and optical coherence tomography angiography (OCTA) [4–7]. This chapter will further discuss the superiority of each modality.

2. An overview of age-related macular degeneration

Age-related macular degeneration is commonly classified based on its characteristics into dry (nonexudative) ARMD and wet (exudative) ARMD [5, 7]. Meanwhile, according the natural course of the disease, it categorizes into early, intermediate, and advanced ARMD [6, 7]. Dry ARMD represents approximately 90% of diagnosed ARMD cases [5, 7]. This type is distinguished by the present drusen accumulation, the absence of choroid neovascularization, and retinal pigment epithelium (RPE) atrophy [8]. The hallmark of wet ARMD is the development of choroidal neovascularization, and this fragile new blood vessel tends to leak forming exudates [9]. It counts for 10% of ARMD cases and has been linked with rapid deterioration toward blindness [7].

Beyond aging process, smoking and ethnicity are the only consistent risk factors related with ARMD documented in studies. A cohort study of 65 years old or older patients found smoking doubles the risk of having ARMD in 5 years compared to nonsmokers [10]. The exact underlying pathophysiology of ARMD is still unknown. Several theories are hypothesized to be the fundamental factors behind ARMD. These include lipofuscin accumulation, drusen accumulation, chronic inflammation, oxidative stress, reduction of antioxidant, mutation of complements, and choroidal neovascularization [10, 11]. The new blood vessels are fragile and generate complications to the surrounding structure causing hemorrhages, exudate, RPE and/or retinal detachment, and scar, hence the progression into the end-stage ARMD, which is exudative ARMD [5, 6, 9, 12].

The identification of ARMD in patients is a crucial aspect in delivering early treatment. Elder patients especially those aged above 40 years are more susceptible to develop ARMD. According to the American Academy of Ophthalmology, it is suggested that individuals aged 40 years and above should be screened for the possible ARMD. Binocular slit-lamp examination with three mirror lens or condensing lens is also needed to disclose drusen, profound signs of CNV such as macular edema, subretinal fluid, hemorrhages, acclivity of retinal pigment epithelium, and RPE atrophy [6]. High-risk individuals are suggested to regularly conduct further comprehensive eye examinations. A comprehensive eye examination includes noninvasive and invasive imaging to detect any subtle changes in the retina structures [6].

3. Multimodal imaging in age-related macular degeneration

Imaging not only holds an important diagnostic tool in ARMD but also provides better understanding of ARMD pathophysiology, determines treatment options, and evaluates the treatment responds and disease progression [7, 13]. Imaging aids clinicians to visualize abnormalities exhibited by ARMD such as lipofuscin, RPE atrophy, drusen deposits, choroidal neovascularization, and subretinal fluid [7, 14, 15]. The characteristics found during the imaging determine the treatment options and prognosis of the patient. The various modalities are color fundus photography, fundus fluorescence angiography (FFA), indocyanine green angiography (ICGA), fundus autofluorescence (FAF), optical coherence tomography (OCT), and OCTA [13]. Despite the various imaging technologies, fluorescein angiography remains as a gold standard for diagnosis of the wet ARMD.

3.1 The role of fundus photography in age-related macular degeneration

Fundus photography (FP) is one of the simplest imaging modalities that can be utilized in detecting ARMD. Fundus photography was found at the end of the nineteenth century. In the 1950s, electronic flash and 35 mm cameras were adapted; thus modern ophthalmic camera was born. This examination uses fundus camera, which projects light into the dilated pupil to illuminate fundus. Fundus camera usually possesses 30—35° optical angle of view conceiving a 2.5 times life size 2D image [13, 15].

This modality is useful to detect both dry and wet ARMD. It can display various ARMD abnormalities consisting lipofuscin, drusen as a yellow deposit, reticular pseudodrusen, well-defined area of RPE atrophy, and choroid neovascularization [14, 15]. In nonexudative ARMD, FP allows visualization of drusen that appears as yellowish round lesion, pigmentary deposit around macula, while atrophic RPE shows a hypopigmentation around the macula. This imaging also enables measurement of drusen characteristics and size. The hard drusen appears as well-defined border yellow deposit, while soft drusen exhibits an ill-defined border yellow deposit [16]. The size of drusen is categorized into small (<63 μm), intermediate (63–124 μm), and large (≥125 μm). **Figure 1A** shows the characteristics of soft and hard drusen. This also contributes to staging of ARMD. Meanwhile, the utilization of color fundus photography in wet ARMD is beneficial in the detection of any exudative complications such as macular edema and macular detachment [7].

Regardless of its convenience, color fundus photography has several disadvantages. First, the image created is in 2D and thus lacks depth and generates problem in visualizing small details. Any abnormalities in the refractive media such as cataract result in lower image clarity [15]. When used as single imaging procedure, fundus photography has lower sensitivity to detect choroidal neovascularization 78% compared to OCT 94% [17]. Fundus photography has better accuracy when in conjunction with other imaging modalities. Ly et al. found that fundus photography has 61% accuracy in diagnosing ARMD and its accuracy was proven by 5% with additional imaging [18]. This was also documented in **Figure 1** that the FP image only shows the presence of drusen but upon OCT examination, subretinal and fibrovascular pigment epithelial detachment is evident. FP alone is inadequate to

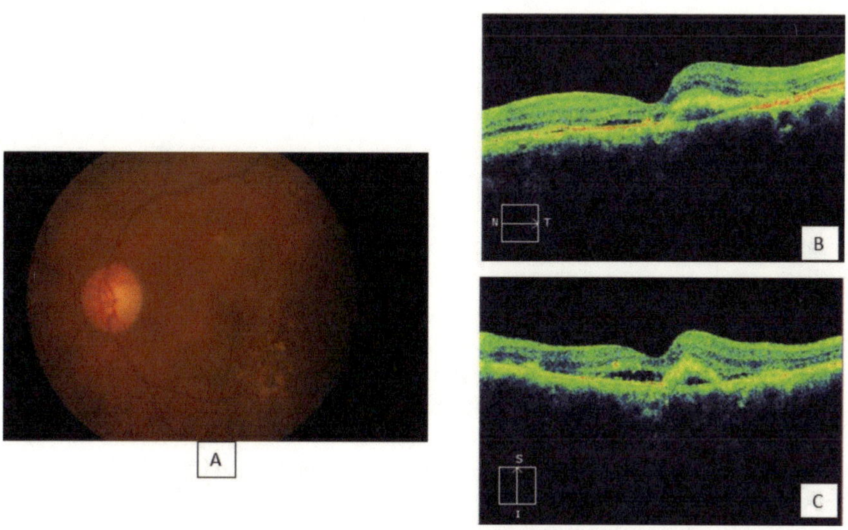

Figure 1.
Drusen appearance on FP and OCT of the same patient. The color fundus photography (FP) shows the presence of soft drusen and hard drusen at the inferior to fovea (A). Upon OCT examination, the presence of drusen is noticeable as a low mounds on the RPE layer. The OCT also shows that subretinal fluid and fibrovascular pigment epithelial detachment are also evident on the OCT (B) and (C) indicating a typical wet ARMD.

diagnose wet ARMD as it underestimates the presence of choroidal neovascularization. Hence, another modality is needed to complement FP limitations.

3.2 The fundus autofluorescence

Fundus autofluorescence (FAF) is an imaging method using a specific wavelength of light to trigger the fundus fluorescent characteristics without the need of contrast [7, 13, 15]. This autofluorescence characteristic is mainly due to lipofuscin, by-product of RPE, with its toxic component biretinoid fluorophore [7, 19, 20]. Specific wavelength of light around 300–500 nm is used to excite the lipofuscin, which then emits 500–700 nm [15]. FAF is done using fundus spectrophotometer, confocal scanning laser ophthalmoscope, or a fundus camera. Confocal scanning laser ophthalmoscope (cSLO) is more superior to others as it has capability to reduce the noise from other autofluorescence sources commonly from anterior segment of the eye [15, 19]. In comparison with color fundus photography, fundus autofluorescence has the ability to detect retinal changes in early and intermediate ARMD that may appear normal in color fundus photography [19].

FAF images have the capability to detect numerous retinal abnormalities such as pigmentary changes, drusen, and reticular pseudodrusen [19]. Lipofuscin deposits in RPE exhibit hyperautofluorescence due to the presence of *N-retinyl-N-retinylidene ethanolamine* (A2E), while RPE atrophy appears hypoautofluorescence. The condition where these hyperautofluorescence and hypoautofluorescence coincide suggests that an area of hyperautofluorescence (lipofuscin) surrounding a hypoautofluorescence could be a predictive tool for enlargement of RPE atrophy and thus useful for monitoring GA progression. This was exhibited by Gobel et al. who discovered enlargement of GA mainly occurred in area of hyperautofluorescence and the size increases four times the original size within 9 years of follow-up [15]. This corresponds to the hypothesis of lipofuscin containing toxic that causes the RPE cell death [20, 21].

Meanwhile, drusen appears in numerous fashions on imaging. In FAF, drusen can appear as hypoautofluorescence, hyperautofluorescence, and normal lesion, owing to the variability of fluorophore components and the size of drusen [19]. Hard drusen, especially small ones, is hard to detect using FAF. Soft drusen under FAF appears as hyperautofluorescence around the edges and slightly hypoautofluorescence in the center. Reticular pseudodrusen resembles as a well-organized network hypoautofluorescence lesion surrounding the normal retina. This is hypothesized due to its subretinal location that obstructs the autofluorescence of lipofuscin in RPE [19, 22].

A patchy pattern, reticular pattern, and linear pattern documented on FAF have been associated with the development of neovascular ARMD. Cohort study by Batioglu et al. discovered that initial findings of patchy pattern were the most associated FAF pattern linked with the development of exudative ARMD with frequency rate of 30.4%, followed by linear pattern and reticular pattern (25 and 20.8%, respectively) during 2.5 years' follow-up, showing that FAF is useful as a prognostic tool to predict the incidence of neovascular ARMD [23]. Similar finding was also exhibited by Cachulo et al., whereas the patchy pattern was the most associated FAF pattern abnormality converted to exudative ARMD (29%) [24].

In neovascular ARMD, FAF images exhibit various FAF pattern. Hemorrhages, scarring, and fibrovascular membranes are hypoautofluorescence lesion. Subretinal fluid appears as hyperautofluorescence. Break in RPE exhibits as reduced autofluorescence [19]. In classic neovascular ARMD, Peng et al. described the FAF findings as reduced FAF at the lesion core with elevated FAF around the lesion border. The author also compared the FAF image with fundus fluorescence angiography; the lesion on FFA appeared smaller than that in FAF showing that FAF has more advantages in detailing the alteration in RPE. In occult neovascular ARMD, FAF images exhibit diverse FAF characteristics with both reduced FAF and elevated patchy FAF [25]. FAF has high sensitivity in detecting neovascular ARMD (93%) but relatively low specificity (37%) in comparison with FFA as the gold standard [24].

Near-infrared autofluorescence (NIA) is another imaging technique that utilizes the other fluorophore characteristics of retina, melanin. Melanin is found predominantly in RPE cell and small amount in choroid. Unlike the ordinary FAF, NIA adapts longer wavelength (diode laser light) for excitation 787 nm and capture specific wavelength above 800 nm. The image is captured using confocal scanning laser ophthalmoscope, producing 30 × 30° images [26, 27]. In visualizing the retina, NIA exhibits comparable retina characteristics taken by FAF. The NIA images show high hyperautofluorescence in the center of fovea owing to the high melanin contents in RPE cells [26]. In dry AMRD patients, both NIA and FAF appear dark in atrophic region, meanwhile the area adjacent to the atrophic region appeared increased intensity. Kellner et al. found that half of their ARMD patients have increased NIA in normal FAF site; the author suggests that there is an increase in melanin activity prior to lipofuscin activity [27]. In wet ARMD, the image appears dark in both NIA and FAF due to obstructed autofluorescence signal by subretinal fluid, hemorrhage, or choroidal neovascularization. However, it was found that FAF (56.5%) is more effective in detailing exudative activity compared to NIA (33.9%) [27]. **Figure 2** shows the comparison of regular fundus autofluorescence and infrared autofluorescence.

Retromode imaging (RM) is another imaging modality employing infrared laser at 790 nm, equipped with a laterally deviated confocal aperture with central stop. The imaging utilizes confocal scanning laser ophthalmoscope, yielding a pseudo-3D appearance of deeper retinal layers and choroid. This imaging modality is found to be useful in identifying pathological structures in dry and wet ARMD. It was found that drusen was more apparent in retromode imaging compared to fundus photography, and even smaller-size drusen is easily detected [28]. In wet ARMD, Pilotto et al. found that RM has a superior intermethod agreement with OCT in visualizing macular edema, but relatively low for RPE detachment and poor for neuroretinal detachment [29].

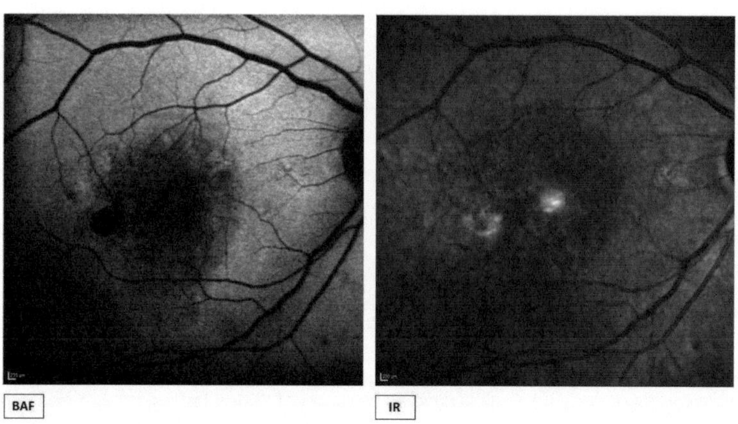

Figure 2.
Fundus autofluorescence of wet ARMD. BluePeak Autofluorescence (BAF) shows a hypoautofluorescence at the fovea and perifovea due to macular detachment accompanied by exudates. Meanwhile in infrared (IR) autofluorescence, the macular detachment and exudates appear as hyperautofluorescence; the reduced IR was blocked due to probable subretinal fluid and hemorrhage.

3.3 Fundus fluorescence angiography

Fundus fluorescence angiography (FFA) is an invasive imaging modality that uses intravenous fluorescent contrast called resorcinolphthalein sodium. FFA serves as the gold standard for neovascular ARMD. It allows visualization of the blood vessel structure and integrity. A camera with a ring-shaped flash 485–500 nm is used to excite the molecule in the contrast. The projected blue light is then reflected back by retina layers. Some light is absorbed by the fluorescein and emits back as green light at wavelength of 520–535 nm. The emitted green light is then captured by 520–535 nm green filter onto digital surface, producing image at 2.5× magnification and 30° of angle view. In FFA, there is early state and late state [14].

Compared to other modalities, FFA excels in detailing the state of choroid neovascularization in its structural and leakage state. Based on the location of CNV, it is classified as extrafoveal, subfoveal, and juxtafoveal. Extrafoveal CNV is neovascular located around 200–2500 μm from the center of foveal avascular zone (FAZ). Subfoveal CNV is located underneath the center of FAZ. Lastly, juxtafoveal CNV is located up to 199 μm from the center of FAZ and some part of FAZ excluding the center portion [14]. Identification of the CNV location is a useful prognostic factor and treatment options.

FFA also provides leakage property of the CNV, which is then further classified into occult CNV (type I), classic CNV (type II), and retinal angiomatous proliferation (type III) [6, 14, 22]. Occult CNV appears as poorly defined mottled and patchy hyperfluorescence in early-phase angiogram and leaks at the later phase of angiogram, forming larger hyperfluorescence dots. The occult CNV is further classified based on its leakage characteristics found upon FFA examinations. Type I occult CNV is fibrovascular PED and is described as stippled hyperfluorescence upon early phase (1–2 minutes after fluorescein dye injection) followed by poorly defined progressive leakage upon late-phase angiogram (**Figure 3**). Type II occult CNV is late leakage from undetermined source and is described as CNV does not appear hyperfluorescence during early phase but shows speckled hyperfluorescence upon mid- to late-phase angiogram (2–5 minutes after dye injection) [30]. Classic CNV presents as well-defined hyperfluorescence network membrane in early phase, followed by progressive leakage in late-phase angiogram [14, 22].

Another neovascularization lesion often found in ARMD patients is retinal angiomatous proliferation (RAP). RAP is recently described as neovascularization arising from intraretinal layer and infiltrating into the choroid layer forming a retinal-choroidal anastomosis (RCA) [22]. According to classification by Yannuzzi et al., there are three stages of RAP. Stage I is intraretinal capillary proliferation rising from deep capillary plexus in paramacular region [31]. Upon FFA examination,

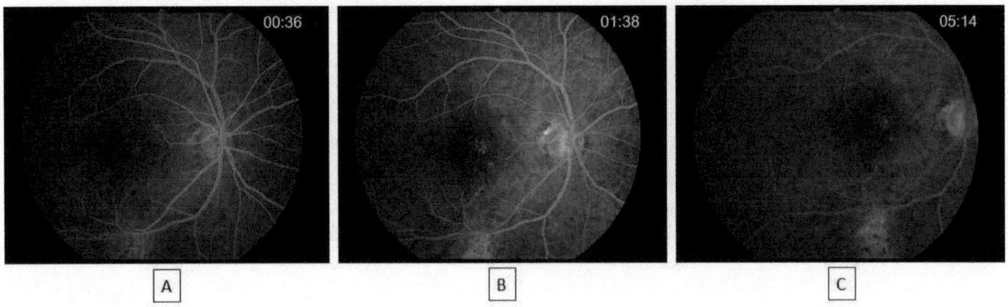

Figure 3.
Fundus fluorescence angiography ((FFA) characteristics of occult CNV, fibrovascular PED type). The early phase (A) shows a stippled hyperfluorescence followed by progressive increase of hyperfluorescence at mid-phase (B) and late-phase angiogram (C).

it appears as well-defined border of hyperfluorescence at the focal area surrounded with intraretinal edema [32]. Stage II is defined as neovascularization that has extended through photoreceptor layer infiltrating into subretinal space [31]. FFA reveals a hyperfluorescence at focal area indicating intraretinal neovascularization and at subretinal spaces followed by subretinal leakage, often interpreted as occult CNV [32]. Stage III is described as the presence of choroid neovascularization (CNV), anastomosis of retina and choroid, and pigment epithelial detachment [31]. On FFA examination, sometimes it is difficult to detect stage III as the detailed layer of subretinal neovascularization, choroid neovascularization, and detached RPE combined into homogenous nonspecific hyperfluorescence [32]. Hence, another imaging technique such as indocyanine green angiography is needed to offer a better visualization of the lesion.

Drawbacks of the FFA procedure are its systemic complication from the injected fluorescent dye. The complications are nausea, allergic reaction, and anaphylaxis reaction. The dye used leaks extensively to the surrounding tissue, which could alter detailing of the CNV. Thus in some cases of type I CNV, PCV, and RAP, ICGA is the more preferable method compared to FFA [33].

3.4 Indocyanine green angiography

Indocyanine green angiography (ICGA) uses indocyanine green dye, a high-molecular weight contrast (775kD), and projects 790 nm infrared light directed into the eyes that allows deep penetration to the RPE structure [14, 22]. The dye used in ICGA binds to plasma proteins and thus leaks less compared to FFA imaging. The ICGA leakage then reabsorbed, thus producing hypercyanescent in the late phase [13, 14]. Similar to FFA, ICGA is an invasive procedure using injection of intravenous dye into the systemic circulation, which could trigger systemic complication such as nausea, vomiting, urticarial, allergic reaction, and anaphylactic reaction [14].

Abnormalities exhibited by ICGA appear as hypercyanescent plaque, focal hot spot, or combination of both. ICGA readings have three timed phase, early phase, mid phase, and late phase. ICGA is well suited in identification of type I CNV or occult CNV, the early phase often showing ill-defined hypercyanescent lesion, progressive intensity in mid phase, and the late-phase hypercyanescent plaque [33, 34]. However, ICGA is less superior in detecting classic CNV; this type of CNV appears as well-defined hypercyanescent [34].

Other types of CNV pivotal in determining the treatment options and outcome are polypoidal choroidal vasculopathy (PCV) and retinal angiomatous proliferation (RAP). Polypoidal choroidal vasculopathy (PCV) is described as branching of abnormal choroidal vascular network with aneurysmal dilatation (polypoidal characteristics) at its edge. The exact origin of PCV is still in dispute; some suggest that PCV arises from choroidal abnormalities, while others speculate that PCV is another type 1 CNV modification [35–37]. Upon FFA imaging, PCV often masks the appearance of occult CNV or classic CNV and thus ICGA serves as the gold standard in identification of PCV as its appearance masked by the RPE layers in FFA. On ICG angiography examination, PCV appears as hypercyanescent hot spot in the early angiogram with a grape-like/polypoid structure (**Figures 4** and **5**) [38]. **Figure 5** is an example where PCV lesion masking an occult CNV on FFA and the ICGA examination revealed hypercyanescent hot spot with polypoid structure upon early, mid, and with "wash out" phenomenon in late-phase angiogram.

The occurrence of PCV has been associated with serosanguineous PED, neurosensory detachment, high recurrent case, and poor visual outcome [38]. It was found that the poor outcome despite the effective treatment of anti-VEGF should always suspect the occurrence of PCV [39].

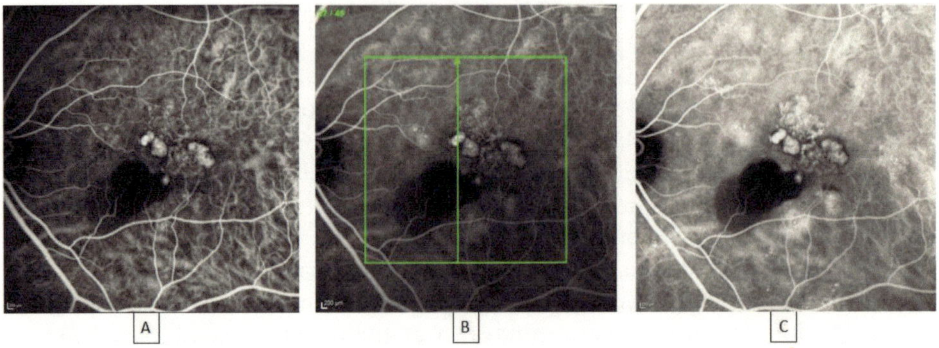

Figure 4.
ICGA examination of a patient (A) early phase at 1 minute 45 seconds shows a well-demarcated hypercyanescent lesion with polypoidal characteristics (B) increasing intensity at mid phase at 3 minute 51 seconds and late phase 5 minute 59 seconds (C) indicating PCV lesion.

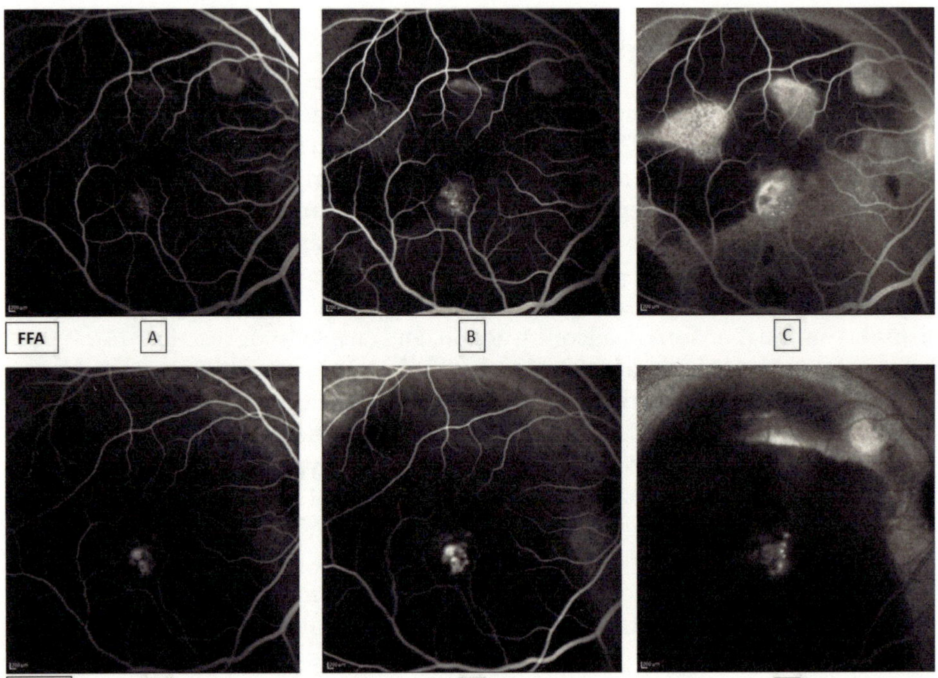

Figure 5.
FFA image shows appearance of what looks like occult CNV. Ill-defined stippled hyperfluorescence is visible upon early phase (A), progressively increasing in intensity during mid-phase (B) and late-phase angiogram (C). However, upon ICGA examination, the lesion appears to have PCV characteristics. "Hot-spot" with polypoid appearance is evident upon early angiography (D) followed by progressive intensity upon mid phase (E) and "wash-out" on late phase (F). The choroidal structure is blocked by the presence of massive submacular hemorrhage, which appears as hypofluorescence background.

Retinal angiomatous proliferation (RAP) is also a type of CNV best visualized by ICGA. This lesion appears as early hyperfluorescence hot spot with apparent retinal artery communication into the CNV, followed by progressive increase in both size and intensity in the late phase [32, 40]. Identification of RAP on one eye has been linked with the increased chance of neovascularization on the other eye reaching almost 100% risk within 3 years of follow-up [41].

As mentioned before, ICGA operates on longer wavelength of infrared compared to FFA, thus allowing deeper penetration to RPE and choroidal structure providing more specific information regarding CNV location [14, 22]. These advantages also allow the image to further penetrate any subretinal fluid or hemorrhages and pigment epithelium detachment that often alter imaging in FFA. Kramer et al. found that upon FFA examination, most of their patients with retinal hemorrhage exhibit ill-defined hyperfluorescence surrounded with area of blocked fluorescence (23/30), while under ICGA, these lesions appear to be hypercyanescent hot spot in 12 cases, plaque in 8 cases, and combination in 8 cases [40]. Thus in the presence of hemorrhage, ICGA image offers more detailed characteristics of CNV in ARMD patients compared to FFA.

3.5 The utilization of optical coherence tomography in age-related macular degeneration

Optical coherence tomography (OCT) is performed by projecting low coherence laser into retina. The image is a product of time delay and backscattered lights resulting in cross section of retina layers [13, 14]. Time domain OCT (TD-OCT) is the first OCT invented and requires longer time to produce image. TD-OCT produces axial and later resolution 15 μm. Spectral domain OCT requires less time to acquire images, resulting in greater density and better image quality (axial 3 μm, transverse resolution 10 μm) [14, 22]. Polarization-sensitive SD-OCT (PS-SD-OCT) is a modified form of SD-OCT in purpose to overcome limitation to detect RPE unity and condition [42]. Lastly, the newly developed swept-source OCT uses longer wavelength and simpler methods and thus enables deeper tissue penetration and shorter duration of image acquisition compared to SD-OCT.

Image produced by OCT is in the form of hyperreflective and hyporeflective bands representing the layer of retina [43]. In clinical practices, there are four hyperreflective bands that are observed in ARMD patients. These hyperreflective bands are presumed to represent external limiting membrane, inner/outer segment of photoreceptor, RPE, and Bruch's membrane [44]. OCT is capable to exhibit ARMD abnormalities such as drusen deposits, pseudodrusen, subretinal fluid, RPE detachment, and choroid neovascularization. In OCT, drusen deposits appear as low mounds underneath RPE layer [22]. Findings of drusen in OCT are found to be significantly correlated with drusen findings in FAF in the study of Landa et al. [45].

Reticular pseudodrusen presents as hyperreflective deposit localized under the retina layer [22]. The presence of pseudodrusen in ARMD patients has been linked with the increased risk for end-stage ARMD, geographic atrophy, or neovascular ARMD. Ueda-Arakawa et al. found that OCT has the highest sensitivity (94.6%) and specificity (98.4%) in detecting the presence of pseudodrusen in comparison with other imaging modalities [46]. The presence of reticular pseudodrusen also alters the choroid function proven by thinning of choroid thickness [47, 48].

In geography atrophy, the RPE atrophy exhibits a feathered-like pattern projected deep into the RPE due to laser beam penetrated into RPE [14]. OCT images also exhibit a progressive loss of retinal bands, which includes external limiting membrane, inner/outer segments of photoreceptor layer, RPE membrane, and outer nuclear membrane [15]. These findings are in concordance with the study of Fleckenstein et al.; the authors discover that the enlargement of the atrophic region was associated with gradual loss of the outer hyperreflective bands and thinning of outer nuclear layer, outer plexiform layer, RPE membrane, and Bruch's membrane during 12 months of follow-up [49, 50]. The authors also discovered that GA was linked with increased of retinal thickness by 14.09 μm [49]. Their other study also found separation of inner and outer parts of band 4, presumed to be RPE/Bruch's membrane [50].

Neovascularization activity is visualized on OCT based on accumulation of fluid in various levels of retina. Subretinal fluid is described as hyporeflective lesion located above the RPE and beneath the retina [14, 22]. RPE detachment appears as dome shaped at RPE layer [14]. The exudative activity is one of determining factors for neovascular ARMD treatment. Increased choroid thickness could represent the possible choroid; however, these cannot differ between classic ARMD and polypoidal choroidal vasculopathy [22]. Another structural abnormality of the retina found in OCT is outer retinal tubule. This lesion appears as hyporeflective center surrounded by hyperreflective border. Outer retinal tubule represents the degenerated photoreceptors and thus does not represent exudative activity for neovascularization and does not need treatment for neovascular ARMD [51].

OCT is one of the most convenience imaging modalities to detect and monitor ARMD. It provides information of retinal changes without an invasive procedure and systemic complication as required in invasive angiographic imaging such as fundus fluorescence angiography (FFA) and indocyanine green angiography (ICGA). OCT is reported to have higher sensitivity in detecting CNV (94%) compared to FP (78%) [17]. However, comparing OCT to FA as the gold standard for CNV, OCT possesses lower sensitivity (40%) and relatively moderate specificity (69%) [52]. Unfortunately, the advancement of OCT still has limitation in detailing and grading CNV. **Figure 6** exhibits the utilization of multimodal imaging in wet ARMD resulting in detailed characteristics of RAP after OCTA successfully provided the appearance of CNV in all retina and choroid layer. This shows that the limitation can be overcome by conducting fundus fluorescence angiography or OCTA in conjunction with OCT when indicated.

3.6 The new advance in retinal imaging for age-related macular degeneration

OCT technology is continuously developed. The previously developed spectral domain OCT (SD-OCT) has limitation in detecting structures under hemorrhage and capturing the integrity of RPE layers. It was then proposed by Ahlers et al. [42],

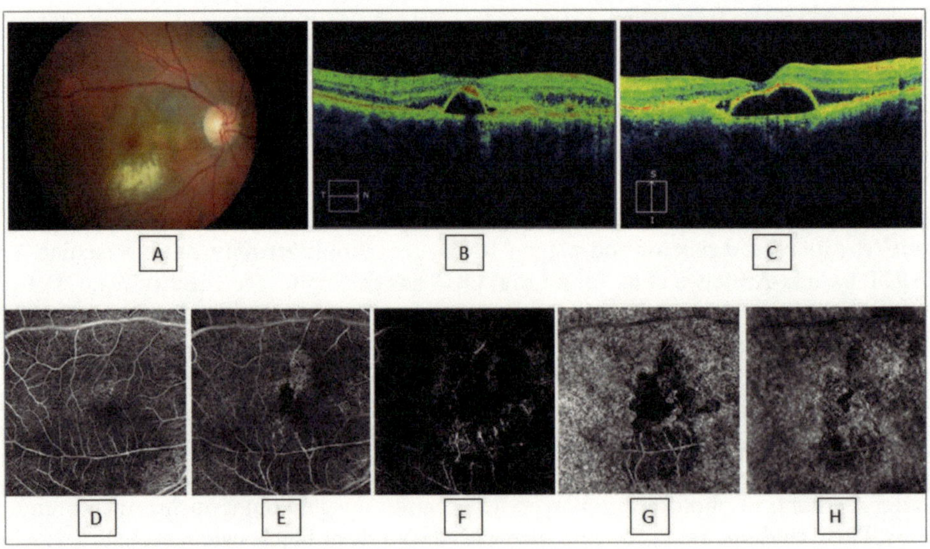

Figure 6.
Multimodal imaging on a neovascular ARMD patient. The color fundus photography exhibits pale macula with the presence of drusen, hard exudate on color fundus photography, and macular detachment (A). Upon OCT examination, pigment epithelial detachment is apparent along with subretinal fluid (B). Meanwhile, on OCTA examination, choroidal neovascularization is evident arising from choroid layer (H), choriocapillaris layer (G), avascular zone (F), extending into deep vascular layer (E) and superficial vascular layer (D), which is a characteristic of typical RAP.

where the SD-OCT was modified adding its capability to detect depolarization characteristics of RPE layers, called polarization-sensitive (PS) SD-OCT. The use of PS-SD-OCT was observed in both dry and wet ARMD. The PS-SD-OCT was successful in visualizing the continuous layer of RPE located under the drusen, larger RPE atrophy area, and focal skip lesions in the RPE layer, which was unable to be visualized using the standard SD-OCT [42].

Another modification of OCT is done by implementation of adaptive optics (AO). OCT has a greater capability in producing high axial resolutions; however, its transverse resolution is limited due to the ocular aberration. This aberration is due to cornea, crystalline lens, and the size of the pupil. AO aids in correction of ocular aberrations, increases lateral resolutions, reduces artifacts, and increases detection to weak reflections [53]. Combining these two techniques enhances OCT capability, thus allowing visualization of cellular structures; hence, early recognition of cellular pathology afore the visual alteration occurs. A comparison of commercial B-scans OCT with AO-OCT resulted higher reflectivity and reduced speckle size in retina images taken with AO-OCT [54]. Utilization of AO-OCT in ARMD has been documented in several studies. One of the studies conducted by Athanasios et al. shows the application of AO-OCT in geographic atrophy patients. The AO-OCT successfully provided detailed extralimiting membrane loss, inner and outer segment loss, and RPE loss in geographic atrophy (GA). In advanced GA, the AO-OCT capable of visualizing calcified drusen and drusenoid pigment epithelial detachment. This modification also allows the clinicians to directly witness the destruction of photoreceptor cell caused by drusen [55].

In 2008, swept-source OCT (SS-OCT) was introduced. This new technique uses tunable laser, which possesses longer wavelength (1050 nm) for deeper tissue penetration and predivided spectrum for simpler mechanisms, hence faster image acquisition [56]. Therefore, SS-OCT is greater in visualizing the choroidal structure and RPE. In comparison to SD-OCT, SS-OCT has greater capability in identifying retinal thickness. It was found that the agreement between these two methods of OCT is low, especially in those with active wet ARMD [57]. The author argues that the active disease, such as hemorrhage and subretinal fluid, obscures the OCT signals in SD-OCT. The superiority of SS-OCT is also supported by Copete et al. [58]; the SD-OCT was unable to identify choroidosclera border in those with thicker choroid (23%) upon SS-OCT examination. The odd ratio of SD-OCT failure is greatest (10.3) at 400 μm of subfoveal choroidal thickness.

Age-related macular degeneration affects elderly; thus the use of fluorescence dye results in worse side effects. However, the visualization of retina and choroidal microvasculature in ARMD detection is crucial in management of ARMD. Thus, the development of noninvasive angiographic imaging technique is essential. The advancement of OCT technology helps in the development of OCTA. The shortened OCT image acquisition allows the development of OCTA as multiple image retrieval is required. The breakthrough in OCTA began after the discovery in OCT signal differences caused by blood flow. This contrast is classified as Doppler phase shift and speckle variance [59]. However, Doppler phase shift is found to be ineffective to visualize retinal and choroidal microvasculature [59]. It was then discovered in 2005 by Barton et al. where the speckle variation in OCT signal arises from scatterer motion. Speckle variation was further classified into phase based and amplitude or intensity.

OCTA is a noninvasive imaging examination that allows visualization of retina and choroid vascular structure. By utilizing the principle of OCT, it detects erythrocyte flow using sequential B-scans to detect the variable amplitudes and signal intensity gradients. This gradient is then processed through full-spectrum or split-spectrum processing [22, 59, 60]. It can produce en face or cross-sectional image displaying neovascular network. En face OCTA is the most commonly utilized technique in clinical practices. This allows visualization of vascular characteristics from retina, superficial vascular, deep vascular, avascular zone, choriocapillaris zone, and choroid zone. However, OCTA does not allow any leakage property of the vascular zone [22, 47].

OCTA is best to describe abnormalities existing in both exudative and nonexudative CNV. In nonexudative CNV, the use of OCTA is beneficial in visualizing choriocapillaris blood flow, especially in atrophy region. Kvanta et al. found a significant decrease in choriocapillaris flow in atrophic zone extending outside the geographic atrophy area. This could potentially describe the choriocapillaris alteration in dry ARMD [61]. OCTA was also used in the study of Toto et al. in which the author found significant decreased vessel density by 9% in dry ARMD patients in both superficial vascular layer and deep vascular layer compared with healthy individuals [48]. However, reading OCTA in dry ARMD should be done in careful manner because the drusen affects the signal, thus lowering image quality especially for area below drusen.

OCTA allows to visualize the neovascular network afore the leakage, hence early detection and prompt treatment. CNV appears as hyperfluorescence high flow network varying on the depth of the retina involvement according to the degree of CNV [22]. OCTA has been proven to have a comparable detection capability in visualizing CNV compared to other imaging such as FFA and ICGA. Type I CNV appears on the choriocapillaris layer penetrating the Brusch's membrane and below the RPE [62]. This CNV appears as a minimal demarcated vascularization arising from choroid, choriocapillaris, and RPE with no evidence of neovascularization in outer retina [63]. A retrospective case series by Roisman et al. found that OCTA exhibits more detailed images in detecting CNV compared to FFA and ICGA in asymptomatic ARMD patients [64]. In their study, the authors discover that CNV, which appears on FFA as a minimal leakage and macular plaques on ICGA, was a type I CNV in OCTA imaging. However, this finding is contradict with the study conducted by Told et al. in which the capability of OCTA to detect occult CNV was found to be less sensitive and specific compared to ICGA [65].

Meanwhile, type II CNV presents as choroidal neovascularization arising into RPE and subretinal space [22]. It appears as a sharp demarcated vascular changes

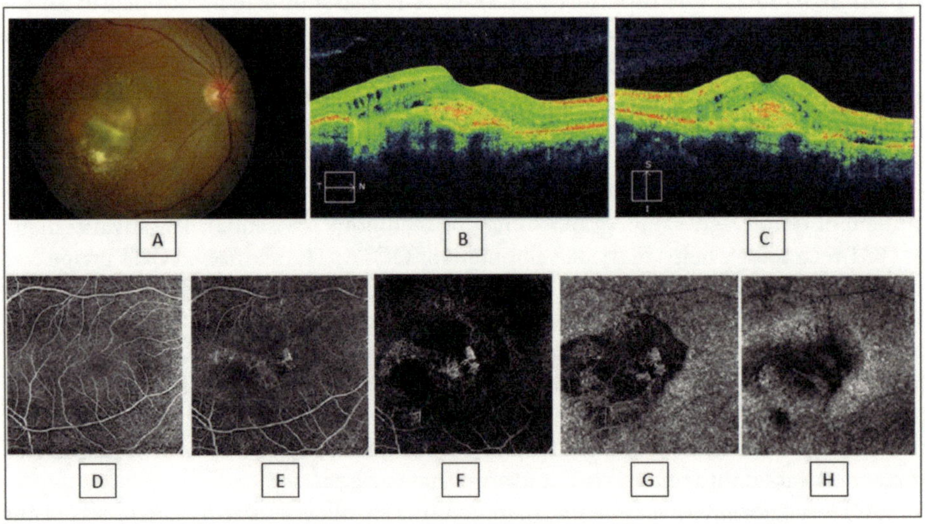

Figure 7.
Color fundus photography shows an appearance of drusen surrounding the macula. The presence of exudates due to subretinal fluid is also evident, showing characteristics of wet ARMD (A). The OCT image shows the presence of macular edema with intraretinal and subretinal fluid; hyperreflective lesion is also noted below the RPE suggesting choroid neovascularization (B). The presence of choroid neovascularization is confirmed by OCTA, arising from choroid (H), choriocapillaris (G), avascular zone (F), into deep vascular layer (E), except superficial vascular layer (D), exhibiting a type III CNV.

at the choroid, choriocapillaris, RPE, and extending to outer retina [63]. Lastly, the appearance of RAP or type III CNV is hyperreflective cluster situated in outer retinal layer with interconnecting vessel with the inner retinal circulation (**Figure 7**) [66]. Comparing OCTA and FFA in detecting exudative ARMD, OCTA has lower sensitivity 81.3% where large subretinal hemorrhage was found on the false-negative patient. The authors argue that the subretinal hemorrhage weakens the OCTA signal to detect CNV [67]. Another limitation of OCTA was documented in Told et al. and Costanzo et al., which OCTA tends to underestimate the CNV size compared to ICGA [33, 65].

The ongoing development of OCT affects greatly in the development of OCTA. The most common OCT system used by OCTA is SD-OCT. However, some suggest that the SS-OCT system provides more superior image quality compared to SD-OCT system in the presence of intraretinal hemorrhage. The longer wavelength used in SS-OCT system is thought to be able to penetrate any obscuring materials such as hemorrhage or subretinal fluid and thus provides more detailed structure on RPE and choroidal layer for ARMD patients. Miller et al. found that the CNV areas appeared to be larger upon SS-OCTA compared with SD-OCTA both on 3×3 and 6×6 mm^2 scans [68].

4. Conclusions

Early diagnosis of age-related macular degeneration has the major role in delaying the progression of advanced ARMD. The advance in technology provides detailed structure of retina alteration in ARMD without the need of invasive procedure. The utilization of multimodal imaging in diagnosis of ARMD results in early detection and comprehensive management of ARMD.

Acknowledgment

This article's publication is supported by the United States Agency for International Development (USAID) through the Sustainable Higher Education Research Alliance (SHERA) Program for Universitas Indonesia's Scientific Modeling, Application, Research and Training for City-centered Innovation and Technology (SMART CITY) Project, Grant #AID-497-A-1600004, Sub Grant #IIE-00000078-UI-1.

Author details

Andi Arus Victor
Department of Ophthalmology, Faculty of Medicine, Cipto Mangunkusumo National General Hospital, Universitas Indonesia, Jakarta, Indonesia

*Address all correspondence to: arvimadao@yahoo.com

References

[1] Friedman DS, O'Colmain BJ, Munoz B, Tomany SC, McCarty C, de Jong PT, et al. Prevalence of age-related macular degeneration in the United States. Archives of Ophthalmology. 2004;**122**(4):564-572

[2] Wong WL, Su X, Li X, Cheung CM, Klein R, Cheng CY, et al. Global prevalence of age-related macular degeneration and disease burden projection for 2020 and 2040: A systematic review and meta-analysis. The Lancet Global Health. 2014;**2**(2):e106-e116

[3] Colijn JM, Buitendijk GHS, Prokofyeva E, Alves D, Cachulo ML, Khawaja AP, et al. Prevalence of age-related macular degeneration in Europe: The past and the future. Ophthalmology. 2017;**124**(12):1753-1763

[4] Schwartz R, Loewenstein A. Early detection of age related macular degeneration: Current status. International Journal of Retina and Vitreous. 2015;**1**:20

[5] Cunningham J. Recognizing age-related macular degeneration in primary care. Journal of the American Academy of Physician Assistants. 2017;**30**(3):18-22

[6] Panel AAoORV. Preferred Practice Pattern Guideline Age-Related Macular Degeneration. San Francisco, CA: American Academy of Opthalmology Retina/Vitreous Panel; 2015

[7] Al-Zamil WM, Yassin SA. Recent developments in age-related macular degeneration: A review. Clinical Interventions in Aging. 2017;**12**:1313-1330

[8] Bowes Rickman C, Farsiu S, Toth CA, Klingeborn M. Dry age-related macular degeneration: Mechanisms, therapeutic targets, and imaging. Investigative Ophthalmology & Visual Science. 2013;**54**(14):ORSF68-ORSF80

[9] Kaszubski P, Ben Ami T, Saade C, Smith RT. Geographic atrophy and choroidal neovascularization in the same eye: A review. Ophthalmic Research. 2016;**55**(4):185-193

[10] Jonasson F, Fisher DE, Eiriksdottir G, Sigurdsson S, Klein R, Launer LJ, et al. Five-year incidence, progression, and risk factors for age-related macular degeneration: The age, gene/environment susceptibility study. Ophthalmology. 2014;**121**(9):1766-1772

[11] Chew EY, Clemons TE, Agron E, Sperduto RD, Sangiovanni JP, Kurinij N, et al. Long-term effects of vitamins C and E, beta-carotene, and zinc on age-related macular degeneration: AREDS report no. 35. Ophthalmology. 2013;**120**(8):1604-11.e4

[12] Nowak JZ. Age-related macular degeneration (AMD): Pathogenesis and therapy. Pharmacological Reports. 2006;**58**(3):353-363

[13] Keane PA, Sim DA, Sadda SR. Advances in imaging in age-related macular degeneration. Current Ophthalmology Reports. 2013;**1**(1):1-11

[14] Gess AJ, Fung AE, Rodriguez JG. Imaging in neovascular age-related macular degeneration. Seminars in Ophthalmology. 2011;**26**(3):225-233

[15] Gobel AP, Fleckenstein M, Schmitz-Valckenberg S, Brinkmann CK, Holz FG. Imaging geographic atrophy in age-related macular degeneration. Ophthalmologica. 2011;**226**(4):182-190

[16] Abdelsalam A, Del Priore L, Zarbin MA. Drusen in age-related macular degeneration: Pathogenesis, natural course, and

laser photocoagulation-induced regression. Survey of Ophthalmology. 1999;**44**(1):1-29

[17] Mokwa NF, Ristau T, Keane PA, Kirchhof B, Sadda SR, Liakopoulos S. Grading of age-related macular degeneration: Comparison between color fundus photography, fluorescein angiography, and spectral domain optical coherence tomography. Journal of Ophthalmology. 2013;**2013**:385915

[18] Ly A, Nivison-Smith L, Zangerl B, Assaad N, Kalloniatis M. Advanced imaging for the diagnosis of age-related macular degeneration: A case vignettes study. Clinical & Experimental Optometry. 2018;**101**(2):243-254

[19] Ly A, Nivison-Smith L, Assaad N, Kalloniatis M. Fundus autofluorescence in age-related macular degeneration. Optometry and Vision Science. 2017;**94**(2):246-259

[20] Suter M, Reme C, Grimm C, Wenzel A, Jaattela M, Esser P, et al. Age-related macular degeneration. The lipofusion component N-retinyl-N-retinylidene ethanolamine detaches proapoptotic proteins from mitochondria and induces apoptosis in mammalian retinal pigment epithelial cells. The Journal of Biological Chemistry. 2000;**275**(50):39625-39630

[21] Sparrow JR, Boulton M. RPE lipofuscin and its role in retinal pathobiology. Experimental Eye Research. 2005;**80**(5):595-606

[22] Talks SJ, Aftab AM, Ashfaq I, Soomro T. The role of new imaging methods in managing age-related macular degeneration. The Asia-Pacific Journal of Ophthalmology. 2017;**6**(6):498-507

[23] Batioglu F, Demirel S, Ozmert E, Oguz YG, Ozyol P. Autofluorescence patterns as a predictive factor for neovascularization. Optometry and Vision Science. 2014;**91**(8):950-955

[24] Cachulo L, Silva R, Fonseca P, Pires I, Carvajal-Gonzalez S, Bernardes R, et al. Early markers of choroidal neovascularization in the fellow eye of patients with unilateral exudative age-related macular degeneration. Ophthalmologica. 2011;**225**(3):144-149

[25] Peng Q, Dong Y, Zhao PQ. Fundus autofluorescence in exudative age-related macular degeneration. Genetics and Molecular Research. 2013;**12**(4):6140-6148

[26] Keilhauer CN, Delori FC. Near-infrared autofluorescence imaging of the fundus: Visualization of ocular melanin. Investigative Ophthalmology & Visual Science. 2006;**47**(8):3556-3564

[27] Kellner U, Kellner S, Weinitz S. Fundus autofluorescence (488 nm) and near-infrared autofluorescence (787 nm) visualize different retinal pigment epithelium alterations in patients with age-related macular degeneration. Retina. 2010;**30**(1):6-15

[28] Acton JH, Cubbidge RP, King H, Galsworthy P, Gibson JM. Drusen detection in retro-mode imaging by a scanning laser ophthalmoscope. Acta Ophthalmologica. 2011;**89**(5):e404-e411

[29] Pilotto E, Sportiello P, Alemany-Rubio E, Vujosevic S, Segalina S, Fregona I, et al. Confocal scanning laser ophthalmoscope in the retromode imaging modality in exudative age-related macular degeneration. Graefe's Archive for Clinical and Experimental Ophthalmology. 2013;**251**(1):27-34

[30] Luis Arias JM. Fluorescein angiography. In: Bandello F, editor. Age-Related Macular Degeneration. Portugal: Grupo De Estudos Da Retina; 2011

[31] Yannuzzi LA, Negrao S, Iida T, Carvalho C, Rodriguez-Coleman H, Slakter J, et al. Retinal angiomatous proliferation in age-related

macular degeneration. Retina. 2001;**21**(5):416-434

[32] Donati MC, Carifi G, Virgili G, Menchini U. Retinal angiomatous proliferation: Association with clinical and angiographic features. Ophthalmologica. 2006;**220**(1):31-36

[33] Costanzo E, Miere A, Querques G, Capuano V, Jung C, Souied EH. Type 1 choroidal neovascularization lesion size: indocyanine green angiography versus optical coherence tomography angiography. Investigative Ophthalmology & Visual Science. 2016;**57**(9):OCT307-OCT313

[34] Eandi CM, Ciardella A, Parravano M, Missiroli F, Alovisi C, Veronese C, et al. Indocyanine green angiography and optical coherence tomography angiography of choroidal neovascularization in age-related macular degeneration. Investigative Ophthalmology & Visual Science. 2017;**58**(9):3690-3696

[35] Yannuzzi LA, Sorenson J, Spaide RF, Lipson B. Idiopathic polypoidal choroidal vasculopathy (IPCV). Retina. 1990;**10**(1):1-8

[36] Yuzawa M, Mori R, Kawamura A. The origins of polypoidal choroidal vasculopathy. The British Journal of Ophthalmology. 2005;**89**(5):602-607

[37] Yannuzzi LA, Wong DW, Sforzolini BS, Goldbaum M, Tang KC, Spaide RF, et al. Polypoidal choroidal vasculopathy and neovascularized age-related macular degeneration. Archives of Ophthalmology. 1999;**117**(11):1503-1510

[38] Maribel Fernandez MG, Gonzalez F, Gomez-Ulla F. Diagnostic usefulness of indocyanine green angiography (ICGA) in age-related macular degeneration (AMD). In: Bandello F, editor. AMD Book. GER Group: Portugal; 2017

[39] Wong CW, Yanagi Y, Lee WK, Ogura Y, Yeo I, Wong TY, et al. Age-related macular degeneration and polypoidal choroidal vasculopathy in Asians. Progress in Retinal and Eye Research. 2016;**53**:107-139

[40] Kramer M, Mimouni K, Priel E, Yassur Y, Weinberger D. Comparison of fluorescein angiography and indocyanine green angiography for imaging of choroidal neovascularization in hemorrhagic age-related macular degeneration. American Journal of Ophthalmology. 2000;**129**(4):495-500

[41] Gross NE, Aizman A, Brucker A, Klancnik JM Jr, Yannuzzi LA. Nature and risk of neovascularization in the fellow eye of patients with unilateral retinal angiomatous proliferation. Retina. 2005;**25**(6):713-718

[42] Ahlers C, Gotzinger E, Pircher M, Golbaz I, Prager F, Schutze C, et al. Imaging of the retinal pigment epithelium in age-related macular degeneration using polarization-sensitive optical coherence tomography. Investigative Ophthalmology & Visual Science. 2010;**51**(4):2149-2157

[43] Karampelas M, Sim DA, Keane PA, Papastefanou VP, Sadda SR, Tufail A, et al. Evaluation of retinal pigment epithelium-Bruch's membrane complex thickness in dry age-related macular degeneration using optical coherence tomography. The British Journal of Ophthalmology. 2013;**97**(10):1256-1261

[44] Pircher M, Gotzinger E, Findl O, Michels S, Geitzenauer W, Leydolt C, et al. Human macula investigated in vivo with polarization-sensitive optical coherence tomography. Investigative Ophthalmology & Visual Science. 2006;**47**(12):5487-5494

[45] Landa G, Rosen RB, Pilavas J, Garcia PM. Drusen characteristics revealed by spectral-domain optical

coherence tomography and their corresponding fundus autofluorescence appearance in dry age-related macular degeneration. Ophthalmic Research. 2012;**47**(2):81-86

[46] Ueda-Arakawa N, Ooto S, Tsujikawa A, Yamashiro K, Oishi A, Yoshimura N. Sensitivity and specificity of detecting reticular pseudodrusen in multimodal imaging in Japanese patients. Retina. 2013;**33**(3):490-497

[47] Cicinelli MV, Rabiolo A, Sacconi R, Carnevali A, Querques L, Bandello F, et al. Optical coherence tomography angiography in dry age-related macular degeneration. Survey of Ophthalmology. 2018;**63**(2):236-244

[48] Toto L, Borrelli E, Di Antonio L, Carpineto P, Mastropasqua R. Retinal vascular Plexuses' changes in dry age-related macular degeneration, evaluated by means of optical coherence tomography angiography. Retina. 2016;**36**(8):1566-1572

[49] Fleckenstein M, Schmitz-Valckenberg S, Adrion C, Kramer I, Eter N, Helb HM, et al. Tracking progression with spectral-domain optical coherence tomography in geographic atrophy caused by age-related macular degeneration. Investigative Ophthalmology & Visual Science. 2010;**51**(8):3846-3852

[50] Fleckenstein M, Schmitz-Valckenberg S, Martens C, Kosanetzky S, Brinkmann CK, Hageman GS, et al. Fundus autofluorescence and spectral-domain optical coherence tomography characteristics in a rapidly progressing form of geographic atrophy. Investigative Ophthalmology & Visual Science. 2011;**52**(6):3761-3766

[51] Zweifel SA, Engelbert M, Laud K, Margolis R, Spaide RF, Freund KB. Outer retinal tubulation: A novel optical coherence tomography finding. Archives of Ophthalmology. 2009;**127**(12):1596-1602

[52] Do DV, Gower EW, Cassard SD, Boyer D, Bressler NM, Bressler SB, et al. Detection of new-onset choroidal neovascularization using optical coherence tomography: The AMD DOC study. Ophthalmology. 2012;**119**(4):771-778

[53] Jonnal RS, Kocaoglu OP, Zawadzki RJ, Liu Z, Miller DT, Werner JS. A review of adaptive optics optical coherence tomography: Technical advances, scientific applications, and the future. Investigative Ophthalmology & Visual Science. 2016;**57**(9):OCT51-OCT68

[54] Kenta Sudo BC, editor. Adaptive optics-assisted optical coherence tomography for imaging of patients with age related macular degeneration. In: Ophthalmic Technologies XXIII: Proceedings of SPIE 8567. 2013; DOI: https://doi.org/10.1117/12.2004165

[55] Panorgias A, Zawadzki RJ, Capps AG, Hunter AA, Morse LS, Werner JS. Multimodal assessment of microscopic morphology and retinal function in patients with geographic atrophy. Investigative Ophthalmology & Visual Science. 2013;**54**(6):4372-4384

[56] Kishi S. Impact of swept source optical coherence tomography on ophthalmology. Taiwan Journal of Ophthalmology. 2016;**6**(2):58-68

[57] Hanumunthadu D, Ilginis T, Balaggan KS, Patel PJ. Agreement of swept-source and spectral-domain optical coherence-tomography retinal thickness measurements in neovascular age-related macular degeneration. Clinical Ophthalmology. 2017;**11**:2121-2123

[58] Copete S, Flores-Moreno I, Montero JA, Duker JS, Ruiz-Moreno JM. Direct

comparison of spectral-domain and swept-source OCT in the measurement of choroidal thickness in normal eyes. The British Journal of Ophthalmology. 2014;**98**(3):334-338

[59] Gao SS, Jia Y, Zhang M, Su JP, Liu G, Hwang TS, et al. Optical coherence tomography angiography. Investigative Ophthalmology & Visual Science. 2016;**57**(9):OCT27-OCT36

[60] Hagag AM, Gao SS, Jia Y, Huang D. Optical coherence tomography angiography: Technical principles and clinical applications in ophthalmology. Taiwan Journal of Ophthalmology. 2017;**7**(3):115-129

[61] Kvanta A, Casselholm de Salles M, Amren U, Bartuma H. Optical coherence tomography angiography of the foveal microvasculature in geographic atrophy. Retina. 2017;**37**(5):936-942

[62] Cohen SY, Creuzot-Garcher C, Darmon J, Desmettre T, Korobelnik JF, Levrat F, et al. Types of choroidal neovascularisation in newly diagnosed exudative age-related macular degeneration. The British Journal of Ophthalmology. 2007;**91**(9):1173-1176

[63] Farecki ML, Gutfleisch M, Faatz H, Rothaus K, Heimes B, Spital G, et al. Characteristics of type 1 and 2 CNV in exudative AMD in OCT-angiography. Graefe's Archive for Clinical and Experimental Ophthalmology. 2017;**255**(5):913-921

[64] Roisman L, Zhang Q, Wang RK, Gregori G, Zhang A, Chen CL, et al. Optical coherence tomography angiography of asymptomatic neovascularization in intermediate age-related macular degeneration. Ophthalmology. 2016;**123**(6):1309-1319

[65] Told R, Sacu S, Hecht A, Baratsits M, Eibenberger K, Kroh ME, et al. Comparison of SD-optical coherence tomography angiography and indocyanine green angiography in type 1 and 2 neovascular age-related macular degeneration. Investigative Ophthalmology & Visual Science. 2018;**59**(6):2393-2400

[66] Chalam KV, Sambhav K. Optical coherence tomography angiography in retinal diseases. Journal of Ophthalmic and Vision Research. 2016;**11**(1):84-92

[67] Faridi A, Jia Y, Gao SS, Huang D, Bhavsar KV, Wilson DJ, et al. Sensitivity and specificity of OCT angiography to detect choroidal neovascularization. Ophthalmology Retina. 2017;**1**(4):294-303

[68] Miller AR, Roisman L, Zhang Q, Zheng F, Rafael de Oliveira Dias J, Yehoshua Z, et al. Comparison between spectral-domain and swept-source optical coherence tomography angiographic imaging of choroidal neovascularization. Investigative Ophthalmology & Visual Science. 2017;**58**(3):1499-1505

Chapter 13

Management Strategies and Visual Results for the Treatment of Neovascular Age-Related Macular Degeneration

Siyang Chaili and Sean D. Adrean

Abstract

The purpose of this chapter is to examine the various treatment strategies used to manage neovascular age-related macular degeneration (nAMD). The chapter will focus on the three main strategies including fixed interval dosing, as needed Pro-Re-Nata (PRN) treatment and Treat-and-Extend (TAE), with its variant the Treat-Extend-Stop (TES) protocol. We will discuss the visual results of randomized clinical trials and retrospective studies using these methodologies and compare their outcomes, the pros and cons of each treatment strategy, as well as the underlying mechanisms that may explain these differences. The results of long-term extension trials following landmark randomized clinical studies and other long-term retrospective studies will also be compared to studies using a fixed interval dosing or the TAE/TES method. We will also focus on the visual results of the TES protocol and examine recurrence rates, proposing a definition of the recurrence of choroidal neovascularization (CNV) versus increased disease activity. These topics discussed will help optimize anti-VEGF treatment regimens for patients with nAMD over the long term.

Keywords: neovascular age-related macular degeneration (nAMD), anti-vascular endothelial growth factor (anti-VEGF), treat-extend-stop (TES), long-term management, recurrence

1. Introduction

Age-related macular degeneration (AMD) continues to be the leading cause of non-preventable blindness in the world and is the most frequent cause of blindness in industrialized nations [1, 2]. With an ever-aging population and age itself as the chief risk factor for the development of AMD, the burden of disease is expected to rise [3, 4]. Advanced AMD is defined by the presence of geographic atrophy or new onset of aberrant vessel growth from the underlying choroid, termed choroidal neovascularization (CNV) [5]. The development of CNV may lead to secondary subretinal or sub-retinal pigmented epithelial (RPE) hemorrhage or serous exudation, followed by fibrosis and scarring [5]. The degenerative form of the disease, "dry macular degeneration", may convert to the neovascularization form, "wet macular degeneration", at a rate of about 10–15% [6]. The natural disease course of nAMD over the long term is poor. Jager et al. demonstrated that at 2 years, patients lost on average 4 Early Treatment Diabetic

Retinopathy Study (ETDRS) lines [6]. They also found at baseline 20% of patients had 20/200 vision or worse, but at the end of 3 years, that percentage had increased to 76% of patients with vision 20/200 or worse [6].

Mitigating aberrant vessel growth and its sequelae have been a focus for treating neovascular AMD (nAMD). The use of argon and krypton photocoagulation on CNV was first evaluated by the Macular Photocoagulation Study Group (MPS studies) [7, 8], followed by photodynamic therapy (PDT) studied by the Treatment of Age-related macular degeneration with Photodynamic therapy (TAP) and Verteporfin in Photodynamic Therapy (VIP) study groups [9, 10].

The isolation and discovery of vascular endothelial growth factor (VEGF) as the main driver of nAMD led to its targeting and inhibition as treatment [11]. This began with intravitreal injections of pegaptanib sodium (Macugen, OSI Pharmaceuticals, Melville, NY), a pegylated $VEGF_{165}$ specific aptamer, which demonstrated promising results in clinical studies and received fast-track approval from the FDA in 2004 [12]. Shortly thereafter, use of other anti-VEGF agents emerged with the positive results of off-label bevacizumab (Avastin, Genentech, San Francisco, CA) described in September 2005 [11, 13], which became a cornerstone of therapy for nAMD, along with its truncated Fab counterpart ranibizumab (Lucentis, Genentech, San Francisco, CA), later available in 2006 [14, 15]. Subsequently, the soluble VEGF decoy receptor, aflibercept (Eylea, Regeneron, Tarrytown, NY) has seen increased usage since its approval in 2011, due to its comparable efficacy to the other agents as well as some perceived advantages in clinical management with the possibility for less frequent dosing [16]. It has also demonstrated variable efficacy in clearing persistent fluid in eyes previously treated with bevacizumab or ranibizumab [17, 18]. Indeed, the use of anti-VEGF agents proved far superior to previous therapies, including laser photocoagulation and photodynamic therapy [7, 10, 15]. These extremely positive results caused a rapid paradigm shift in the management of nAMD and anti-VEGF agents quickly became the standard of care.

Although the anti-VEGF agent class is clearly superior, there are instances when PDT or thermal laser used in combination with anti-VEGF agents is appropriate. A commonly reported draw-back of thermal laser in the management of CNV is the high incidence of disease recurrence [19–21]. However, Adrean et al. have demonstrated in a case series of five eyes with peripapillary CNV, with subfoveal extension of exudate and fluid, that anti-VEGF therapy pretreatment may better help define the CNV area receiving laser treatment by first limiting the size of the CNV then causing resolution of the hemorrhage and exudate [22]. Following laser treatment, a subsequent anti-VEGF injection is given 1 week later to inhibit pathological CNV growth in response to the thermal laser [22]. This robust treatment method demonstrated that all study eyes were free of recurrence at a mean follow-up time of 24 months with average vision improving from 20/50 to 20/30 ($p = 0.0232$) [22].

Newer studies are underway examining other therapeutic options for the management of nAMD [23, 24].

2. Anti-VEGF treatment protocols and visual results

Three main treatment strategies have been developed to manage nAMD. The first method is fixed interval dosing, a mainstay of randomized clinical trials (RCT), where patients receive treatments on a monthly, bimonthly or quarterly interval based on the anti-VEGF agent. Shortly thereafter, the Pro-Re-Nata (PRN) method was introduced, where patients were treated as needed based on optical coherent tomography (OCT) status, usually preceded by three monthly anti-VEGF loading doses. Another method developed was the Treat-and-Extend regimen (TAE). Patients are typically treated until a dry macula is obtained, and then the time interval between injections is gradually increased, usually by one to two-week intervals. These distinct treatment methods produce comparable visual and anatomic outcomes in the short term (≤1–2 years). However, in the long term (≥3 years), small differences in these outcomes are substantially amplified.

2.1 Fixed interval dosing

The treatment of nAMD using anti-VEGF therapy began with fixed interval dosing, which is the mainstay of the initial, landmark RCTs. Subjects with CNV typically have scheduled examinations with SD-OCT and receive intravitreal injections every 4 to 6 weeks. Patients may also get fundus photos (FF) and fluorescein angiography (FA) initially and at other predetermined time intervals [14].

This treatment strategy is the initial treatment regimen that demonstrated superior efficacy compared with previous methods such as thermal laser and verteporfin, as well as a largely positive safety profile, in RCTs and clinical practice. In the seminal anti-VEGF RCTs, namely the Ranibizumab for Neovascular Age-Related Macular Degeneration (MARINA), Ranibizumab versus Verteporfin for Neovascular Age-Related Macular Degeneration (ANCHOR), and Twelve and Twenty-four-month efficacy and safety of 0.5 mg or 2.0 mg ranibizumab in patients with subfoveal neovascular age-related macular degeneration (HARBOR) trials, treatment arms with monthly ranibizumab injection demonstrated an average visual improvement of +6.5 to +11.3 ETDRS letters [14, 15, 25, 26]. Subsequent trials such as the ranibizumab and bevacizumab for treatment of neovascular age-related macular degeneration (CATT) and alternative treatments to inhibit VEGF in age-related choroidal neovascularization (IVAN) trials reported, at minimum, similar clinical efficacy of ranibizumab and bevacizumab in each of the treatment arms (Δ = 1.4 letters CATT 24 months; Δ = 1.3 letters IVAN 24 months) [27–30]. Intravitreal aflibercept reported a composite 8.4 ETDRS letter gain at 52 weeks in the VIEW 1 and VIEW 2 RCTs and met non-inferiority criteria when compared with ranibizumab treatment arms [16]. Yet one study, the PIER study, evaluated fixed interval dosing with ranibizumab, at a greater time interval between injections and showed poorer overall outcomes compared to monthly treatments. Patients were randomized 1:1:1 to receive 0.3 mg ranibizumab, 0.5 mg ranibizumab, and sham injections, respectively, at quarterly intervals [31]. At the end of the first year, patients in each of the treatment groups had already experienced visual declines below baseline vision [31], and by the end of the second year, visual loss was even more dramatic (e.g. −0.2 at 1 year and −2.3 letters at 2 years for 0.5 mg ranibizumab vs. onset study vision) [32]. While better than sham injections, these results were strikingly worse compared to monthly fixed dosing in previous RCTs (+6.5 to +11.3 ETDRS letters vs. baseline). Study patients were subsequently rolled-over to monthly injections, and although some vision was able to be recovered (+2.9 to +4.3 ETDRS letters), visual acuity (VA) was never able to be restored to levels consistent with monthly dosing [32]. This was one of the first examples that reduced treatment in a RCT had decreased visual outcomes and that more frequent dosing of anti-VEGF agents resulted in better visual outcomes.

Then multiple retrospective studies describing the success of monthly dosed anti-VEGF injections were published, with certain retrospective studies demonstrating efficacy over the long term [33, 34]. For example, Peden et al. retrospectively reported average visual results of 14.0 letters, 12.2 letters and 12.1 letters at an average treatment duration of 5, 6 and 7 years, respectively, using a fixed monthly injection regimen averaging 10.5 injections per year [34]. However, due to the treatment and potential economic burden, injection fatigue to both patient and physician, as well as the concern for systemic arteriothrombotic events (ATEs), other treatment strategies have been developed.

2.2 Pro-Re-Nata (PRN) dosing

The first response to fixed interval dosing was the development of a treat as needed (PRN) dosing regimen, which gained rapid acceptance after initial RCTs evaluating its efficacy at 1–2 years compared favorably to monthly fixed dosing. Patients receiving this strategy typically receive loading injections, most commonly once per month for 3 months, and then injections are given or held based on exam. If patients' vision and disease stabilize, then injections are held. If there is persistent fluid or exudate, anti-VEGF therapy is continued monthly until a "dry" macula occurs, typically determined on SD-OCT. Otherwise, changes such as decreased vision, new onset fluid or growth of lesion size, among others, as demonstrated by clinical exam, OCT, FA or other diagnostic methods typically drive renewal of treatment [27, 28].

The HARBOR and CATT trials reported clinically comparable visual gains between monthly fixed dosing and PRN study arms at year one [25, 27]. Although in the Harbor trial, examining ranibizumab, the PRN arm was unable to meet the pre-specified, non-inferiority outcomes even at 1 year compared to fixed-monthly injections [25]. On the other hand, even though the CATT study reported worse vision in the PRN group in both the bevacizumab or ranibizumab arms, it met the non-inferiority criteria compared to fixed monthly dosing [27]. Interestingly, these two landmark RCTs had different non-inferiority criteria, differing by only one letter [25, 27]. Regardless, by the end of year two, visual outcomes in the PRN treatments arms was significantly worse than the fixed monthly dosed groups in both studies ($p < 0.05$) [26, 28]. In fact, the HARBOR study concluded that at the end of 12 months, monthly dosing of ranibizumab proved superior over PRN dosing [26]; and, the CATT study likewise summarized that "[PRN] resulted in less gain in VA, whether instituted at enrollment or after 1 year of monthly treatment [28]." The IVAN study, later conducted in the United Kingdom, concluded that visual outcomes using the PRN method were "equivalent" to continuous treatment (−0.4 letters, 95% Cl, −2.40 to 1.70) in the first year of evaluation [29]. However, by the end of the second year, they reported that the "reduction in the frequency of retreatment resulted in a small loss of efficacy irrespective of drug," and demonstrated that discontinuous treatment resulted in 1.6 letters lost compared to monthly fixed dosing, although this was not statistically significant ($p = 0.18$) [30]. These, arguably small, differences were further amplified when this treatment methodology was continued over the long term. Two landmark extension studies of RCTs demonstrated this effect: The Five-Year Outcomes with Anti-Vascular Endothelial Growth Factor Treatment of Neovascular Age-Related Macular Degeneration (CATT-5) trial and the Seven-year Outcomes in Ranibizumab-treated Patients in ANCHOR, MARINA, and HORIZON: a Multicenter Cohort Study (SEVEN-UP). In these two studies, most patients were transitioned or maintained on a PRN schedule following the conclusion of their respective RCTs. By the end of year 5 of the CATT-5 study, patients on average lost 3 ETDRS letters from baseline and 11 letters from the 2-year endpoint of the original CATT study [35]. Moreover, 20% of eyes had vision 20/200 or worse compared to only 6% at study baseline, which improved to 5% in years 1 and 2 [35]. Overall, 36.4% of eyes lost ≥5 letters from baseline and 54.6% of eyes lost ≥5 letters from the end of year 2 [35]. In fact, nearly 24% of eyes lost ≥15 letters baseline and 29% lost ≥15 letters from the original study conclusion [35]. In the SEVEN-UP study, 37% of eyes had vision 20/200 or worse at the end of

7 years, with 34% of eyes losing ≥15 letters for an average decline of 8.6 letters from ANCHOR or MARINA baseline [36]. Strikingly, this was a change of −19.8 letters from the peak vision obtained at the end of the ANCHOR and MARINA trials [36]. In fact, most eyes lost vision at the end of the SEVEN-UP study when compared to any of the presenting or exiting vision of its preceding studies (56.9% vs. MARINA or ANCHOR entry; 84.6% vs. MARINA or ANCHOR exit) [36]. Similar trends have been observed in clinical practice and documented in multiple retrospective studies, demonstrating good clinical outcomes in the near term which deteriorated over time, commonly below baseline levels. In a study by Rasmussen et al., 192 eyes receiving PRN injections had an improvement of 3.4 letter above baseline at the end of 1 year, which regressed to 1.4 letters at the end of year 4 [37]. This was one of the few PRN studies that demonstrated an average final vision above baseline, although this was still not statistically significant [37]. Others, such as those by Gillies et al. [38], Zhu et al. [39], Haddad et al. [40], the PACORES study group [41] and Westborg et al. [42] recorded average visual losses from as little as −4.3 letters to as much as −25.4 letters from peak visual gains, when studied over the long term.

2.3 Treat-and-Extend (TAE) and Treat-Extend-Stop (TES) methods

Although initially well received, small deficiencies in visual and anatomic outcomes under the PRN strategy were amplified both in RCTs and clinical practice, particularly when patients required anti-VEGF injections over the long term. Thus, in response, a graduated treatment protocol, termed "Treat-and-Extend" (TAE), along with its variation, the "Treat-Extend-Stop" regimen developed by Adrean et al. [43], was created to improve patient outcomes while keeping the benefits of reduced treatment burden. Due to the success of this method, it is currently the most widely used treatment protocol of retinal specialists in the United States [44]. Patients treated with this strategy are typically treated with a minimum of 3 monthly loading doses until there is clinical resolution of fluid and SD-OCT demonstrates a "dry" macula [43]. Treatments are then lengthened by 1–2-weeks based on evaluation at each visit [43]. If a "dry" macula is maintained on SD-OCT, then the time interval is increased to a typical maximum of 10–12 weeks [43]. If at any time patients experience a decrease in vision or increase in exudation as quantified on SD-OCT, then treatment intervals are adjusted, usually decreasing by 1–2 weeks, to adequately control the disease process [43]. Some patients can reach maximum extension, and therefore continue receiving treatment every 10–12 weeks indefinitely; other patients never reach maximal extension, but instead require constant adjustment or continuous treatment at shorter intervals [43]. If patients are determined to be failing one anti-VEGF agent after 3–6 intravitreal injections, the anti-VEGF agent is typically changed.

The TES strategy was developed for patients achieving a maximal extension to further decrease treatment burden [43]. Using the TES method, patients who reached a maximum extension of 12 weeks then receive 2 additional injections, each 12 weeks apart, with an FA performed at the second 12-week visit to evaluate the CNV [43]. Patients are then examined 12 weeks later [43]. If the macula was "dry" at that point, as determined by SD-OCT, patients are then considered to be in disease remission and further injections are held [43]. Next, patients are carefully monitored for any signs of disease recurrence with a monitoring phase beginning 4 weeks later [43]. Evaluation intervals are then progressively lengthened at 2-week intervals until 12 weeks are reached, at which time patients are then monitored indefinitely at quarterly intervals [43]. If at any time, patients notice decreased vision or an increase in metamorphopsia, they are instructed to return immediately to the clinic for re-initiation of treatment, and the TES protocol is restarted from the beginning [43].

In RCTs and clinical practice, the TAE method has demonstrated visual outcomes similar to monthly fixed dosing at a decreased increased injection frequency, and superior to those reported using the PRN method. In the Comparison of Ranibizumab and Bevacizumab for Neovascular Age-Related Macular Degeneration Accord to LUCAS Treat-and Extend Protocol (LUCAS) trial by Berg et al., bevacizumab and ranibizumab were found to be equivalent with an average of 7.9 and 8.2 letters gained, respectively, at the end of the first year [45]. In the second year, bevacizumab and ranibizumab continued to demonstrate efficacy with average visual improvements of 7.4 and 6.6 letters from baseline, respectively [45]. Interestingly, a greater number of injections were given in the bevacizumab group than in the ranibizumab group [45]. Around the same time, Wykoff et al. published a Prospective Trial of Treat-and-Extend versus Monthly Dosing for Neovascular Age-Related Macular Degeneration [46]. Wykoff et al. demonstrated at the end of 1 year that TAE dosing of 0.5 mg ranibizumab resulted in similar outcomes compared to fixed monthly dosing, with average visual gains of 10.5 and 9.2 letters respectively [46]. The comparative efficacy between TAE and fixed monthly administration has also been described in numerous other studies, both retrospectively and prospectively. For example, Chen et al. demonstrated in a retrospective analysis that eyes undergoing monthly vs. TAE treatment at 1 year on average had a visual difference of −0.5 letters ($p = 0.81$) [47]. Additionally, Abedi et al. demonstrated in a prospective cohort study of 120 eyes, average visual gains of 9.5 letters and 8.0 letters at 12 and 24 months, respectively, which were comparable to those of the pivotal clinical trials [48]. These visual outcomes may also be maintained over the long term. For example, in a retrospective cohort study by Mrejen et al., 210 study eyes, with a retention rate of 62.9%, at an average of 3.5 years, had visual improvement of 20/90 from study baseline to 20/75, or approximately one line of improvement ($p < 0.05$) with an average of 8.3 injections per year [49]. Perhaps the longest studies evaluating this method are those performed by Adrean et al., specifically using the TES variation. In one study, patients received TES treatment for an average of nearly 3 years until the disease was controlled to remission, and patients were transitioned to quarterly follow up, as described previously, without injections [43]. At this point, the average visual improvement was approximately +7.5 ETDRS letters, improving from 20/70 to 20/50, with 60% of eyes achieving 20/40 vision or better [43]. At study conclusion, accounting for CNV disease recurrence and re-initiation of treatment, a total of 38.1% of eyes gained 3 or more lines of vision, whereas only 2 eyes of a single patient (4.8%) lost 3 lines of vision due to development of geographic atrophy [43]. In another study, Adrean et al. demonstrated that long-term treatment of 71 study eyes with nAMD, using the TES protocol, resulted in average visual gains of 9.7 letters over an average treatment period of 6.5 years [50]. Notably, this visual improvement was maintained over an average follow-up period of 8 years, with only a slight decrease to a final average visual improvement of 8.7 letters [50]. The percentage of eyes gaining 3 or more lines of vision at final follow-up in this study at 8 years, was 35.2%; conversely, 9.9% of eyes lost 3 or more lines [50]. In fact, these visual outcomes are similar to the proportion of eyes gaining at least 3 lines of vision found in monthly fixed dosing RCTs, such as MARINA (33.3% with 0.5 mg ranibizumab) [14], ANCHOR (41% with 0.5 mg ranibizumab) [15], and HARBOR (34.5% with 0.5 mg ranibizumab) [26] at the final study endpoint of only 2 years.

Both RCTs and retrospective studies using the TAE/TES method have demonstrated superior visual outcomes compared to PRN studies. In a systematic review by Rufai et al., which included the assessment of 748 eyes undergoing the TAE protocol, the one-year BCVA improvement was 8.9 letters, compared to the 3.5 letters reported by Chin-Yee et al. in a separate systematic review regarding the PRN method [51]. Head to head studies, such as those by Chin-Yee et al., demonstrated an average 10.4

letter improvement in the TAE group vs. 5.4 letters in the PRN group at 12 months, with the TAE group receiving about 3.5 more injections on average [52]. Likewise, in a study by Oubraham et al., average visual acuity was greater in TAE treated eyes compared to PRN treated eyes by 8.5 letters with an average of 2.7 more injections [53]. Interestingly, the number of follow-up visits was similar (8.5 vs. 8.8, TAE vs. PRN, p = 0.2085) [53]. The most interesting studies might be those conducted by Hatz et al. and Cohen et al. As with the rescue effect observed in the patients rolled-over from PRN to monthly dosing in the PIER trials, patients transitioning from the PRN to the TAE method demonstrated improved vision despite having a greater number of office visits in the PRN group [54, 55]. Although there is no long-term head-to-head comparison study between TAE/TES vs. PRN treatment methods in RCTs or private practice, a comparison of these outcomes individually reveals that the TAE/TES method is superior. RCTs, such as the CATT-5 and SEVEN-UP studies, along with many retrospective studies employing the PRN method beyond an average follow-up time of 3 years (up to 7 years) have demonstrated average visual changes of +1.4 to −19.3 letters from baseline vision [35–42]. Conversely, prospective and retrospective data have reported visual increases of 5–9.7 letters for similar time intervals in eyes managed by a TAE/TES strategy [43, 49, 50].

3. Potential mechanisms of management strategies for disease and visual outcomes

Various factors have been implicated in the variation of visual outcomes for eyes with nAMD managed by anti-VEGF therapy [6]. For example, older age or male gender has been associated with increased exudative disease and the need for retreatment [56]. However, recent studies have suggested that some factors, such as initial presenting vision, are predictive of the long-term visual gains [57]. Additionally, other groups have examined CNV lesion type and demonstrated that there was a differential response to anti-VEGF therapy and visual outcomes [14, 15, 49]. Therefore, it appears that the optimization of these factors may lead to more favorable responses in patients' visual outcomes, especially over the long term.

Shah and Del Priore in a large meta-analysis described that patients' presenting vision contributed to as much as 90% of the final visual outcomes obtained using anti-VEGF therapy [57]. Poorer presenting vision was typically due to longer delays before the initial presentation to the physician, with patients reporting a longer duration of symptoms before seeking care [57]. The greater the delay was prior to initiating anti-VEGF therapy, the worse the final achievable vision [57]. Interestingly, they also noted that patients with worse initial vision also had greater amounts of active exudation and more commonly presented with type-2 classic CNV [57]. It is generally accepted that in the typical course of the disease, if left untreated, type-1 occult lesions often progress to mixed and, subsequently, classic CNV [58]. Over time, uncontrolled disease activity and exudation perpetually cause damage to the neurosensory retina and RPE, ultimately leading to subretinal fibrosis and irreversible vision loss.

Distinct lesions respond differently to anti-VEGF therapy. Early RCTs, for example, when comparing the results achieved from monthly dosing of 0.5 mg ranibizumab in the MARINA study for minimally classic or occult lesions to the predominantly classic lesions evaluated in the ANCHOR trials, demonstrated that visual gains were greater in the classical CNV study [14, 15]. While this seems to contradict the findings of Shah and Del Priore [57], this is because patients with subretinal fibrosis or signs of advanced macular degeneration were excluded. Additionally, patients' baseline vision in the ANCHOR trial had to be better than

20/320 to be included in the trial, which limited many patients with advanced exudative disease [15]. While visual gains were better realized in the ANCHOR study, possibly due to poorer presenting vision, a ceiling effect was likely encountered in the MARINA study. For example, the average presenting vision of the 0.5 mg ranibizumab arm of the ANCHOR study was 47.1 ± 13.2 letters [15], whereas it was 53.7 ± 12.8 letters in MARINA [14], a difference of nearly 7 letters. At the end of year one, the study eyes in the ANCHOR study had gained an average of 11.3 letters in the 0.5 mg ranibizumab group [15] compared to 7.2 letters in the MARINA study [14], for average final VA of 58.4 vs. 60.9 letters respectively [14, 15]. Other reasons, such as the location of the CNV or exudation in relation to the fovea may also play a factor. Classic lesions outside of the fovea with subfoveal leakage and exudate may have better visual outcomes since the CNV itself is not subfoveal. As the fluid and exudate dissipate with therapy, the subfoveal architecture remains largely intact with preservation of the central photoreceptors and retinal pigment epithelium, allowing for increased visual gains.

As described previously, there are relatively few studies examining the long-term treatment results of anti-VEGF therapy. Those describing the PRN strategy have been the most numerous, while those examining the TAE/TES or monthly dosing regimens are substantially fewer. There are even fewer studies that characterize lesion type or subtype and their response to anti-VEGF therapy over 2–3 years. One study, by Mrejen et al., examined the response of anti-VEGF treatment administered using a TAE strategy in eyes with different CNV lesion subtypes [49]. Occult lesions were found to have the best initial presenting vision, which was maintained throughout 4 years, although these patients also received an average of 0.6–2.2 more injections compared to other groups ($p < 0.05$) [49]. Preservation of vision tends to be greater in occult or mixed lesions as opposed to classic lesions [49]. These results were replicated in a similar study by Berg et al., which demonstrated that longer-term anti-VEGF therapy using a TAE method resulted in better visual maintenance in eyes with occult or mixed lesions over classic lesions or retinal angiomatous proliferation (RAP) [59]. Together with the evidence described above, reporting that eyes with delayed initial presentation and worse baseline vision having greater evidence of active exudation as well as the progression from type-1 occult to type-2 classic lesions, it is apparent that early diagnosis and thorough control of nAMD should result in the best possible visual outcomes. Otherwise, a CNV left untreated or inadequately treated may lead to progressive retinal damage, which generally manifests as increased fluid or exudation, which then leads to end-stage disease such as atrophic and fibrovascular scarring, ultimately resulting in decreased vision.

As we have previously noted, slightly worse vision due to PRN treatment in short-term studies has resulted in substantially worse vision over the long term when compared to monthly fixed or TAE/TES dosing strategies, even when baseline characteristics are otherwise comparable. This may be, in fact, due to the reactive nature of the PRN strategy, leading to considerable delays in recognition of increased disease leading to suboptimal treatment. Due to the inherent difficulty in scheduling office visits and the unreliability of patients to report increased disease (caused by several factors, such as the subtlety of symptoms confounded by the vision in the fellow eye), by the time the patient presents for follow-up, even if scheduled ahead of time, new onset or progression of active disease may have already occurred. It may be, in fact, that the fewer injection numbers reported by PRN studies, particularly in the long term, are not a result of better disease control, but are instead demonstrative of missed opportunities for adequate disease control.

Indeed, the number of injections is a key factor associated with final visual outcomes [60]. This may be due to greater numbers of injections maintaining a therapeutic level of VEGF inhibition in the eye. In a study by Lumbroso et al., vessel proliferative cycling of CNV in the presence of anti-VEGF activity was examined [61]. The proliferation of aberrant vessels in CNV appears to cycle through a series of predictable stages after anti-VEGF inhibition [61]. Pruning begins within 24 h of initial anti-VEGF injection and progresses to maximal inhibition at 6–12 days [61]. As anti-VEGF levels fall, the sprouting of new vessels and angiogenic leakage may then develop anywhere from 20 to 50 days later [61]. Interestingly, with increasing numbers of anti-VEGF injections, likely maintaining steady inhibitory concentrations within the eye, the time between each proliferative cycle lengthens [61]. Neovascular vessel burden decreases and, instead, the central vessels from which they sprout and open increase in size [61]. This process may also explain why untreated occult disease may eventually progress to type-2 lesions, followed by fibrovascular scarring and irreversible vision damage. Due to the reactive nature of the PRN strategy described above, poor inhibition on this mechanism of neovascular proliferation likely occurs. For example, after transitioning all original treatment groups in the CATT, MARINA and ANCHOR trials to the PRN method for long-term treatment, the number of eyes with residual fluid at the end of the CATT-5 and SEVEN-UP trials was 68 and 83%, respectively [35, 36]. Moreover, 24.5% of CATT-5 study eyes were found to have leakage on FA [35]. Likewise, 48% of eyes had active or probable leakage of FA in the SEVEN-UP study [36]. Interestingly, despite 68% of eyes having intraretinal or subretinal fluid, and nearly half of eyes with leakage on FA, only 46% of eyes were receiving ongoing treatment at the end of the SEVEN-UP study [36]. Although it is unclear which of the factors described above may have contributed to the visual decline of the study patients in these two RCTs, the mismatch between eyes with active disease or persistent fluid/exudation and those that were receiving active treatment suggests that adequate disease follow-up and control may not have been well established. Moreover, this is complicated by the fact that, as reported in both SEVEN-UP and CATT-5 studies, the subretinal fluid itself was not significantly associated with decreased vision, while intra-retinal fluid was [35, 36]. However, the SEVEN-UP study group suggested that subretinal fluid may be relevant in the context of generally uncontrolled neovascular disease progression [62]. Along with hemorrhage and exudation, permanent damage to the neurosensory retina and surrounding structures may also lead to macular atrophy, one of the strongest drivers of decreased vision in the long-term treatment of nAMD [62]. The CATT study group, on the other hand, proposed that subretinal fluid may, in fact, be protective against the development of geographic atrophy [63]. However, these two studies differ in their respective definitions of atrophic disease. The CATT study group suggested that the atrophic macular lesions they describe may be clinically indistinguishable from those arising from non-neovascular origins, mainly geographic atrophy [63]. Macular atrophy may be a separate entity since it lacks the classic anatomical features of geographic atrophy [62]. Thus far, it appears that timeliness and greater numbers of injections generally lead to better anatomical and visual outcomes. Future studies further elucidating these factors may help better optimize treatment strategies.

When comparing the number of injections patients received, the average number of injections received was greatest in the monthly dosed regimens, followed by the TAE/TES method, and finally PRN. For example, Peden et al. reported an average of 10.5 injections per year at 7 years, using the monthly fixed interval dosing [34]. Adrean et al. in their consistent long-term anti-VEGF study, utilizing the TES strategy, were performing 9.6 injections per year at 6.5 years and 8.1 injections per year at the final follow-up at 8 years [50]. Conversely, RCTs utilizing the PRN method reported an average of 5.1 injections per year in the CATT-5 study [35] and 2 injections per year in the SEVEN-UP study after exit from the HORIZON follow-up trial [36]. Interestingly, in a subgroup of patients that received more injections (3.2 per year) in the SEVEN-UP trial, their vision was significantly better than other study participants [36]. As described earlier, the number of injections has been demonstrated to be an independent factor positively contributing to visual improvement. Again, this phenomenon may be explained in the context of increased injections leading to maintenance of adequate inhibition of VEGF, which in turn, inhibits vessel growth and increases the time for neovascular vessel proliferation cycles. While some studies demonstrate that the PRN method has fewer injections than TAE/TES dosing at a 1-year endpoint, they have similar number of visits, with poorer visual outcomes [64].

Taken together, these lines of evidence suggest that the improper timing of the PRN method to detect and treat disease, as well as the subtherapeutic dosing of anti-VEGF agents due to less frequent injections, leads to a greater exudation, hemorrhage, and progressive macular damage, ultimately resulting in poorer vision. Monthly dosing, on the other hand, is superior for controlling disease. However, this method may not scale as the population ages and the incidence of nAMD rises. Fixed monthly dosing may lead to overtreatment, injection fatigue, as well as increased costs and the potential for increased risk of adverse events. The TAE/TES method, with progressively lengthening treatment and observation times, individualized to each patient, may maintain adequate intravitreal anti-VEGF levels which allows for the lengthening of neovascular vessel proliferation cycles. The long-term visual outcomes of the TAE/TES method compare favorably to the fixed dosing method, with fewer office visits and injections. Future therapeutic advancements may further optimize nAMD management.

4. Dosing strategy and effect on disease activity, recurrence and visual outcomes

Various studies have attempted to define characteristics of disease control and make better assessments for when to continue treatments consistently or possibly discontinue treatment. The most commonly used characteristics are changes in visual acuity and the presence or absence of retinal fluid, typically based on SD-OCT data regardless of the dosing strategy utilized [65, 66].

A consensus article by Amoaku et al. attempts to characterize the degree of response eyes have to anti-VEGF therapy [66]. Eyes are categorized as good, partial, poor or non-responders. Good responders are free of fluid or have a central retinal thickness (CRT) reduced by >75% following the initial loading phase of therapy, typically the first 3 monthly injections. Visually, these eyes demonstrate an improvement of >5 ETDRS letters or achieve greater than 70 total ETDRS letters, if a ceiling effect is present. Partial responders have less CRT reduction (25–75%) and may have some persistent subretinal or intraretinal fluid. Visual improvement is generally limited to 1–4 letters gained. Poor responders have even less CRT reduction (0–25%) as well as persistent fluid on SD-OCT. Visual acuity is typically unchanged from baseline to a loss of −4 letters. Finally, non-responders have unchanging or increasing CRT, fluid or pigmented epithelial detachment (PED), with eyes losing 5 or more letters. Management of nAMD can be stratified based on these characteristics. For example, good and partial responders may continue their current anti-VEGF regimen if their vision or morphology is maintained. If there is decreased vision or indicators of poorer morphology, the time interval between treatment should be reduced, and if treatment has been maintained at 4-week intervals without an improvement in morphology, a switch in anti-VEGF agents is needed. Other studies have characterized response based on lesion type, concluding that occult and mixed lesions generally respond better to anti-VEGF therapy than classic or RAP lesions [49, 59]. Moreover, not all retinal fluid is equal, as some groups have suggested that subretinal fluid is protective against geographic atrophy [63]. Nonetheless, many agree that achieving a dry macula is necessary to prevent retinal damage over the long term and is essential for the improvement and preservation of vision.

When considering the dosing regimen, Amoaku et al. suggested that more frequent dosing tends towards improved visual outcomes, likely due to proactive disease control that is not realized in PRN methods which often result in under-treatment [66]. Other factors such as antibody neutralization and tachyphylaxis may also affect the success of anti-VEGF treatment regardless of factors such as presenting vision or morphology [66]. Therefore, it appears that a patient's response to anti-VEGF therapy is a complex interplay between multiple factors that are attributable intrinsically to the patient as well as their treatment history.

One key factor in a patient's treatment history affecting visual outcomes is the degree of disease control. However, there is loose language surrounding the topic of active disease progression or disease recurrence. Many studies have described recurrence as any new onset of fluid or exudation regardless of time, thus implicitly suggesting that active disease is controlled as soon as the macula is deemed "dry". Other studies use the term "disease recurrence" to mean new onset CNV or exudation after disease remission, for example, a minimum time criterion of 4 months with no evidence of fluid or exudation ("active disease") [40, 43]. At present, there is no formal definition accepted. This is problematic because, as discussed earlier, neovascular vessel proliferative cycling times may be lengthened with successive anti-VEGF injections, leading to clearing of fluid, but the underlying disease may not be entirely controlled. Thus, those that conclude active disease is controlled after the fluid has been eliminated from the macula after a single injection may be mistaken, and the clearing of fluid observed may be short-lived. Indeed, this fact is most concerning for patients undergoing anti-VEGF treatment with a PRN regimen, as follow-up visits which demonstrate "absence" of disease and subtle visual changes may ultimately cause delays in treatment and progressive retinal damage. This phenomenon is less likely to be present in TAE/TES or monthly fixed dosing strategies since injections are more frequent and scheduled. However, a lack of consensus definition confuses the reported outcomes in literature and serves to make comparisons between studies more challenging. Given that previous in vitro studies have demonstrated that new pathologic vessels may develop after a single anti-VEGF injection of up to 62 days later [61], true disease remission logically should be at minimum outside of this time. Thus, disease remission may be defined as no fluid recurrence within 4 months and that at this point the disease is considered quiescent. If fluid occurs outside of the 4-month period, it is likely that a true recurrence of nAMD has occurred. However, any increase of subretinal or intraretinal fluid that occurs during active treatment in the TAE/TES protocol should be defined as an increase in disease activity and the time interval should be decreased accordingly, depending on the amount of increased disease activity. If patients are in the loading or maintenance phase of a TAE/TES protocol and are in the 5–8 week treatment range, then the time interval between injections should be reduced by 1–2 weeks. If patients are being treated at the 10–12 week range and there is a small amount of increased exudation, then the time interval again may be reduced by 2 weeks. However, if there is a significant increase in disease activity, then the time interval should be reduced more aggressively, potentially even restarting the TAE/TES protocol. If patients continue to have increased exudation and the time interval between anti-VEGF injections has been decreased to the 4–6 week range, then likely the anti-VEGF agents needs to be switched [43, 45, 50]. If patients are being treated with a PRN methodology, and there is increased fluid at a time interval of less than 4 months without treatment, again this should be considered increased disease activity. If increased exudation occurs outside of 4 months, this should be considered a true recurrence.

Reports on true CNV disease recurrence are currently limited. Two retrospective studies have reported this phenomenon. In the first, Haddad et al. utilized a PRN dosing method in 132 eyes over an average follow-up of 7.75 years [40]. Eighty-three (63%) eyes experienced long-term remission without requiring treatment for 1 year at least one time during the duration of the study [40]. However, among them, 42 (51%) eyes experienced a true recurrence of CNV [40]. The average vision of the entire cohort improved 5.0 letters after 1 year compared to baseline [40]. However, by the end of 7.75 years, this visual improvement was not maintained and decreased to −3.4 letters below baseline, a total loss of 8.4 letters [40]. Conversely, in a study by Adrean et al., 143 of 385 eyes (37.3%), treated with a TES protocol, experienced long-term disease remission with a minimum treatment cessation period of 4 months [43]. Prior to this time, these eyes were treated with a TES protocol for an average of 33 months [43]. The average initial presenting vision was 20/70 and improved to 20/50 at the completion of the treatment phase, or approximately 7.5 ETDRS letters [43]. The average time to true disease recurrence was 14 months later and occurred in 42/143 (29.4%) eyes [43]. At this point, average vision decreased to 20/60, with 54.8% of eyes experiencing a recurrence without a decrease in vision [43]. However, once eyes were restarted on the TES protocol, average vision recovered to 20/50 and was maintained throughout the remaining average 27 months of follow-up [43]. Although the criteria for remission of disease are different between these two studies, the average time observed of quiescent disease not requiring treatment was around 1 year [40, 43]. Notably different, however, is that the final vision of eyes treated with the more robust TES method was better and was able to be salvaged should a recurrence occur [40, 43]. This is likely due to the undertreatment of active disease that is commonly experienced from PRN methods, even if eyes demonstrate signs of good response [66]. Eyes demonstrating good response under a PRN method may require more vigilant monitoring over a greater period of time before one may conclude that active disease has been controlled. On the other hand, eyes that have received more robust treatment under the TES method may be carefully monitored at longer intervals if good response has been demonstrated throughout the course of treatment for active disease.

5. Conclusion

In this chapter, the three main treatment strategies to treat nAMD were presented and discussed. The first strategy examined was the fixed dose treatment method, where anti-VEGF agents are given on a routine basis, typically monthly or bimonthly after an initial loading phase. The advantage of this method is that it has been proven successful in multiple landmark clinical trials and patients may expect potentially the best visual outcomes. Fixed dosing disadvantages include the lack of individualized treatment with potentially no endpoint and the possibility of being overtreated. There is a potential for more episodes of endophthalmitis with more injections given and the chance for systemic effects, although this is still debated. The next treatment strategy presented was the PRN methodology, where patients are typically given a loading dose of three monthly anti-VEGF injections and then monitoring is begun once the macula is dry. Patients are then treated only after the detection of new-onset decreased vision or increased fluid. The advantage of this treatment methodology is that patients receive fewer injections with potentially fewer systemic and ocular side effects. However, there is the potential for delayed detection of decreased visual or anatomic damage, increasing the risk for undertreatment with this methodology. Visual results of this method have definitely proven inferior compared to other dosing regimens, particularly over the long term. The final treatment strategy presented was the treat-and-extend regimen with its variant treat-extend-stop. After three loading doses of anti-VEGF therapy for nAMD, patients are then extended by 2-week intervals once a dry macular is achieved. In some patients, the therapy is stopped after patients are given two injections 12 weeks apart and held at the third 12-week interval, after which careful monitoring of patients' visual function and macular changes is begun. This personalized anti-VEGF regimen offers the greatest potential for success. The TAE/TES regimen may be the best choice for managing patients with nAMD, particularly over the long term, regardless of the choice of the anti-VEGF agent. The TAE/TES method provides comparable visual results to monthly fixed interval dosing, however at a decreased treatment burden and has the potential for decreased adverse events. This proactive and patient-specific method also has many benefits over the PRN strategy, including but not limited to greater visual improvement, better maintenance of visual improvement over the long term, increased potential for disease remission, fewer rates of CNV recurrence, and the ability for recovery of vision after recurrence.

This chapter also discussed the definition of recurrence versus increased disease activity. Increased disease activity was defined as increased intraretinal or subretinal fluid with potentially decreased vision and increased metamorphopsia that occurred during active treatment. If patients fail to respond to any one agent after 4–6 monthly anti-VEGF injections and still have worsening subretinal or intraretinal fluid, these patients may meet the definition of primary treatment failure and the anti-VEGF agent can be switched. If patients are in the extension part of the TAE/TES protocol and there is increased fluid and exudation, the time interval between treatments should be reduced by 1–2 weeks if there is minimally increased exudation. If there is a significant increase in exudation or hemorrhage, then the time interval should be decreased more aggressively, potentially restarting the TAE/TES protocol. Patients with nAMD likely require at least 1 year of therapy, extended to 12-week treatment intervals, before treatment cessation is considered since there is a subset of patients of whom are delayed responders and may demonstrate increased vision over a longer time frame. A true disease recurrence would be defined as one where a CNV shows increased exudation and hemorrhage after 4 months of no treatment and careful monitoring. This true recurrence rate was found to be 29% in the TES protocol and patients with a true recurrence had overall visual outcomes comparable to their vision at treatment cessation after re-initiation of anti-VEGF treatment. It is likely that partial, poor or non-responders are more inclined to receive consistent treatment at time intervals in the 4–8 week range, and these patients' visual acuity over the long run may be best maintained with this dosing interval. This conservative calibration strategy thus strives to proactively optimize the treatment regimen to the patients' response.

Additional studies, particularly prospective randomized clinical trials evaluating the response of various treatment methodologies over the long term as well as those exploring the mechanisms underlying clinical outcomes, will help further optimize anti-VEGF therapy and spur the development of novel methods for the treatment of nAMD.

Conflict of interest

None.

Notes/thanks/other declarations

None.

Author details

Siyang Chaili and Sean D. Adrean*
Retina Consultants of Orange County, Fullerton, CA, USA

*Address all correspondence to: seadrean@yahoo.com

References

[1] Age-Related Macular Degeneration (AMD) [Internet]. 2018. Available from: https://nei.nih.gov/eyedata/amd [Accessed: 01 July 2018]

[2] Causes of blindness and visual impairment. [Internet]. 2018. Available from: http://www.who.int/blindness/causes/en/ [Accessed: 01 July 2018]

[3] Klein R, Klein BEK, Linton KLP. Prevalence of age-related maculopathy: The beaver dam eye study. Ophthalmology. 1991;**99**:933-943

[4] Hm L, Krueger DE, Maunder LR, et al. The Framingham eye study monograph. Survey of Ophthalmology. 1980;**24**:335-610

[5] Coleman HR, Chan CC, Ferris FL III, Chew EY. Age-related macular degeneration. Lancet. 2008;**372**(9652):1835-1845

[6] Jager RD, Mieler WF, Miller JW. Age-related macular degeneration. The New England Journal of Medicine. 2008;**358**(24):2606-2617

[7] Argon laser photocoagulation for neovascular maculopathy. Five-year results from randomized clinical trials. Macular Photocoagulation Study Group. Archives of Ophthalmology. 1991;**109**(8):1109-1114

[8] Krypton laser photocoagulation for neovascular lesions of age-related macular degeneration. Results of a randomized clinical trial. Macular Photocoagulation Study Group. Archives of Ophthalmology. 1990;**108**(6):816-824

[9] TAP Study Group. Photodynamic therapy of subfoveal choroidal neovascularization in age-related macular degeneration with verteporfin: One-year results of 2 randomized clinical trials–TAP report. Treatment of age-related macular degeneration with photodynamic therapy (TAP) Study Group. Archives of Ophthalmology. 1999;**117**(10):1329-1345

[10] Verteporfin in Photodynamic Therapy Study Group. Verteporfin therapy of subfoveal choroidal neovascularization in age-related macular degeneration: Two-year results of a randomized clinical trial including lesions with occult with no classic choroidal neovascularization–verteporfin in photodynamic therapy report 2. American Journal of Ophthalmology. 2001;**131**(5):541-560

[11] Miller JW. VEGF: From discovery to therapy: The Champalimaud award lecture. Translational Vision Science and Technology. 2016;**5**(2):9

[12] VEGF Inhibition Study in Ocular Neovascularization (V.I.S.I.O.N.) Clinical Trial Group. Year 2 efficacy results of 2 randomized controlled clinical trials of pegaptanib for neovascular age-related macular degeneration. Ophthalmology. 2006;**113**(9):1508.e1-1508.25

[13] Rosenfeld PJ, Moshfeghi AA, Puliafito CA. Optical coherence tomography findings after an intravitreal injection of bevacizumab (avastin) for neovascular age-related macular degeneration. Ophthalmic Surgery, Lasers & Imaging. 2005;**36**(4):331-335

[14] Rosenfeld PJ, Brown DM, Heier JS, et al. Ranibizumab for neovascular age-related macular degeneration. NEJM. 2006;**355**:1419-1431

[15] Brown DM, Michels M, Kaiser PK, et al. Ranibizumab versus verteporfin photodynamic therapy for neovascular age-related macular degeneration: Two-year results of the ANCHOR study. Ophthalmology. 2009;**116**(1):57-65.e5

[16] Heier JS, Brown DM, Chong V, et al. Intravitreal aflibercept (VEGF trap-eye) in wet age-related macular degeneration. Ophthalmology. 2012;**119**(12):2537-2548

[17] Cho H, Shah CP, Weber M, Heier JS. Aflibercept for exudative AMD with persistent fluid on ranibizumab and/or bevacizumab. The British Journal of Ophthalmology. 2013;**97**(8):1032-1035

[18] Kumar N, Marsiglia M, Mrejen S, Fung AT, Slakter J, et al. Visual and anatomical outcomes of intravitreal aflibercept in eyes with persistent subfoveal fluid despite previous treatments with ranibizumab in patients with neovascular age-related macular degeneration. Retina. 2013;**33**(8):1605-1612

[19] Macular Photocoagulation Study Group. Recurrent choroidal neovascularization after argon laser photocoagulation for neovascular maculopathy. Archives of Ophthalmology. 1986;**104**(4):503-512

[20] Macular Photocoagulation Study Group. Persistent and recurrent neovascularization after krypton laser photocoagulation for neovascular lesions of age-related macular degeneration. Archives of Ophthalmology. 1990;**108**(6):825-831

[21] Macular Photocoagulation Study Group. Persistent and recurrent neovascularization after laser photocoagulation for subfoveal choroidal neovascularization of age-related macular degeneration. Macular photocoagulation study group. Archives of Ophthalmology. 1994;**112**(4):489-499

[22] Adrean SD, Grant S, Chaili S. Bevacizumab (Avastin) and thermal laser combination therapy for peripapillary choroidal neovascular membranes. Journal of Ophthalmology. 2017;**2017**:4802690

[23] Dugel P, et al. HAWK & HARRIER: 48-week results of 2 multi-centered, randomized, double-masked trials of brolucizumab versus aflibercept for neovascular AMD. In: Presented at: The American Academy of Ophthalmology 2017 Annual Meeting on November 10, 2017; New Orleans

[24] Dugel P, et al. A comparison of the anatomical efficacy of brolucizumab and aflibercept in neovascular age-related macular degeneration (nAMD): An analysis over 16 weeks of matched treatment in the HAWK and HARRIER studies. In: Presented at: The Association for Research in Vision and Ophthalmology (ARVO) 2018 Annual Meeting; Honolulu, HI

[25] Busbee BG, Ho AC, Brown DM, et al. Twelve-month efficacy and safety of 0.5 mg or 2.0 mg ranibizumab in patients with subfoveal neovascular age-related macular degeneration. Ophthalmology. 2013;**120**(5):1046-1056

[26] Ho AC, Busbee BG, Regillo CD, et al. Twenty-four-month efficacy and safety of 0.5 mg or 2.0 mg ranibizumab in patients with subfoveal neovascular age-related macular degeneration. Ophthalmology. 2014;**121**(11):2181-2192

[27] CATT Research Group, Martin DF, Maguire MG, et al. Ranibizumab and bevacizumab for neovascular age-related macular degeneration. The New England Journal of Medicine. 2011;**364**(20):1897-1908

[28] CATT Research Group, Martin DF, Maguire MG, et al. Ranibizumab and bevacizumab for treatment of neovascular age-related macular degeneration: Two-year results. Ophthalmology. 2012;**119**(7):1388-1398

[29] Study Investigators IVAN, Chakravarthy U, Harding SP, Rogers CA, Downes SM, et al. Ranibizumab versus bevacizumab to treat neovascular age-related macular

degeneration: One-year findings from the IVAN randomized trial. Ophthalmology. 2012;**119**(7):1399-1411

[30] Chakravarthy U, Harding SP, Rogers CA, Downes SM, Lotery AJ, et al. Alternative treatments to inhibit VEGF in age-related choroidal neovascularisation: 2-year findings of the IVAN randomised controlled trial. Lancet. 2013;**382**(9900):1258-1267

[31] Regillo CD, Brown DM, Abraham P, et al. Randomized, double-masked, sham-controlled trial of ranibizumab for neovascular age-related macular degeneration: PIER Study year 1. American Journal of Ophthalmology. 2008;**145**(2):239-248

[32] Abraham P, Yue H, Wilson L. Randomized, double-masked, sham-controlled trial of ranibizumab for neovascular age-related macular degeneration: PIER study year 2. American Journal of Ophthalmology. 2010;**150**(3):315-324

[33] Do DV. Implications of the comparisons of age-related macular degeneration treatments trials on clinical practice: What have we learned? Ophthalmology. 2013;**120**(5 Suppl):S8-S10

[34] Peden MC, Suñer IJ, Hammer ME, et al. Long-term outcomes in eyes receiving fixed-interval dosing of anti-vascular endothelial growth factor agents for wet age-related macular degeneration. Ophthalmology. 2015;**122**(4):803-808

[35] Maguire MG, Martin DF, Ying GS, et al. Five-year outcomes with anti-vascular endothelial growth factor treatment of neovascular age-related macular degeneration: The comparison of age-related macular degeneration treatments trials. Ophthalmology. 2016;**123**(8):1751-1761

[36] Rofagha S, Bhisitkul RB, Boyer DS, et al. Seven-year outcomes in ranibizumab-treated patients in Anchor, Marina, and Horizon: A multicenter cohort study (SEVEN-UP). Ophthalmology. 2013;**120**(11):2292-2299

[37] Rasmussen A, Bloch SB, Fuchs J, et al. A 4-year longitudinal study of 555 patients treated with ranibizumab for neovascular age-related macular degeneration. Ophthalmology. 2013;**120**:2630-2636

[38] Gillies MC, Campain A, Barthelmes D, et al. Long-term outcomes of treatment of neovascular age-related macular degeneration: Data from an observational study. Ophthalmology. 2015;**122**(9):1837-1845

[39] Zhu M, Chew JK, Broadhead GK. Intravitreal ranibizumab for neovascular age-related macular degeneration in clinical practice: Five-year treatment outcomes. Graefe's Archive for Clinical and Experimental Ophthalmology. 2015;**253**(8):1217-1225

[40] Haddad WM, Minous FL, Legeai J, et al. Long-term outcomes and incidence of recurrence of neovascularization in treated exudative age-related macular degeneration. Retina. 2017;**37**(5):951-961

[41] Arevalo JF, Lasave AF, Wu L, et al. Intravitreal bevacizumab for choroidal neovascularization in age-related macular degeneration: 5-year results of the Pan-American Collaborative Retina Study Group. Retina. 2015;**36**:859-867

[42] Westborg I, Granstam E, Rosso A, Albrecht S, Karlsson N, et al. Treatment for neovascular age-related macular degeneration in Sweden: Outcomes at seven years in the Swedish Macula Register. Acta Ophthalmologica. 2017;**95**(8):787-795

[43] Adrean SD, Chaili S, Grant S, Pirouz A. Recurrence rate of choroidal neovascularization in neovascular

age-related macular degeneration managed with a treat–extend–stop protocol. Ophthalmology Retina. 2018;**2**(3):225-230

[44] American Society of Retina Specialists. PAT survey. 2016. Available from: https://www.asrs.org/international/global-trends-in-retina [Accessed: 01 July 2018]

[45] Berg K, Pedersen TR, Sandvik L, Bragadóttir R. Comparison of ranibizumab and bevacizumab for neovascular age-related macular degeneration according to LUCAS treat-and-extend protocol. Ophthalmology. 2015;**122**(1):146-152

[46] Wykoff CC, Croft DE, Brown DM, et al. Prospective trial of treat-and-extend versus monthly dosing for neovascular age-related macular degeneration: TREX-AMD 1-year results. Ophthalmology. 2015;**122**(12):2514-2522

[47] Chen YN, Powell AM, Mao A, Sheidow TG. Retrospective review of lucentis "treat and extend" patterns and outcomes in age-related macular degeneration. Retina. 2016;**36**(2):272-278

[48] Abedi F, Wickremasinghe S, Islam AF, Inglis KM, Guymer RH. Anti-VEGF treatment in neovascular age-related macular degeneration: A treat-and-extend protocol over 2 years. Retina. 2014;**34**(8):1531-1538

[49] Mrejen S, Jung JJ, Chen C, Patel SN, Gallego-Pinazo R, et al. Long-term visual outcomes for a treat and extend anti-vascular endothelial growth factor regimen in eyes with neovascular age-related macular degeneration. Journal of Clinical Medicine. 2015;**4**(7):1380-1402

[50] Adrean SD, Chaili S, Ramkumar H, Pirouz A, Grant S. Consistent long-term therapy of neovascular age-related macular degeneration managed by 50 or more anti-VEGF injections using a treat-extend-stop protocol. Ophthalmology. 2018;**125**:1047-1053

[51] Rufai SR, Almuhtaseb H, Paul RM, Stuart BL, Kendrick T. A systematic review to assess the 'treat-and-extend' dosing regimen for neovascular age-related macular degeneration using ranibizumab. Eye (London, England). 2017;**31**(9):1337-1344

[52] Chin-Yee D, Eck T, Fowler S, Hardi A, Apte RS. A systematic review of as needed versus treat and extend ranibizumab or bevacizumab treatment regimens for neovascular age-related macular degeneration. The British Journal of Ophthalmology. 2016;**100**(7):914-917

[53] Oubraham H, Cohen SY, Samimi S, Marotte D, Bouzaher I. Inject and extend dosing versus dosing as needed: A comparative retrospective study of ranibizumab in exudative age-related macular degeneration. Retina. 2011;**31**(1):26-30

[54] Hatz K, Prünte C. Changing from a pro re nata treatment regimen to a treat and extend regimen with ranibizumab in neovascular age-related macular degeneration. The British Journal of Ophthalmology. 2016;**100**(10):1341-1345

[55] Cohen SY, Dubois L, Ayrault S, et al. Ranibizumab for exudative AMD in a clinical setting: Differences between 2007 and 2010. Graefe's Archive for Clinical and Experimental Ophthalmology. 2013;**251**(11):2499-2503

[56] Kuroda Y, Yamashiro K, Miyake M, Yoshikawa M, Nakanishi H. Factors associated with recurrence of age-related macular degeneration after anti-vascular endothelial growth factor treatment: A retrospective cohort study. Ophthalmology. 2015;**122**(11):2303-2310

[57] Shah AR, Del Priore LV. Natural history of predominantly classic, minimally classic, and occult subgroups in exudative age-related macular degeneration. Ophthalmology. 2009;**116**(10):1901-1907

[58] Schneider U, Gelisken F, Inhoffen W. Natural course of occult choroidal neovascularization in age-related macular degeneration: Development of classic lesions in fluorescein angiography. Acta Ophthalmologica Scandinavica. 2005;**83**(2):141-147

[59] Berg K, Roald AB, Navaratnam J, Bragadóttir R. An 8-year follow-up of anti-vascular endothelial growth factor treatment with a treat-and-extend modality for neovascular age-related macular degeneration. Acta Ophthalmologica. 2017;**95**(8):796-802

[60] Pedrosa AC, Sousa T, Pinheiro-Costa J, Beato J, Falcão MS, et al. Treatment of neovascular age-related macular degeneration with anti-VEGF agents: Predictive factors of long-term visual outcomes. Journal of Ophthalmology. 2017;**2017**:4263017

[61] Lumbroso B, Rispoli M, Savastano MC, et al. Optical coherence tomography angiography study of choroidal neovascularization early response after treatment. Developments in Ophthalmology. 2016;**56**:77-85

[62] Bhisitkul RB, Mendes TS, Rofagha S, Enanoria W, Boyer DS, et al. Macular atrophy progression and 7-year vision outcomes in subjects from the ANCHOR, MARINA, and HORIZON studies: The SEVEN-UP study. American Journal of Ophthalmology. 2015;**159**(5):915-24.e2

[63] Grunwald JE, Pistilli M, Daniel E, Ying GS, Pan W, et al. Incidence and growth of geographic atrophy during 5 years of comparison of age-related macular degeneration treatments trials. Ophthalmology. 2017;**124**(1):97-104

[64] Eldem BM, Muftuoglu G, Topbaş S, Çakir M, Kadayifcilar S, et al. A randomized trial to compare the safety and efficacy of two ranibizumab dosing regimens in a Turkish cohort of patients with choroidal neovascularization secondary to AMD. Acta Ophthalmologica. 2015;**93**(6):e458-e464

[65] Brown DM, Regillo CD. Anti-VEGF agents in the treatment of neovascular age-related macular degeneration: Applying clinical trial results to the treatment of everyday patients. American Journal of Ophthalmology. 2007;**144**(4):627-637

[66] Amoaku WM, Chakravarthy U, Gale R, et al. Defining response to anti-VEGF therapies in neovascular AMD. Eye (London, England). 2015;**29**(6):721-731

Chapter 14

Diabetic Retinopathy and Blindness: An Epidemiological Overview

Maya Georgieva Pandova

Abstract

Prevalence of diabetes is rising worldwide. In the course of the last 20 years, blindness and low vision due to diabetic eye complications have increased in large regions in Eastern Europe, North Africa/Middle East, Asia, Latin America, and Oceania. The magnitude and trends of vision-threatening disease are presented. Systemic risk factors for progression to sight-threatening disease are reviewed. The impact of economic and cultural background on early diagnosis and adherence to treatment is highlighted. Current management of diabetic macular edema, proliferative diabetic retinopathy, neovascular glaucoma, and cataract surgery of diabetic patients is outlined, and its contribution to preventing vision loss is reviewed.

Keywords: diabetic retinopathy, trends, blindness, risk factors, treatment, visual outcome

1. Introduction

> *"It is a truism that each solution brings its own problems. Diabetic retinopathy in survivors of longstanding diabetes...represents the price paid for conquests that are not quite complete. The prolongation of life without corresponding prolongation of health, is loaded with intractable problems." commented Arnold Sorsby on the "striking increase" of blindness from diabetes for both men and women between 1948 and 1962. [1]*

The next six decades saw intensive research in the pathogenesis and epidemiology of diabetic eye disease and the introduction of laser photocoagulation in the early treatment of diabetic retinopathy, pars plana vitrectomy for traction, and rhegmatogenous retinal detachment and intravitreal pharmacotherapy in the management of diabetic macular edema (DME), all addressing prevention of vision loss in these patients.

2. Magnitude of blindness due to diabetic eye disease

Reports on the vision loss attributable to diabetes in the 1980s and 1990s vary greatly in their methodology—some have derived clinical information from hospital series, and others have reviewed the registry forms of certified disabled persons from the records of societies of the blind; there are reviews on patients referred to low vision rehabilitation centers and finally some present data from population-based observational studies. Each source has its shortcomings. Definitions in registry databases depend on the national disability legislation and often differ from the categories for blindness and low vision in the International Classification of Diseases (ICD)—Ninth and Tenth Revisions—that were in use at that time. Many authors stress on the difficult task of identifying the onset and the main cause of vision loss in diabetic patients with multiple ophthalmic comorbidities, especially in their final stages. For a long period, well into the 1980s, non-ophthalmic professionals were allowed to certify blind persons for registration that raises reservations regarding the accuracy of the cause. A common concern is the inability to determine the number of underreported and unregistered diabetic persons with vision loss as registration is voluntary, and it depends on clinical, social, and cultural factors; many authors have noted a rise in the incidence rates of DR with the arrival of more consultants in the area, after upgrade in the financial benefits and social support for legally blind or following campaigns to improve public awareness and reduce stigmatization.

Hospital series analyze clinical data collected in specialized diabetic units over long periods in a consistent manner and provide reliable estimate on the severity and progression of vision loss; however, extrapolations of their findings for the population beyond their urban region are seldom possible.

Publications from the UK, Denmark, and Sweden demonstrate a decrease in the incidence of new blindness from DR in the 1980s and 1990s [2–5]; however it remained unchanged between 1967 and 1991 in Italy and Avon, UK [6, 7]. In their review on the trends in blindness in Singapore, See et al. [8] present a sharp increase in the prevalence of diabetes in the age between 15 and 69 from 1.99% in 1975 to 8.6% in 1992 and a rise in the proportion of blindness from diabetic complications from 5% in the 1950s to 47.3% in the 1980s.

Global data on blindness [9, 10], a review report of the WHO programme for prevention of blindness, summarized available information from population-based assessment of visual loss and its causes. DR was not among the four major causes for blindness and low vision globally and ranked between the first and fourth only in Western Europe, the former socialist economies of Europe, North America, Latin America, and Oceania. The authors note the lack of relevant epidemiological data for some specific causes of blindness; however they emphasize that this disease is "generally recognized to be the leading cause of blindness among those in working age in developed countries and rapidly emerging in urban areas of the developing world."

An update on the estimates of global and regional blindness and low vision was published in 2004 presenting results of new population-based studies and other sources of information. The proportion of DR rose to 4.8% globally, and it was ranked fifth as a cause of blindness, with significant regional variations reaching 17% for North America and Australia, 17–15% in Europe, and 3–7% in the rest of the world where the majority of vision loss was due to cataract, glaucoma, and corneal opacities as complications of trachoma [11].

A meta-analysis of all available population-based studies performed worldwide from 1990 to 2010 [12] estimated that 833,690 people were blind and 3.7 million were visually impaired globally in 2010 due to DR. The highest number of blind diabetic patients was in South Asia, 295,000; North Africa/Middle East, 108,000; Eastern sub-Saharan Africa, 50,000; and Western sub-Saharan Africa, 66,000. The age-standardized prevalence of blindness from diabetic retinopathy in people over the age of 50 years was 0.05% globally, reaching 0.19% in Western sub-Saharan Africa, 0.16% in North Africa/Middle East, 0.14% in Eastern sub-Saharan Africa, and 0.12% in Southeast and East Asia. Moderate and severe vision impairment due to DR affected 3174 million, and the largest number of them were in South Asia, 1450 million, followed by North Africa/Middle East, 336,000; Eastern Asia, 279,000; Western Europe, 225,000; Western sub-Saharan Africa, 193,000; Eastern Europe, 166,000; Eastern sub-Saharan Africa, 128,000; and Central Latin America, 109,000. The age-standardized prevalence of moderate and severe vision impairment due to DR in people over the age of 50 years was 1.9% globally and was highest—0.51%—in South Asia, 0.50% in Western sub-Saharan Africa, 0.44% in North Africa/Middle East, 0.36% in Southern Latin America, 0.33% in Central sub-Saharan Africa, 0.32% in Andean Latin America, 0.31% in Eastern sub-Saharan Africa, and 0.26% in Oceania [13]. From 1990 to 2010, the number of blind diabetics had increased by 27% and those with visual impairment by 64% globally. Globally, age-standardized prevalence of blindness and vision impairment of diabetics over the age of 50 years was relatively unchanged in the course of these 20 years. It reduced by half in high-income Pacific Asia, Europe, Australasia, and North America; however it remained high in large, densely populated regions of Africa and Asia with rapidly increasing prevalence of diabetes.

A continuation of this systematic review and meta-analysis of data from 261 population-based studies published till 2014 [14] observed that while blindness to all causes reduced between 1990 and 2015, DR was the only one with prevalence that increased by 7.7% for blindness and by 28.6% for impairment. The proportion of vision loss attributable to diabetes ranked seventh in 2015 at 1.06% (0.15–2.38) globally and was highest in Eastern Europe, 4.91%, followed by Australasia, high-income North America, high-income Pacific Asia, and Central Asia. The contribution of DR to moderate and severe vision impairment was 1.30% (0.20–2.93) and reached 5.06% in Eastern Europe, followed by Australasia, high-income North America, high-income Pacific Asia, and Central Asia. The same regions were leading in the percentage of blindness and low vision due to DR for people over the age of 50 years. The age-standardized prevalence of blindness from DR across all ages was relatively low, in the range of 0.00–0.01 (0.00–0.02), and was considerably higher for vision impairment, 0.03% (0.00–0.13), with Eastern Europe ranking first at 0.11%, Central Asia, 0.09%; Southern Latin America, 0.08%; and North Africa/Middle East and Australasia, 0.07%. The age-standardized prevalence of blindness of diabetics over the age of 50 was 0.02% (0.00–0.07) and was highest in North Africa/Middle East, Eastern Europe, and Central Asia. The age-standardized prevalence of low vision in the same age group was 0.13% (0.01–0.48), and the same regions were most affected. For the first time, this report presented data on the gender differences in the cause and magnitude of vision loss and demonstrated that the relative risk of blindness and vision impairment in diabetic women as compared to men was 2.52. The number of people with blindness due to diabetic retinopathy was estimated at 400,000 (0–1.5 million) and low vision 2.6 million (0.2 million—9.9 million), both almost doubled since 1990. The projections for diabetic complications for 2020 are for further increase, and the largest number of people are expected to reside in North Africa/Middle East, 73,000 blind and 4,480,000 with low vision; Eastern Europe, 47,000 blind and 362,000 with low vision; Western Europe, 46,000 blind and 422,000 with low vision; East Asia, 41,000 blind and 400,000 with low vision; and Southeast Asia, 30,000 blind and 216,000 with low vision. The authors point out that the prevalence of any DR and sight-threatening DR was similar in men and women, whereas their analysis suggested female preponderance for vision-impairing DR. They attribute this discrepancy to the use of aggregated data for both genders combined in some of the studies and highlight the need for further research into the gender differences. There are considerable regional variations in the blindness and low vision due to DR, and they are related to the prevalence of diabetes in the population and the life expectancy of the diabetic patients. In the Middle East, Kuwait, for example, the prevalence of diabetes has reached 20–25% of the whole population and over 50% after the age of 60 years. In some regions, in particular in South Asia, the life expectancy of diabetic individuals is reduced, they do not have the chance to develop retinopathy as sequela of the disease, and the prevalence of debilitating retinopathy is low despite the high proportion of diabetes.

A detailed meta-analysis of the trends in vision loss in high-income countries in Pacific Asia, Australasia, North and Latin America and Western Europe, as well as Central and Eastern Europe from 1990 to 2015 [15] presented a relatively low and stable prevalence of blindness due to DR for all ages in the range of 0.01–0.02% in the whole super-region; however the rates for moderate and severe visual impairment varied in the range from 0.6–0.7% in most of the high-income countries to 1.6% in Eastern Europe and Australasia. The crude prevalence of blindness among diabetics over 50 years was in the range of 0.02–0.03% in the high-income countries, 0.04% in Central Europe, and 0.06–0.07% in Eastern Europe, and visual impairment was lowest in Western and Central Europe and Pacific Asia, followed by North America and Australasia and highest in Eastern Europe. The projections for 2020 were for stable or slightly reduced prevalence of blindness and gradual increase of patients with visual impairment in the super-region.

Vision loss in the multiethnic population of Singapore over the age of 40 years was investigated in a series of population-based studies that demonstrated relatively high prevalence of diabetes in the sample—29.5%; DR was the second leading cause of vision impairment and blindness, and Indians and Malays were more affected than the Chinese. The authors point out that DR-related blindness in these three ethnicities in Singapore was less than the mainland Southern Indians, mainland Han Chinese, and peninsula Malays, and they attribute this to better access to qualified eye screening and care in Singapore. Diabetes was a significant contributing factor for visual impairment generally and increased the risk by 2.96 for people below the age of 60 years and 12.70 times for those over 60, particularly for females and patients with cognitive impairment and deafness, a tendency that was consistently observed across Malays, Indians, and Chinese. Diabetes in combination with other comorbidities, hypertension, hyperlipidemia, cardiovascular, or renal disease, was associated with higher risk of vision loss, up to 9.51 for people younger than 60 years and 26.56 for those older than 60, particularly for Indians, and an interaction effect for concomitant diabetes and renal diseases [16].

Vision-threatening DR (VTDR) is a compound term used in the literature for the presence of proliferative disease grading over level 60 by EDTRS scale and its modification and/or macular edema in its various stages [17, 18], and its magnitude is essential for planning the life-long management of these patients and prevention of blindness. The prevalence and risk factors of VTDR were estimated in a large meta-analysis of 38 population-based studies from Australia, the USA, Europe, and Asia involving 42,091 participants from 20 to 79 years with diabetes. There was no discernible sex difference in the age-standardized prevalence of VTDR, 11.7%; it was highest among African Americans, 16.89%; followed by Caucasians, 15.45%; and Hispanics, 10.35, and was lowest in South Asians—5.2%. Duration of diabetes (DM) was associated with rapidly increasing prevalence from 3.53% for DM less than 10 years to 17.78% for 10–20 years and up to 87% for more than 20 years.

Metabolic control, estimated by the levels of HbA1c, directly affected the extent of VTDR—the disease doubled in patients with levels between 7.1 and 8.0% and tripled among those with more than 9.0%. Elevated blood pressure over 140/90 and hypercholesterolemia over 4.0 mMol/L elevated the risk of VTDR twice, particularly for macular edema. Individuals with type 1 diabetes for more than 20 years were 15 times more likely to have proliferative diabetic retinopathy (PDR) (15.3 [11.3–20.8]), 5 times more likely to have DME (4.83 [3.71–6.30]), and 8.7 times more likely to have VTDR (8.69 [7.10–10.63]) than those with type 2 diabetes for less than 10 years. On a positive note, the prevalence of VTDR reduced from 15.62% in studies where the fundus photographs were taken before the year 2000 to 7.86% in the studies with assessment of the patients after 2000.

This pivotal work highlighted the importance and cutoff levels of the systemic factors associated with progression of DR to sight-threatening stage and the need for close collaboration with the treating diabetology team. It outlined the profile of the patients at risk of vision loss with their features—type and duration of diabetes, levels of metabolic control, hypertension, and hypercholesterolemia. The role of ethnicity was limited to the populations studied, and the authors note the absence of studies from Middle East, Africa, and South America that could affect the accuracy of their global estimates. The differences in the rates of VTDR in the various populations could be due to both genetic factors and access to health care. Ethnicity itself is multidimensional, and it may not be possible to differentiate its effect from the risk associated with remoteness, urbanization, lifestyle, education, health awareness, and individual income.

3. Social and economic risk factors

Social and economic factors have a fundamental impact on the visual prognosis of diabetic eye disease. A number of studies have investigated the negative influence of deprivation on the prevalence of diabetes, access to evaluation and care, level of metabolic control, and rate of complications and were reported in systematic reviews for type 1 [19] and type 2 diabetes [20]. Remoteness [odds ratio (OR) 2.02] and diabetes in combination with never having had an eye examination (OR 14.47) were among the main risk factors for vision loss in indigenous Australians, and blindness prevalence was 2.8 times higher among them than in non-indigenous Australians after age and gender adjustment [21]. The presence of PDR was associated with low income (OR = 3.6 for developing PDR if income was less than $20000) in the Proyecto VER Study in the USA involving 4774 Hispanics over the age of 40, after controlling for other factors [22]. Deprivation, as a comprehensive measure of income, employment, health and disability, education, crime, barriers to housing, services, and living environment at the level of small geographic areas, was developed in the UK as a numerical index per residential code and used in a large national database study of 79,775 diabetic patients to highlight its effect on visual acuity and need for early treatment at first hospital presentation [23]. The OR of presenting with "sight impairment" at first visit to the hospital eye service was gradually decreasing from 1.29 in the most deprived group to 0.77 in the least deprived one, and OR for "severely sight impaired" was 1.17 in the most deprived decile versus 0.88 in the least deprived one. The risk of sight-threatening maculopathy and vitreous hemorrhages showed little variations across the deprivation range, and tractional retinal detachment was less likely in the two least deprived deciles. The large scale of the study and use of "real-world" multicenter in-hospital dataset provided statistical strength to the conclusion that the impact of deprivation extends to late presentation of retinopathy, significant loss of vision at presentation, and a pattern of advanced retinal complications that affect the treatment these patients receive. Financial factors are often self-reported by diabetic patients who are missing screening appointments and treatment sessions. However a study in Tanzania revealed that the reasons for poor compliance are more complicated. The clarity of referral process and ease of navigation through the unfamiliar hospital environment are essential, particularly for the elderly and less educated patients from remote areas [24]. Another formidable obstacle is the widespread complacency and fatalistic resignation with the notion that retinopathy will inevitably end up with blindness. Constant assurance and encouragement that diabetic eye disease is a treatable condition with good prognosis is a practical strategy to prevent delays in diagnosis of sight-threatening complications. Lack of education greatly affects the health awareness and adherence with retinopathy management. In Kuwait, 16% of the men and 46% of the women over 65 years are illiterate, and 20% of the men and 24% of the women in the same age group can only read and write [25]. This is a significant barrier to in-depth understanding and compliance with recommended treatment and lifestyle and eventually compromises the visual outcome despite the high economic standard of the Kuwaiti nationals and availability of services in the country. Family support greatly improves the continuum of care and is essential for the regular attendance of the patients, especially females from a more conservative background.

Progression of nonproliferative to proliferative disease was investigated in several large cohort studies [26, 27]. Disease severity was estimated by the EDTRS classification and taken separately for each eye or concatenated as the bilateral grade, and progression was defined as the increase of two or more steps in severity. The rate of progression to PDR varied greatly—it was from 4 to 9.9% in the first 4–5 years and 8–12% in the next 5 years and reached a cumulative level of 31% after 16 years and 42% after 25 years in type 1 and type 2 diabetics. There are differences between the populations and methodology applied in the hospital-based and community-based studies as more patients with severe disease that required active management were probably referred to tertiary care centers [28–32].

The diagnosis of diabetic macular edema has evolved with the introduction of stereoscopic photography of the posterior pole and optical coherence tomography (OCT). The presence of any edema and clinically significant edema (CSME) by the modified EDTRS classification has been investigated in multiple hospital series and population-based studies. Detection of DME in non-stereoscopic fundus photographs is less sensitive to milder forms with recent onset, and probably the reported prevalence covers the more severe chronic stage. The prevalence of CSME in type 1 patients was from 5.73% in Spain to 9.4% in Brazil [33, 34]. Among patients with type 2 diabetes, it was in the range from 1.4% in Portugal to 12.8% in Denmark [35, 36]. There are reports indicating that the prevalence of DME in Central and Eastern Europe [37], North Africa, and Middle East [38] is considerably higher, and further research on the magnitude of CSME and risk factors for its progression will contribute to the estimates of sight-threatening retinopathy globally.

4. Diabetic nephropathy

Diabetic nephropathy (DN), the primary cause of chronic kidney disease, is significantly associated with incidence and progression of diabetic retinopathy as demonstrated in Brazilian [39], Spanish [40], Korean [41], Taiwanese Chinese [42], and Australian [43] patients. The presence of chronic kidney impairment had adjusted a hazard ratio of 5.01 for nonproliferative and 9.7 for proliferative disease as compared to patients without nephropathy. At 5-year follow-up, the hazard ratio of progression to PDR was 2.26 in patients with DN, and it was related to the levels of microalbuminuria and estimated glomerular filtration rate with cutoff below 60 mL/min/1.73 m^2 [44]. Hypertension and DN in patients with chronic kidney disease increased the risk of progression to proliferative disease; however diabetic nephropathy did not significantly affect the development or progression of DME. Among the Taiwanese Chinese patients, diabetic macular edema had high crude hazard ratio association with cerebrovascular accidents and lesser one for hypertension and use of statins; however the significance was lost after controlling for age, sex, comorbidities, and medications.

5. Pregnancy in diabetic patients

Diabetes affects 17% of pregnancies worldwide and can be pre-existing type 1, gestational, or type 2, in some of the patients—previously undiagnosed. The highest rate of diabetes in pregnancy is recorded in Southeast Asia, 25%, and the prevalence of pre-existing diabetes is highest among women from the Middle East and North Africa—3.1%. Australian mothers who were born in high diabetes risk areas such as Polynesia, Asia, and the Middle East are 1.4 times more likely to have type 2 diabetes during pregnancy [45]. Similarly, in the USA and UK, patients belonging to Black, Asian, Hispanic, and Pacific Island ethnic minorities had higher proportion of pre-existing diabetes and pre-existing type 2 DM. Progression of retinopathy during pregnancy is related to the level of diabetic retinopathy prior to conception and was noted in 58% of the patients with moderate or more severe DR at baseline. Duration of diabetes type 1 greater than 15 years and type 2 more than 6 years was significantly associated with higher rate of progression of retinopathy in patients with pre-existing proliferative disease. Poor glycemic control prior and during pregnancy was an independent risk factor for retinopathy progression; however tight control and rapid optimization of metabolic control in such patients were associated with worsening of retinopathy. As the long-term benefits of proper glycemic management outweigh the short-term risk of deteriorating retinopathy, optimal control is currently recommended prior to and as soon as possible after conception for the health of the mother and fetus. Progression of retinopathy during pregnancy was significantly higher in diabetic patients with preeclampsia, with sight-threatening complications in 50% of the diabetic women with preeclampsia compared to 8% without it [46]. Other risk factors for deteriorated retinopathy during pregnancy include young age of type 1 onset, insulin treatment in type 2 prior to pregnancy, low vision at baseline, and pre-existing macular edema at baseline [47].

6. Diabetic foot syndrome

Diabetic foot syndrome is one of the important consequences of long-term uncontrolled diabetes, which occurs due to a combination of peripheral neuropathy and microvasculopathy in the lower extremities. It may vary from a minor ulceration to necrosis of tissues, sometimes warranting amputation [48]. Several hospital series demonstrated the presence of retinopathy in 90–95% and proliferative disease and severe nonproliferative changes in 39–55% in such patients independent of the ulcer severity [49]. Diabetic foot syndrome in type 1 and type 2 diabetic patients with retinopathy was associated with higher levels of HbA1c, serum creatinine, older age, and lower hematocrit, particularly elevated in the subgroup with proliferative disease—all characteristics of concomitant chronic kidney disease and neuropathy in poorly controlled, long-lasting diabetes. Despite the lack of data on macular edema, the presence of any stage of diabetic foot ulcer is emerging as a predictor for retinopathy deterioration [50, 51].

7. Depression and anxiety

The overall prevalence of depressive symptoms in diabetic patients with retinopathy is estimated in the range of 35% in China to 50% in African Americans and is more prevalent in type 2 [52, 53]. The association between depressive symptoms, diabetes, and diabetic retinopathy is likely to be bidirectional: the impairment and burden of diabetes and its complications can precipitate depression and vice versa, and depression can impair diabetes control through various biological and behavioral pathways [54, 55]. Depression aggregates negative attitudes toward treatment and often leads to poorer glycemic control, less adherence to treatment, higher risk for PDR, greater morbidity and mortality, and higher costs [56]. Low income has been implicated in some research from the USA; however it was not found significant in a large cross-sectional study from Australia. Patients with longer duration of diabetes, worse glycemic control, lower educational level, and severe vision impairment below 20/63 were associated with greater depression symptoms. Symptoms of anxiety were associated with type 1 diabetes, presence of myocardial infarction/ angina, arrhythmia, stroke, asthma, anemia, arthritis or osteoporosis, younger age, and female gender [57]. Severe NPDR and PDR, but not macular edema, were independently associated with depressive symptoms, and the authors suggest that severity of retinopathy could be an indicator to prompt monitoring of depression in at-risk diabetic individuals. Antidepressant medications have been associated with slowing the progression of retinopathy in diabetic patients. However the outcome was limited to subjects with elevated C-reactive protein over 0.3 mg/dL. Selective serotonin reuptake inhibitor users had significantly lower risk of developing severe retinopathy than non-SSRI users [58]. The results of longitudinal studies show that the speed of cognitive decline in type 2 diabetic patients is up to twice as fast as that of normal aging individuals and diabetic patients have an increased risk of mild cognitive impairment (MCI). In addition, type 2 diabetic patients had an almost twofold higher risk of developing Alzheimer's disease than age-matched nondiabetic subjects. This increased risk was maintained even after adjusting for vascular risk factors. The annual conversion rate from MCI to dementia ranges between 10 and 30% in the general population, but this is much higher in the type 2 diabetic population. The impact of cognitive impairment on the compliance with lifelong retinopathy treatment and its outcome needs further evaluation; however clinical practice indicates the need for personalized multidisciplinary approach.

8. Progression to vision-threatening retinopathy

The variability in the rate of progression to vision-threatening retinopathy and particularly in the response to treatment was noted from the onset of clinical and epidemiological studies in diabetic patients and has been attributed to the effect of genetic predisposition together with systemic and socioeconomic factors. Single-nucleotide polymorphisms [58–60] and genome-wide associations [61–63] have been investigated in patients with proliferative disease and macular edema, and the results so far are inconclusive mainly due to the size of the samples and the inclusion of cases with coexisting proliferations and edema in the cohorts. Detailed assessment in the polymorphisms of the VEGF gene revealed that some of them are related to higher susceptibility to severe retinopathy, but not to the outcome of ranibizumab intravitreal injections [64] in contrast to an earlier report on the response to bevacizumab [65]. In order to confirm the association of several novel genetic loci with severe retinopathy, replication studies and extension in additional cohorts and ethnic groups have been recommended [66]. Research of systemic and retinal inflammation as risk factors for DR and DME [67, 68], upregulated leptin [69, 70] and adiponectin [71], oxidative stress [72], and vitamin D deficiency [73] has provided significant associations. Reliable and accessible markers of these factors can be important predictors of the disease severity and progression and thus provide early guidance in personalizing the monitoring and treatment of the patients at risk of vision loss.

9. Management of DME

The introduction of intravitreal anti-VEGF drugs and corticosteroid implants revolutionized the management of DME. Prospective randomized clinical trials have addressed the efficacy and safety of different types of agents and administration regimens and have shown wide variations in terms of visual acuity gain. In the DRCR.net trial, after 2 years of treatment, approximately 98% of the patients maintained their visual acuity and attained visual gain in 37% of the patients on ranibizumab, 35% of those on bevacizumab, and 39% of those on aflibercept [74]. Stratified analysis of RESTORE in DME, RETAIN, and Protocol I demonstrated that the most significant gain in number of EDTRS letters after 12–36 months was in patients with baseline BCVA 60 and less letters in the range of 8.6–10.36 letters, versus the gain for patients with baseline BCVA 61–71 letters who achieved 7.96–4.36 letters, and the least gain of 5.42–4.2 letters was in the group with baseline BCVA better that 73 letters [75]. Thus, the patients with most severe vision deterioration and baseline BCVA in the range of 20/320–20/63 who responded favorably to 2 years of intensive therapy improved to BCVA from 20/160 to 20/40. High visual acuity in the range of 20/40–20/32 was achieved only in patients with baseline BCVA over 20/30 despite the small number of gained EDTRS letters. The range and stability of this visual improvement depended on increasing age, level of glycemic control, and previous panretinal photocoagulation [76]. OCT markers of better functional outcome after anti-VEGF treatment were the presence of intact ellipsoid zone and lack of hyperreflective spots or disruption of the inner retinal layers, which are seen in patients with more recent onset of the edema and no previous macular grid laser [77]. Patients with chronic macular edema had considerably better functional and structural results after treatment with steroid implants. Visual gain of more than 15 letters was achieved in 22% after 3 years on intravitreal dexamethasone [78] and in 34% after 3 years on fluocinolone acetonide [79]. Eyes with submacular fluid, no hyperreflective foci, and a continuous IS-OS layer responded better to dexamethasone implants with gain of 10 or more letters after 2 and 4 months [80]. The adverse effects of both implants included the formation of cataract, 13–50% after 1 year on dexamethasone and 82% after 3 years on fluocinolone acetonide, and intraocular pressure rise over 25 mmHg in 42% of the eyes with dexamethasone and 38% with fluocinolone acetonide; however a small percentage required glaucoma surgery—0.5% of the eyes with dexamethasone and 4.8% with fluocinolone acetonide. Patients with poorly controlled diabetes and DME, severe nonproliferative or proliferative disease, epimacular membranes, myopia, glaucoma, and various degrees of cataract are excluded from the randomized clinical trials; however such cases are predominant in real-world practice and add new dimensions to the challenge of visual rehabilitation. Analysis of large electronic medical record databases from the USA [81] and Korea [82] demonstrated visual outcomes that are meaningfully inferior to those in the clinical trials and were attributed to undertreatment and lack of close monitoring. A sizable group of DME patients were lost to follow-up in the initial stages of anti-VEGF treatment—25% were reported from a single retina practice in the USA and the main risk factors were being Hispanic, Black, or a Pacific islander; low income, AGI less than $50,000; and decreasing baseline visual acuity [83]. In a study of European DME patients, 46% had at least one break-off in their anti-VEGF treatment for more than 100 days, and the most common reason for poor compliance was comorbidity. In 60% of these cases, the visual acuity deteriorated significantly after the break [84]. Prevention of vision loss from diabetic macular edema is achievable with the current therapeutic modalities; however it requires very early identification at stages with relatively high visual acuity and needs the introduction of best-corrected visual acuity and OCT in the screening protocol. As shown in the Protocol G—Subclinical DME study of the DRCR.net that involved a longitudinal assessment of eyes that had retinal thickening on OCT without thickening on clinical exam, a progression to clinically apparent DME was seen in 23–58% of eyes within 2 years.

10. Management of proliferative disease

Vision loss in approximately 25% of patient with diabetic retinopathy is associated with complications of proliferative disease. An estimated 17 million diabetic people worldwide have PDR [17], and without treatment more than half of the patients with high-risk PDR will be blind within 5 years. Panretinal photocoagulation was established as an effective treatment to reduce by 50% the incidence of severe vision loss, if performed prior to the development of vitreous hemorrhages and tractional retinal detachment [85]. Still, the EDTRS has shown that 5% of patients with PDR will require vitreous surgery despite having received adequate PRP [86]. The Diabetic Retinopathy Vitrectomy Study validated the superiority of vitrectomy over observation; however despite the fact that the trial did not include patients with macula, involving traction, the visual outcome was low. Subsequent studies on vitrectomy for PDR reported that between 10 and 20% of the patients did not improve their visual acuity above hand motion or less [87]. Favorable factors for visual rehabilitation after vitrectomy for macula-involving tractional retinal detachment included short duration of detachment, previous panretinal photocoagulation, and lack of severe neovascularization and vitreous hemorrhage. Predictors of poor visual results were iris neovascularization and neovascular glaucoma, papillo-vitreal traction, baseline visual acuity below 20/200, initial macular detachment, intraoperative iatrogenic break, or use of heavy silicone oil [88–90]. Functional outcome was significantly affected in patients with postoperative macular ischemia, recurrent vitreous hemorrhage, optic atrophy, epiretinal membranes, and recurrent retinal detachment [91, 92]. The introduction of small-gauge vitrectomy instruments and trans-scleral cannulas enabled the fast and effective removal of most fibrovascular membranes with the vitrectomy probe applying the lift and shave technique [93]. Visual outcomes were poorer in older age group, tractional retinal detachments involving macula and eyes with extensive membranes and with silicone oil as tamponade; however both 23-gauge and 25-gauge groups were comparable in relation to visual improvement, anatomical success, and intraoperative and postoperative complications [94]. The integration of swept-source optical coherence tomography and digital displays can provide important guidance during surgery for PDR complications and facilitate decision-making [95]; however further research will show whether these technological advances will translate into better postoperative visual outcome.

Medical treatment for PDR has had minimal advancement over the past 40 years since the wide acceptance of panretinal photocoagulation in the early management of the disease. Regression of proliferative activity was noted in eyes treated with anti-VEGF for concomitant macular edema [96] and that lead to a series of trials on aflibercept and ranibizumab versus panretinal photocoagulation in the management of PDR. Both drugs were superior to PRP in 1 [97] and 2 years [98] in terms of visual acuity and visual field sensitivity. Assessment of the peripapillary retinal nerve fiver layer thickness in patients treated with ranibizumab revealed reduction that was due to decreased edema rather than loss of axons [99]. Patients with mild and moderate vitreous hemorrhages treated with ranibizumab had significantly less need for vitrectomy, less recurrences of hemorrhage, and better visual acuity on all follow-up visits than the patient under observation or operated for non-resolving or aggravated hemorrhages [100]. However, despite the improvement in retinopathy severity on color photographs, the retinal perfusion did not improve on wide-field fluorescein angiography that revealed no reperfusion of small vessels in areas of previous capillary non-perfusion [101]. Diabetic patients are prone to significant loss to follow up due to illness, financial hardship, and lack of compliance. The rate of complications and loss of vision after unintentional interruptions for more than 6 months in PDR patients treated only on anti-VEGF was considerably higher than the eyes that received PRP, with a significantly higher number of eyes with tractional retinal detachment and neovascularization of the iris [102]. In a retrospective review of 13 eyes treated exclusively with anti-VEGF for PDR with or without macular edema or severe NPDR with macular edema, with hiatus of 12 months, 9 presented with vitreous hemorrhage, 5 with neovascular glaucoma, and 4 with tractional retinal detachment. Despite the aggressive treatment of the complications, 10 eyes lost more than 3 lines of vision, and 2 had final vision hand motions [103]. So, while anti-VEGF proved to be effective for PDR in the clinical trials, in real-world the unclear long-term advantages of pharmacological monotherapy over PRP, the increased cost, and treatment burden are not optimal for many diabetic patients.

Neovascular glaucoma is a late complication of proliferative disease with chronic ischemia in the posterior segment and development of a fibrovascular membrane on the anterior surface of the iris and iridocorneal angle of anterior chamber, and usually its onset correlates with poor glycemic control. In the early stages, iris neovascularization can be found without elevated IOP. Panretinal photocoagulation remains the mainstay in controlling the neovascular drive and should be considered in all cases of neovascularization of the anterior segment when retinal ischemia is present. After panretinal photocoagulation, complete regression of retinal neovascularization can be reached in 67–77% of cases, visual loss can be prevented in 59–73%, and IOP reduction can be achieved in 42% [104]. Anti-VEGF injections can lead to regression of both iris and angle neovascularization and improve intraocular pressure control when the angle remains open. However, the effects of anti-VEGF agents seemed to induce only a temporary regression of new vessels in the anterior chamber angle and IOP reduction, generally lasting between 4 and 6 weeks [105]. Glaucoma drainage devices are usually considered the first treatment option for refractory glaucoma. Neovascular glaucoma patients are at greater risk for surgical failure after glaucoma valve surgery compared with non-neovascular glaucoma controls. A recent retrospective, comparative, case series of 163 eyes of 151 patients with neovascular glaucoma included 99 treated without and 64 treated with intravitreal bevacizumab. IOP decreased to 18.3 ± 13.8 mmHg in the non-bevacizumab group and 15.3 ± 8.0 mmHg in the bevacizumab group. Panretinal photocoagulation substantially reduced the need for glaucoma surgery ($P < 0.001$) in bevacizumab-treated eyes. Therefore, although bevacizumab delayed the need for glaucoma surgery, panretinal photocoagulation was the most important factor that reduced the need for surgery. Vision and IOP in eyes with neovascular glaucoma treated with bevacizumab showed no long-term differences when compared with eyes that were not treated with bevacizumab. Thus, intravitreal anti-VEGF drugs serve as an effective temporizing treatment but are not a replacement for close monitoring and definitive treatment of neovascular glaucoma [106, 107].

Impairment of vision in diabetic patients is not limited to retinopathy—the leading causes of deteriorated vision and progression of vision loss in a cohort from South India were cataracts and uncorrected refractive errors [108]. The introduction of phacoemulsification significantly reduced the surgical trauma and leads to a growing tendency toward earlier cataract surgery in diabetic patients [109]. This approach facilitates panretinal photocoagulation and allows for the identification and adequate treatment of diabetic macular edema before and after cataract surgery. Preexisting macular edema can increase the risk of edema progression by 20–50%, and intravitreal anti-VEGF agents are recommended perioperatively [110]. Steroids, on the other hand, have been shown to be effective for persistent or refractory diabetic macular edema prior to and after cataract procedures. Dexamethasone implants and fluocinolone implants resulted in significant improvement in clinically significant macular edema and visual outcomes [111]. Despite the advancement in phacoemulsification technology, poor visual acuity following cataract extraction is still common in patients with diabetes. Posterior capsule opacification, postoperative cystoid macular edema, diabetic macular edema [112], and worsening of the DR are the main complications seen in diabetic patients. According to the Early Treatment of Diabetic Retinopathy Study, the presence of clinically significant diabetic macular edema at the time of cataract surgery was significantly associated with poor visual acuity and was a predictor of final visual acuity worse than 20/200 following uncomplicated phacoemulsification [113]. The severity of DR at the time of cataract surgery is also a significant determinant of postoperative VA; more severe retinopathy seems to be associated with an increased prevalence of macular ischemia or edema and a reduced tendency for spontaneous resolution of postoperative macular edema with associated poor postoperative VA. Treatment-naïve PDR before cataract surgery may progress to vitreous hemorrhage and tractional retinal detachment following phacoemulsification, thus threatening good visual outcome [114].

In conclusion, vision loss due to diabetic complications in the eye is growing worldwide despite availability of screening programs, advanced diagnostic tools, pharmacotherapy, and rapidly evolving surgical technology. Prevention requires:

- Identification of the social groups and individuals at high risk of vision-threatening diabetic complications

- Coverage with diabetic retinopathy screening with introduction of AI tools, wide-field retinal assessment, telemedicine, and OCT of the posterior segment

- Outreach of qualified management closer to the diabetic patients' communities

- Early, intensive management before significant vision loss

- Lifetime, highly qualified monitoring and early management of complications

- Close, continuous collaboration with the treating diabetology team
- Involvement of the family, community, diabetic patients' organizations, and social media in patient care, adherence to treatment, prevention of physical and mental disability, and improvement of quality of life

Author details

Maya Georgieva Pandova
KOC Ahmadi Hospital, Ahmadi, Kuwait

*Address all correspondence to: mpandova@kockw.com; mayapandova@gmail.com

References

[1] Sorsby A. The Incidence and Causes of Blindness in England and Wales. London: Her Majesty's Stationary Office; 1966. p. 6

[2] Hovind P, Tarnow L, Rossing K, Rossing P, Eising S, Larsen N, et al. Decreasing incidence of severe diabetic microangiopathy in type 1 diabetes. Diabetes Care. 2003;**26**(4):1258-1264

[3] Aclimandos WA, Galloway NR. Blindness in the city of Nottingham (1980-1985). Eye (London, England). 1988;**2**(Pt 4):431-434

[4] Thompson JR, Du L, Rosenthal AR. Recent trends in the registration of blindness and partial sight in Leicestershire. The British Journal of Ophthalmology. 1989;**73**(2):95-99

[5] Bäcklund LB, Algvere PV, Rosenqvist U. New blindness in diabetes reduced by more than one-third in Stockholm County. Diabetic Medicine. 1997;**14**(9):732-740

[6] Porta M, Tomalino MG, Santoro F, Ghigo LD, Cairo M, Aimone M, et al. Diabetic retinopathy as a cause of blindness in the province of Turin, north-west Italy, in 1967-1991. Diabetic Medicine. 1995;**12**(4):355-361

[7] Grey RH, Burns-Cox CJ, Hughes A. Blind and partial sight registration in Avon. The British Journal of Ophthalmology. 1989;**73**(2):88-94

[8] See JL, Wong TY, Yeo KT. Trends in the pattern of blindness and major ocular diseases in Singapore and Asia. Annals of the Academy of Medicine, Singapore. 1998;**27**(4):540-546

[9] Thylefors B, Négrel AD, Pararajasegaram R, Dadzie KY. Global data on blindness. Bulletin of the World Health Organization. 1995;**73**(1):115-121

[10] Thylefors B, Négrel AD, Pararajasegaram R, Dadzie KY. Available data on blindness (update 1994). Ophthalmic Epidemiology. 1995;**2**(1):5-39

[11] Resnikoff S, Pascolini D, Etya'ale D, Kocur I, Pararajasegaram R, Pokharel GP, et al. Global data on visual impairment in the year 2002. Bulletin of the World Health Organization. 2004;**82**(11):844-851 [Epub Dec 14, 2004]

[12] Leasher JL, Bourne RR, Flaxman SR, Jonas JB, Keeffe J, Naidoo K, et al., Vision Loss Expert Group of the Global Burden of Disease Study. Global estimates on the number of people blind or visually impaired by diabetic retinopathy: A meta-analysis from 1990 to 2010. Diabetes Care. 2016;**39**(9):1643-1649

[13] Flaxman SR, Bourne RRA, Resnikoff S, Ackland P, Braithwaite T, Cicinelli MV, et al., Vision Loss Expert Group of the Global Burden of Disease Study. Global causes of blindness and distance vision impairment 1990-2020: A systematic review and meta-analysis. The Lancet Global Health. 2017;**5**(12):e1221-e1234. DOI: 10.1016/S2214-109X(17)30393-5 [Epub Oct 11, 2017]

[14] GBD 2017 Disease and Injury Incidence and Prevalence Collaborators. Global, regional, and national incidence, prevalence, and years lived with disability for 354 diseases and injuries for 195 countries and territories, 1990-2017: A systematic analysis for the Global Burden of Disease Study 2017. Lancet. 2018;**392**(10159):1789-1858. DOI: 10.1016/S0140-6736(18)32279-7 [Epub Nov 8, 2018]

[15] RRA B, Jonas JB, Bron AM, Cicinelli MV, Das A, Flaxman SR, et al., Vision Loss Expert Group of

the Global Burden of Disease Study. Prevalence and causes of vision loss in high-income countries and in Eastern and Central Europe in 2015: magnitude, temporal trends and projections. The British Journal of Ophthalmology. 2018;**102**(5):575-585. DOI: 10.1136/bjophthalmol-2017-311258 [Epub Mar 15, 2018]

[16] Wong TY, Tham YC, Sabanayagam C, Cheng CY. Patterns and risk factor profiles of visual loss in a multi-ethnic asian population: The Singapore epidemiology of eye diseases study. American Journal of Ophthalmology. 2019. DOI: 10.1016/j.ajo.2019.05.006. pii: S0002-9394(19)30226-0 [Epub ahead of print]

[17] Yau JW, Rogers SL, Kawasaki R, Lamoureux EL, Kowalski JW, Bek T, et al., Meta-Analysis for Eye Disease (META-EYE) Study Group. Global prevalence and major risk factors of diabetic retinopathy. Diabetes Care. 2012;**35**(3):556-564. DOI: 10.2337/dc11-1909 [Epub Feb 1, 2012]

[18] Wu L, Fernandez-Loaiza P, Sauma J, Hernandez-Bogantes E, Masis M. Classification of diabetic retinopathy and diabetic macular edema. World Journal of Diabetes. 2013;**4**(6):290-294. DOI: 10.4239/wjd.v4.i6.290

[19] Lindner LME, Rathmann W, Rosenbauer J. Inequalities in glycaemic control, hypoglycaemia and diabetic ketoacidosis according to socio-economic status and area-level deprivation in Type 1 diabetes mellitus: a systematic review. Diabetic Medicine. 2018;**35**(1):12-32. DOI: 10.1111/dme.13519 [Epub Nov 3, 2017]

[20] Grintsova O, Maier W, Mielck A. Inequalities in health care among patients with type 2 diabetes by individual socio-economic status (SES) and regional deprivation: A systematic literature review. International Journal for Equity in Health. 2014;**13**:43. DOI: 10.1186/1475-9276-13-43

[21] Foreman J, Xie J, Keel S, van Wijngaarden P, Sandhu SS, Ang GS, et al. The prevalence and causes of vision loss in indigenous and non-indigenous Australians: The National Eye Health Survey. Ophthalmology. 2017;**124**(12):1743-1752. DOI: 10.1016/j.ophtha.2017.06.001 [Epub Jul 6, 2017]

[22] West SK, Munoz B, Klein R, Broman AT, Sanchez R, Rodriguez J, et al. Risk factors for Type II diabetes and diabetic retinopathy in a mexican-american population: Proyecto VER. American Journal of Ophthalmology. 2002;**134**(3):390-398

[23] Denniston AK, Lee AY, Lee CS, Crabb DP, Bailey C, Lip PL, et al., UK DR EMR Users Group. United Kingdom Diabetic Retinopathy Electronic Medical Record (UK DR EMR) Users Group: Report 4, real-world data on the impact of deprivation on the presentation of diabetic eye disease at hospital services. The British Journal of Ophthalmology. 2019;**103**(6):837-843. DOI: 10.1136/bjophthalmol-2018-312568 [Epub Sep 29, 2018]

[24] Mtuya C, Cleland CR, Philippin H, Paulo K, Njau B, Makupa WU, et al. Reasons for poor follow-up of diabetic retinopathy patients after screening in Tanzania: A cross-sectional study. BMC Ophthalmology. 2016;**16**:115. DOI: 10.1186/s12886-016-0288-z

[25] Pandova MG, Al-Merjan JI, Sadeq NA. Registered blindness in Kuwait—15 Years of dynamic changes. Ophthalmic Epidemiology. 2019;**26**(2):75-83. DOI: 10.1080/09286586.2018.1521981 Epub 2018 Oct 4

[26] Tam VH, Lam EP, Chu BC, Tse KK, Fung LM. Incidence and

progression of diabetic retinopathy in Hong Kong Chinese with type 2 diabetes mellitus. Journal of Diabetes and its Complications. 2009;**23**(3):185-193. DOI: 10.1016/j.jdiacomp.2008.03.001

[27] Jones CD, Greenwood RH, Misra A, Bachmann MO. Incidence and progression of diabetic retinopathy during 17 years of a population-based screening program in England. Diabetes Care. 2012;**35**(3):592-596. DOI: 10.2337/dc11-0943

[28] Broe R, Rasmussen ML, Frydkjaer-Olsen U, Olsen BS, Mortensen HB, Peto T, et al. The 16-year incidence, progression and regression of diabetic retinopathy in a young population-based Danish cohort with type 1 diabetes mellitus: The Danish cohort of pediatric diabetes 1987 (DCPD1987). Acta Diabetologica. 2014;**51**(3):413-420. DOI: 10.1007/s00592-013-0527-1

[29] Varma R, Choudhury F, Klein R, Chung J, Torres M, Azen SP. Four-year incidence and progression of diabetic retinopathy and macular edema: the Los Angeles Latino Eye Study. American Journal of Ophthalmology. 2010;**149**(5):752-761. DOI: 10.1016/j.ajo.2009.11.014

[30] Klein R, Knudtson MD, Lee KE, Gangnon R, Klein BE. The Wisconsin Epidemiologic Study of Diabetic Retinopathy: XXII the twenty-five-year progression of retinopathy in persons with type 1 diabetes. Ophthalmology. 2008;**115**(11):1859-1868. DOI: 10.1016/j.ophtha.2008.08.023

[31] Cikamatana L, Mitchell P, Rochtchina E, Foran S, Wang JJ. Five-year incidence and progression of diabetic retinopathy in a defined older population: The Blue Mountains Eye Study. Eye (London, England). 2007;**21**(4):465-471

[32] Leske MC, Wu SY, Hennis A, Nemesure B, Schachat AP, Hyman L, et al. Nine-year incidence of diabetic retinopathy in the Barbados eye studies. Archives of Ophthalmology. 2006;**124**(2):250-255. DOI: 10.1001/archopht.124.2.250

[33] Pedro RA, Ramon SA, Marc BB, Juan FB, Isabel MM. Prevalence and relationship between diabetic retinopathy and nephropathy, and its risk factors in the North-East of Spain: A population-based study. Ophthalmic Epidemiology. 2010;**17**(4):251-265. DOI: 10.3109/09286586.2010.498661

[34] Esteves JF, Kramer CK, Azevedo MJ, Stolz AP, Roggia MF, Larangeira A, et al. Prevalence of diabetic retinopathy in patients with type 1 diabetes mellitus. Revista da Associação Médica Brasileira. 2009;**55**(3):268-273. DOI: 10.1590/S0104-42302009000300017

[35] Dutra Medeiros M, Mesquita E, Papoila AL, Genro V, Raposo JF. First diabetic retinopathy prevalence study in Portugal: RETINODIAB Study-Evaluation of the screening programme for Lisbon and Tagus Valley region. The British Journal of Ophthalmology. Oct 2015;**99**(10):1328-1333. DOI: 10.1136/bjophthalmol-2015-306727. [Epub 2 Apr 2015]

[36] Knudsen LL, Lervang HH, Lundbye-Christensen S, Gorst-Rasmussen A. The north Jutland county diabetic retinopathy study: Population characteristics. The British Journal of Ophthalmology. 2006;**90**(11):1404-1409. DOI: 10.1136/bjo.2006.093393

[37] Jaki Mekjavić P, Jūratė Balčiūnienė V, Ćeklić L, Ernest J, Jamrichova Z, Zsolt Nagy Z, et al. The burden of macular diseases in Central and Eastern Europe-implications for healthcare systems. Value in Health Regional Issues. 2019;**19**:1-6. DOI: 10.1016/j.vhri.2018.11.002

[38] Al Ghamdi AH, Rabiu M, Hajar S, Yorston D, Kuper H, Polack S. Rapid

assessment of avoidable blindness and diabetic retinopathy in Taif, Saudi Arabia. The British Journal of Ophthalmology. 2012;**96**(9):1168-1172. DOI: 10.1136/bjophthalmol-2012-301874

[39] Boelter MC, Gross JL, Canani LH, Costa LA, Lisboa HR, Três GS, et al. Proliferative diabetic retinopathy is associated with microalbuminuria in patients with type 2 diabetes. Brazilian Journal of Medical and Biological Research. 2006;**39**(8):1033-1039

[40] López M, Cos FX, Álvarez-GuisasolaF, FusterE. Prevalence of diabetic retinopathy and its relationship with glomerular filtration rate and other risk factors in patients with type 2 diabetes mellitus in Spain. DM2 HOPE study. Journal of Clinical & Translational Endocrinology. 2017;**9**:61-65. DOI: 10.1016/j.jcte.2017.07.004. eCollection 2017 Sep

[41] Park YH, Shin JA, Han JH, Park YM, Yim HW. The association between chronic kidney disease and diabetic retinopathy: the Korea National Health and Nutrition Examination Survey 2008-2010. PLoS ONE. 2015;**10**(4):e0125338. DOI: 10.1371/journal.pone.0125338 (eCollection 2015)

[42] Wat N, Wong RL, Wong IY. Associations between diabetic retinopathy and systemic risk factors. Hong Kong Medical Journal. 2016;**22**(6):589-599 [Epub Oct 24, 2016]

[43] Jeng CJ, Hsieh YT, Yang CM, Yang CH, Lin CL, Wang IJ. Diabetic retinopathy in patients with diabetic nephropathy: Development and progression. PLoS ONE. 2016;**11**(8):e0161897. DOI: 10.1371/journal.pone.0161897 (eCollection 2016)

[44] Man RE, Sasongko MB, Wang JJ, MacIsaac R, Wong TY, Sabanayagam C, et al. The association of estimated glomerular filtration rate with diabetic retinopathy and macular edema. Investigative Ophthalmology & Visual Science. 2015;**56**(8):4810-4816. DOI: 10.1167/iovs.15-16987

[45] Morrison JL, Hodgson LA, Lim LL, Al-Qureshi S. Diabetic retinopathy in pregnancy: A review. Clinical & Experimental Ophthalmology. 2016;**44**(4):321-334. DOI: 10.1111/ceo.12760 [Epub May 17, 2016]

[46] Lövestam-Adrian M, Agardh CD, Aberg A, Agardh E. Pre-eclampsia is a potent risk factor for deterioration of retinopathy during pregnancy in Type 1 diabetic patients. Diabetic Medicine. 1997;**14**(12):1059-1065

[47] Vestgaard M, Ringholm L, Laugesen CS, Rasmussen KL, Damm P, Mathiesen ER. Pregnancy-induced sight-threatening diabetic retinopathy in women with Type 1 diabetes. Diabetic Medicine. 2010;**27**(4):431-435. DOI: 10.1111/j.1464-5491.2010.02958.x

[48] Alavi A, Sibbald RG, Mayer D, Goodman L, Botros M, Armstrong DG, et al. Diabetic foot ulcers: Part I. Pathophysiology and prevention. Journal of the American Academy of Dermatology. 2014;**70**(1):1.e1-1.e18; quiz 19-20

[49] Hwang DJ, Lee KM, Park MS, Choi SH, Park JI, Cho JH, et al. Association between diabetic foot ulcer and diabetic retinopathy. PLoS ONE. 2017;**12**(4):e0175270. DOI: 10.1371/journal.pone.0175270 (eCollection 2017)

[50] Karam T, Kamath YS, Rao LG, Rao KA, Shenoy SB, Bhandary SV. Diabetic retinopathy in patients with diabetic foot syndrome in South India. Indian Journal of Ophthalmology. 2018;**66**(4):547-550. DOI: 10.4103/ijo.IJO_1000_17

[51] Harris Nwanyanwu K, Talwar N, Gardner TW, Wrobel JS, Herman WH.

Stein JD Predicting development of proliferative diabetic retinopathy. Diabetes Care. 2013;**36**(6):1562-1568

[52] Chen X, Lu L. Depression in diabetic retinopathy: A review and recommendation for psychiatric management. Psychosomatics. 2016;**57**(5):465-471. DOI: 10.1016/j.psym.2016.04.003 [Epub Apr 22, 2016]

[53] Rees G, Xie J, Fenwick EK, Sturrock BA, Finger R, Rogers SL, et al. Association between diabetes-related eye complications and symptoms of anxiety and depression. JAMA Ophthalmology. 2016;**134**(9):1007-1014. DOI: 10.1001/jamaophthalmol.2016.2213

[54] Yekta Z, Xie D, Bogner HR, Weber DR, Zhang X, Harhay M, et al. The association of antidepressant medications and diabetic retinopathy among people with diabetes. Journal of Diabetes and its Complications. 2015;**29**(8):1077-1084. DOI: 10.1016/j.jdiacomp.2015.06.009 [Epub Jun 26, 2015]

[55] Nicolau J, Rivera R, Francés C, Chacártegui B, Masmiquel L. Treatment of depression in type 2 diabetic patients: effects on depressive symptoms, quality of life and metabolic control. Diabetes Research and Clinical Practice. 2013;**101**(2):148-152. DOI: 10.1016/j.diabres.2013.05.009 [Epub Jun 22, 2013]

[56] Simó-Servat O, Hernández C, Simó R. Diabetic retinopathy in the context of patients with diabetes. Ophthalmic Research. 2019;**24**:1-7. DOI: 10.1159/000499541 [Epub ahead of print]

[57] Liao JL, Xiong ZY, Yang ZK, Hao L, Liu GL, Ren YP, et al. An association of cognitive impairment with diabetes and retinopathy in end stage renal disease patients under peritoneal dialysis. PLoS ONE. 2017;**12**(8):e0183965. DOI: 10.1371/journal.pone.0183965 (eCollection 2017)

[58] Dong L, Lv XY, Wang BJ, Wang YQ, Mu H, Feng ZL, et al. Association of monocyte chemoattractant protein-1 (MCP-1)2518A/G polymorphism with proliferative diabetic retinopathy in northern Chinese type 2 diabetes. Graef's Archive for Clinical and Experimental Ophthalmology. 2014;**252**(12):1921-1926. DOI: 10.1007/s00417-014-2651-1 [Epub May 9, 2014]

[59] Dong L, Bai J, Jiang X, Yang MM, Zheng Y, Zhang H, et al. The gene polymorphisms of IL-8(−251T/A) and IP-10(-1596C/T) are associated with susceptibility and progression of type 2 diabetic retinopathy in northern Chinese population. Eye (London, England). 2017;**31**(4):601-607. DOI: 10.1038/eye.2016.287 [Epub Dec 9, 2016]

[60] Kaidonis G, Gillies MC, Abhary S, Liu E, Essex RW, Chang JH, et al. A single-nucleotide polymorphism in the MicroRNA-146a gene is associated with diabetic nephropathy and sight-threatening diabetic retinopathy in Caucasian patients. Acta Diabetologica. 2016;**53**(4):643-650. DOI: 10.1007/s00592-016-0850-4 [Epub Mar 21, 2016]

[61] Kaidonis G, Burdon KP, Gillies MC, Abhary S, Essex RW, Chang JH, et al. Common sequence variation in the VEGFC gene is associated with diabetic retinopathy and diabetic macular edema. Ophthalmology. 2015;**122**(9):1828-1836. DOI: 10.1016/j.ophtha.2015.05.004 [Epub Jun 11, 2015]

[62] Grassi MA, Tikhomirov A, Ramalingam S, Below JE, Cox NJ, Nicolae DL. Genome-wide meta-analysis for severe diabetic retinopathy. Human Molecular Genetics. 2011;**20**(12):2472-2481. DOI: 10.1093/hmg/ddr121 [Epub Mar 26, 2011]

[63] Graham PS, Kaidonis G, Abhary S, Gillies MC, Daniell M, Essex RW, et al.

Genome-wide association studies for diabetic macular edema and proliferative diabetic retinopathy. BMC Medical Genetics. 2018;**19**(1):71. DOI: 10.1186/s12881-018-0587-8

[64] Tetikoğlu M, Yüksel Z, Aktas S, Sağdik HM, Özcura F. VEGF-A gene polymorphisms and responses to intravitreal ranibizumab treatment in patients with diabetic macular edema. International Ophthalmology. 2018;**38**(6):2381-2388. DOI: 10.1007/s10792-017-0738-5 [Epub Oct 13, 2017]

[65] El-Shazly SF, El-Bradey MH, Tameesh MK. Vascular endothelial growth factor gene polymorphism prevalence in patients with diabetic macular oedema and its correlation with anti-vascular endothelial growth factor treatment outcomes. Clinical & Experimental Ophthalmology. 2014;**42**(4):369-378. DOI: 10.1111/ceo.12182 [Epub Sep 24, 2013]

[66] Grassi MA, Tikhomirov A, Ramalingam S, Lee KE, Hosseini SM, Klein BE, et al. Replication analysis for severe diabetic retinopathy. Investigative Ophthalmology & Visual Science. 2012;**53**(4):2377-2381. DOI: 10.1167/iovs.11-8068

[67] Tang J, Kern TS. Inflammation in diabetic retinopathy. Progress in Retinal and Eye Research. 2011;**30**(5):343-358. DOI: 10.1016/j.preteyeres.2011.05.002 [Epub May 25, 2011]

[68] Sasongko MB, Wong TY, Jenkins AJ, Nguyen TT, Shaw JE, Wang JJ. Circulating markers of inflammation and endothelial function, and their relationship to diabetic retinopathy. Diabetic Medicine. 2015;**32**(5):686-691. DOI: 10.1111/dme.12640 [Epub Dec 9, 2014]

[69] Dossarps D, Petit JM, Guiu B, Cercueil JP, Duvillard L, Bron AM, et al. Body fat distribution and adipokine secretion are not associated with diabetic retinopathy in patients with type 2 diabetes mellitus. Ophthalmic Research. 2014;**51**(1):42-45. DOI: 10.1159/000355323 [Epub Nov 2013]

[70] Sari R, Balci MK, Apaydin C. The relationship between plasma leptin levels and chronic complication in patients with type 2 diabetes mellitus. Metabolic Syndrome and Related Disorders. 2010;**8**(6):499-503. DOI: 10.1089/met.2009.0127 [Epub Aug 17, 2010]

[71] Yilmaz MI, Sonmez A, Acikel C, Celik T, Bingol N, Pinar M, et al. Adiponectin may play a part in the pathogenesis of diabetic retinopathy. European Journal of Endocrinology. 2004;**151**(1):135-140

[72] Peng JJ, Xiong SQ, Ding LX, Peng J, Xia XB. Diabetic retinopathy: Focus on NADPH oxidase and its potential as therapeutic target. European Journal of Pharmacology. 2019;**853**:381-387. DOI: 10.1016/j.ejphar.2019.04.038 [Epub Apr 19, 2019]

[73] Zhang J, Upala S, Sanguankeo A Relationship between vitamin D deficiency and diabetic retinopathy: A meta-analysis Canadian Journal of Ophthalmology 2017;52 Suppl 1:S39-S44. doi: 10.1016/j.jcjo.2017.09.026

[74] Cai S, Bressler NM. Aflibercept, bevacizumab or ranibizumab for diabetic macular oedema: recent clinically relevant findings from DRCR.net Protocol T. Current Opinion in Ophthalmology. 2017;**28**(6):636-643. DOI: 10.1097/ICU.0000000000000424

[75] Dugel PU, Hillenkamp J, Sivaprasad S, Vögeler J, Mousseau MC, Wenzel A, et al. Baseline visual acuity strongly predicts visual acuity gain in patients with diabetic macular edema following anti-vascular endothelial growth factor treatment across trials. Clinical Ophthalmology. 2016;**10**:1103-1110. DOI: 10.2147/OPTH.S100764 (eCollection 2016)

[76] Bressler SB, Odia I, Maguire MG, Dhoot DS, Glassman AR, Jampol LM, et al., Diabetic Retinopathy Clinical Research Network. Factors associated with visual acuity and central subfield thickness changes when treating diabetic macular edema with anti-vascular endothelial growth factor therapy: An exploratory analysis of the Protocol T randomized clinical trial. JAMA Ophthalmology. 1 Apr 2019;**137**(4):382-389. DOI: 10.1001/jamaophthalmol.2018.6786 [Epub ahead of print]

[77] Campos A, Campos EJ, do Carmo A, Caramelo F, Martins J, Sousa JP, et al. Evaluation of markers of outcome in real-world treatment of diabetic macular edema. Eye and Vision (Lond). 2018;**5**:27. DOI: 10.1186/s40662-018-0119-9 (eCollection 2018)

[78] Boyer DS, Yoon YH, Belfort R Jr, Bandello F, Maturi RK, Augustin AJ, et al., Ozurdex MEAD Study Group. Three-year, randomized, sham-controlled trial of dexamethasone intravitreal implant in patients with diabetic macular edema. Ophthalmology. 2014;**121**(10):1904-1914. DOI: 10.1016/j.ophtha.2014.04.024 [Epub Jun 4, 2014]

[79] Chakravarthy U, Yang Y, Lotery A, Ghanchi F, Bailey C, Holz FG, et al. Clinical evidence of the multifactorial nature of diabetic macular edema. Retina. 2018;**38**(2):343-351. DOI: 10.1097/IAE.0000000000001555

[80] Zur D, Iglicki M, Busch C, Invernizzi A, Mariussi M, Loewenstein A, et al., International Retina Group. OCT biomarkers as functional outcome predictors in diabetic macular edema treated with dexamethasone implant. Ophthalmology. 2018;**125**(2):267-275. DOI: 10.1016/j.ophtha.2017.08.031 [Epub Sep 19, 2017]

[81] Ciulla TA, Bracha P, Pollack J, Williams DF. Real-world outcomes of anti-vascular endothelial growth factor therapy in diabetic macular edema in the United States. Ophthalmology Retina. 2018;**2**(12):1179-1187. DOI: 10.1016/j.oret.2018.06.004 [Epub Jul 29, 2018]

[82] Park KH, Kim YY, Jo YJ, Oh J, Lee JE, Lee JE, et al. Healthcare utilization and treatment patterns in diabetic macular edema in Korea: A retrospective chart review. Journal of Korean Medical Science. 2019;**34**(15):e118. DOI: 10.3346/jkms.2019.34.e118

[83] Gao X, Obeid A, Aderman CM, Talcott KE, Ali FS, Adam MK, et al. Loss to follow-up after intravitreal anti-vascular endothelial growth factor injections in patients with diabetic macular edema. Ophthalmology Retina. 2019;**3**(3):230-236. DOI: 10.1016/j.oret.2018.11.002 [Epub Nov 10, 2018]

[84] Weiss M, Sim DA, Herold T, Schumann RG, Liegl R, Kern C, et al. Compliance and adherence of patients with diabetic macular edema to intravitreal anti-vascular endothelial growth factor therapy in daily practice. Retina. 2018;**38**(12):2293-2300. DOI: 10.1097/IAE.0000000000001892

[85] Photocoagulation treatment of proliferative diabetic retinopathy: The second report of diabetic retinopathy study findings. The diabetic retinopathy study research group. Ophthalmology. 1978;**85**(1):82-106

[86] Flynn HW Jr, Chew EY, Simons BD, Barton FB, Remaley NA, Ferris FL 3rd. Pars plana vitrectomy in the early treatment diabetic retinopathy study. ETDRS report number 17. The Early Treatment Diabetic Retinopathy Study Research Group. Ophthalmology. 1992;**99**(9):1351-1357

[87] Yang CM. Surgical treatment for diabetic retinopathy: 5-Year experience. Journal of the Formosan Medical Association. 1998;**97**(7):477-484

[88] Sakamoto M, Hashimoto R, Yoshida I, Ubuka M, Maeno T. Risk factors for neovascular glaucoma after vitrectomy in eyes with proliferative diabetic retinopathy. Clinical Ophthalmology. 2018;**12**:2323-2329. DOI: 10.2147/OPTH.S184959 (eCollection 2018)

[89] Ramezani A, Ahmadieh H, Rozegar A, Soheilian M, Entezari M, Moradian S, et al. Predictors and outcomes of vitrectomy and silicone oil injection in advanced diabetic retinopathy. Korean Journal of Ophthalmology. 2017;**31**(3):217-229. DOI: 10.3341/kjo.2016.0018 [Epub May 12, 2017]

[90] Yorston D, Wickham L, Benson S, Bunce C, Sheard R, Charteris D. Predictive clinical features and outcomes of vitrectomy for proliferative diabetic retinopathy. The British Journal of Ophthalmology. 2008;**92**(3):365-368. DOI: 10.1136/bjo.2007.124495

[91] Flaxel CJ, Dustin L, Kim J, Bekendam P, Row P. Outcome of diabetic vitrectomy in Latino population. Retina. 2007;**27**(9):1274-1278

[92] Abunajma MA, Al-Dhibi H, Abboud EB, Al Zahrani Y, Alharthi E, Alkharashi A, et al. The outcomes and prognostic factors of vitrectomy in chronic diabetic traction macular detachment. Clinical Ophthalmology. 2016;**10**:1653-1661. Published online Aug 26, 2016. DOI: 10.2147/OPTH.S98555

[93] Berrocal MH. All-probe vitrectomy dissection techniques for diabetic tractional retinal detachments: Lift and shave. Retina. 2018;**38**(Suppl 1):S2-S4. DOI: 10.1097/IAE.0000000000001884

[94] Shroff CM, Gupta C, Shroff D, Atri N, Gupta P, Dutta R. Bimanual microincision vitreous surgery for severe proliferative diabetic retinopathy: Outcome in more than 300 eyes. Retina. 2018;**38**(Suppl 1):S134-S145. DOI: 10.1097/IAE.0000000000002093

[95] Gabr H, Chen X, Zevallos-Carrasco OM, Viehland C, Dandrige A, Sarin N, et al. Visualization from intraoperative swept-source microscope-integrated optical coherence tomography in vitrectomy for complications of proliferative diabetic retinopathy. Retina. 2018;**38**(Suppl 1):S110-S120. DOI: 10.1097/IAE.0000000000002021

[96] Bressler SB, Odia I, Glassman AR, Danis RP, Grover S, Hampton GR, et al. Changes in diabetic retinopathy severity when treating diabetic macular edema with ranibizumab: DRCR.net Protocol I: 5-Year report. Retina. 2018;**38**(10):1896-1904. DOI: 10.1097/IAE.0000000000002302

[97] Sivaprasad S, Prevost AT, Vasconcelos JC, Riddell A, Murphy C, Kelly J, et al., Clarity Study Group. Clinical efficacy of intravitreal aflibercept versus panretinal photocoagulation for best corrected visual acuity in patients with proliferative diabetic retinopathy at 52 weeks (CLARITY): A multicentre, single-blinded, randomised, controlled, phase 2b, non-inferiority trial. Lancet. 2017;**389**(10085):2193-2203. DOI: 10.1016/S0140-6736(17)31193-5 [Epub May 7, 2017]

[98] Bressler SB, Beaulieu WT, Glassman AR, Gross JG, Melia M, Chen E, et al., Diabetic Retinopathy Clinical Research Network. Photocoagulation versus ranibizumab for proliferative diabetic retinopathy: Should baseline characteristics affect choice of treatment? Retina. 2019. DOI: 10.1097/IAE.0000000000002377 [Epub ahead of print]

[99] Jampol LM, Odia I, Glassman AR, Baker CW, Bhorade AM, Han DP, et al., Diabetic Retinopathy Clinical Research Network. Panretinal photocoagulation

versus ranibizumab for proliferative diabetic retinopathy: Comparison of peripapillary retinal nerve fiber layer thickness in a randomized clinical trial. Retina. 2019;**39**(1):69-78. DOI: 10.1097/IAE.0000000000001909

[100] Chelala E, Nehme J, El Rami H, Aoun R, Dirani A, Fadlallah A, et al. Efficacy of intravitreal ranibizumab injections in the treatment of vitreous hemorrhage related to proliferative diabetic retinopathy. Retina. 2018;**38**(6):1127-1133. DOI: 10.1097/IAE.0000000000001673

[101] Bonnin S, Dupas B, Lavia C, Erginay A, Dhundass M, Couturier A, et al. Ranti–vascular endothelial growth factor therapy can improve diabetic retinopathy score without change in retinal perfusion. Retina. 2019;**39**(3):426-434. Published online Jan 3, 2019. DOI: 10.1097/IAE.0000000000002422

[102] Obeid A, Su D, Patel SN, Uhr JH, Borkar D, Gao X, et al. Outcomes of eyes lost to follow-up with proliferative diabetic retinopathy that received panretinal photocoagulation versus intravitreal anti-vascular endothelial growth factor. Ophthalmology. 2019;**126**(3):407-413. DOI: 10.1016/j.ophtha.2018.07.027 [Epub Aug 2, 2018]

[103] Wubben TJ, Johnson MW, Anti-VEGF Treatment Interruption Study Group 1. Anti-VEGF therapy for diabetic retinopathy: consequences of inadvertent treatment interruptions. American Journal of Ophthalmology. 2019. DOI: 10.1016/j.ajo.2019.03.005. pii: S0002-9394(19)30103-5 [Epub ahead of print]

[104] Lang GE. Laser treatment of diabetic retinopathy. Developments in Ophthalmology. 2007;**39**:48-68. DOI: 10.1159/000098499

[105] Horsley MB, Kahook MY. Anti-VEGF therapy for glaucoma. Current Opinion in Ophthalmology. 2010;**21**(2):112-117

[106] Wang JW, Zhou MW, Zhang X, Huang WB, Gao XB, Wang W, et al. Short-term effect of intravitreal ranibizumab on intraocular concentrations of vascular endothelial growth factor-A and pigment epithelium-derived factor in neovascular glaucoma. Clinical & Experimental Ophthalmology. 2015;**43**(5):415-421

[107] Olmos LC, Sayed MS, Moraczewski AL, et al. Long-term outcomes of neovascular glaucoma treated with and without intravitreal bevacizumab. Eye (London, England). 2016;**30**(3):463-472. DOI: 10.1038/eye.2015.259

[108] Srinivasan S, Raman R, Ganesan S, Roy R, Natarajan V, Sharma T. Four-year incidence and progression of visual impairment in a South Indian population with diabetes. Indian Journal of Ophthalmology. 2017;**65**(7):589-595. DOI: 10.4103/ijo.IJO_520_16

[109] Chew EY, Benson WE, Remaley NA, Lindley AA, Burton TC, Csaky K, et al. 3rd Results after lens extraction in patients with diabetic retinopathy: early treatment diabetic retinopathy study report number 25. Archives of Ophthalmology. 1999;**117**:1600-1606

[110] Diabetic Retinopathy Clinical Research Network Authors/Writing Committee, Baker CW, Almukhtar T, Bressler NM, Glassman AR, Grover S, et al. Macular edema after cataract surgery in eyes without preoperative central-involved diabetic macular edema. JAMA Ophthalmology. 2013;**131**:870-879

[111] Danis RP, Sadda S, Li XY, Cui H, Hashad Y, Whitcup SM. Anatomical effects of dexamethasone intravitreal implant in diabetic macular oedema: a

pooled analysis of 3-year phase III trials. The British Journal of Ophthalmology. 2016;**100**:796-801

[112] Greenberg PB, Tseng VL, Wu WC, Liu J, Jiang L, Chen CK, et al. Prevalence and predictors of ocular complications associated with cataract surgery in United States veterans. Ophthalmology. 2011;**118**:507-514

[113] Egan C, Zhu H, Lee A, Sim D, Mitry D, Bailey C, et al., UK AMD and DR EMR Users Group. The United Kingdom Diabetic Retinopathy Electronic Medical Record Users Group, Report 1: Baseline characteristics and visual acuity outcomes in eyes treated with intravitreal injections of ranibizumab for diabetic macular oedema. The British Journal of Ophthalmology. 2017;**101**(1):75-80

[114] Liao SB. Ku WC Progression of diabetic retinopathy after phacoemulsification in diabetic patients: a three-year analysis. Chang Gung Medical Journal. 2003;**26**(11):829-834

Section 4

Low Vision, Blindness and Rehabilitation

Chapter 15

The Role of Vision on Spatial Competence

Giulia Cappagli and Monica Gori

Abstract

Several pieces of evidence indicate that visual experience during development is fundamental to acquire long-term spatial capabilities. For instance, reaching abilities tend to emerge at 5 months of age in sighted infants, while only later at 10 months of age in blind infants. Moreover, other spatial skills such as auditory localization and haptic orientation discrimination tend to be delayed or impaired in visually impaired children, with a huge impact on the development of sighted-like perceptual and cognitive asset. Here, we report an overview of studies showing that the lack of vision can interfere with the development of coherent multisensory spatial representations and highlight the contribution of current research in designing new tools to support the acquisition of spatial capabilities during childhood.

Keywords: blindness, visual impairment, child development, rehabilitation, innovation

1. Introduction

Spatial competence is essential in everyday life for numerous human activities, as it entails the ability to understand and internalize the representation of the structure, entities, and relations of space with respect to one's own body [1, 2]. Despite the fact that spatial competence encompasses a diverse set of skills, research in the field has generally focused on identifying the developmental steps that are necessary to acquire from an early age the ability to reason about spatial properties of the environment.

There is a general consensus on the crucial role of visual experience in guiding the maturation of spatial competence [3]. Vision takes advantages respect to other senses in encoding spatial information because it ensures the simultaneous perception of multiple stimuli in the environment despite the apparent motion of the array on the retina during locomotion enabling us to extract more invariant spatial properties from the surrounding layout [4, 5]. Indeed psychophysical data indicate that when sensorial conflict occurs, audition and touch are strongly biased by simultaneously presented visuospatial information, suggesting that sighted people tend to organize spatial information according to a visual frame of reference [6–12]. Neurophysiological data further confirm the view by suggesting that the visual feedback is fundamental for spatial learning [13–18], i.e., visual experience allows the alignment and thus the integration of auditory and visuospatial cortical maps [19–22]. Thus, research on sighted individuals suggests that vision typically provides the most accurate and reliable information about the spatial properties

IntechOpen

of the external world, therefore it dominates spatial perception. Consequently, if visual experience is necessary to adequately represent spatial information, we would expect blind people to perform worse than sighted people in spatial tasks. This would be especially true if the visual impairment emerges at birth, when multisensory communication is fundamental for the sensorimotor feedback loop that contributes to the development of spatial representations [23, 24].

Despite valuable insights into the important guiding role of vision on spatial development, contrasting results indicate that visually impaired people can manifest or enhanced either impaired skills depending on the spatial aspects investigated, leading to the hypothesis that vision could have an essential or facilitating role depending on the nature of the spatial task that individuals carry out [14]. A clearer definition of the underlying processes involved in spatial competence enhancements and deficits caused by visual loss is important not only to quantify to what extent the perceptual consequences of early blindness translate to real-world settings but also to develop effective rehabilitation tools and technologies to improve their spatial skills [25]. Indeed, scientific findings related to spatial competence development in the absence of visual experience have important implications for clinical outcomes and for the design of new rehabilitation activities meant to activate compensatory strategies since an early age.

2. Development of spatial competence with vision

The first developmental theory of spatial competence was proposed by Jean Piaget and his colleagues [26–28], who hypothesized that spatial understanding gradually improves with age thanks to a progressively more conscious interaction with the external world that permits to accumulate sensorimotor experiences such as reaching. Nonetheless, the identification of the starting points for spatial development remains one of the most debated topics within the literature of spatial competence.

While some researchers argue for innate knowledge of spatial understanding in humans [29] by reporting impressive spatial abilities in infants, other researchers advocate for a gradual acquisition of spatial competence during childhood [30] by reporting significant limitation of early spatial skills during infancy. For instance, several studies have demonstrated that already at 3 months infants are able to represent categorical spatial information by distinguishing between above vs. below and left vs. right [31, 32] and that by 5 months of age babies are sensitive to metric properties of space being able to code spatial object dimensions such as height [33–35], distance location [36], and angles [37]. Conversely, other studies indicate that while sensitivity to spatial properties appears in early infancy, further refinement of spatial accuracy emerges later during development. For instance, coding of categorical and metrical information improves through the primary school years [38–40] as well as capabilities of estimating and reproducing object size and location [41, 42].

The question of whether spatial capabilities are innate or acquired is of central importance to understand if an early sensory deprivation can negatively impact on the acquisition of adult-like competences. In the case of blindness, a key developmental acquisition is the ability to code auditory and tactile spatial properties of the environment in order to independently orient and navigate in space. Research on auditory spatial perception has shown that sighted infants already possess the ability to differentiate acoustic information and perform adequate actions in different dimensions [43]. Indeed they can turn their heads toward a sound from the moment they are born [44, 45] and at the age of 4–5 months, head-orientation movements become even faster and more precise than in the neonatal period. Further improvements in the ability to code the location of sonorous objects in space manifest at 6 months of age, when infants are sensitive to changes in the location of sounds as small as 13–19 degrees [46, 47]. Nonetheless, this reflexive orientation to sound sources is present at birth but disappears during the first month if large movements of the head are required [48] to appear again at 4–5 months of age: for this reason, it has been hypothesized that the early orientation reflex represents the activity of lower brain stem and provides an initial stage to acquire spatial competence [49] that is later consolidated through concrete experience.

In the spatial cognition domain, two main distinctions can be made about spatial representations of the environment [50]. The first distinction is between the egocentric and allocentric frame of reference which indicates the strategy to code location of objects, respectively, in a viewer-dependent or a viewer-independent manner. While the egocentric representation is tied to the observer and can be used either when the observer remains stationary or when the observer moves keeping track of the movement (dead reckoning or path integration), the allocentric representation does not depend on the viewer's current position but on external landmarks that can be adjacent (cue learning) or distal (place learning). Although early spatial representations were originally described as purely egocentric [51], several studies indicated that infants can make use of both intrinsic and external features of the environment to locate objects. There is evidence that infants can update egocentric representations by keeping track of their movement and thus locate objects from novel positions within the first year of life: indeed by 9 months, infants can compensate for simple changes in their position, such as translation along a straight line [52] or rotational movements [53]. Nonetheless, for more complex displacements, infants manifest a general difficulty in keeping track of their changing relation to target location. For example, at 12 months of age, they start to solve complex problems involving both translation and rotation but they perform better when they can make use of adjacent landmarks embedded in the environment [54], and this ability seems to show little improvement between 16 and 36 months [55]. Moreover, previous research has shown that sighted infants reach for sounding objects in the absence of visual clues [47, 56–59], implying that a sense of auditory space is well consolidated at this stage since sounding objects are localized in relation to one's body. The allocentric strategy seems to emerge quite early in the development together with the egocentric strategy, but with different maturational rates for cue learning and place learning types of coding. Indeed, studies employing paradigms where the direction of looking from a novel position indicate where infants expect to see an engaging stimulus demonstrate that by 8.5 months of age, infants use an adjacent salient landmark to locate the stimulus, whereas only at 12 months of age, they consistently use relational information of distal landmarks [54]. Several studies confirm the idea that egocentric and allocentric strategies continue to refine during childhood by showing that at 18–24 months of age, toddlers become able to use geometrical cues such as shape to orient themselves [60, 61]. Nonetheless, an important milestone such as the ability to integrate different reference frames within a common system of spatial representation in order to increase accuracy and reduce the variability of spatial judgments emerge only later during the development. Indeed, children aged between 4 and 8 years old are not able to use both self-motion and external landmarks as egocentric and allocentric information, respectively, to reproduce object location because they alternated both strategies instead of combining them as adults usually do [62].

The second distinction in the spatial cognition domain is between categorical and metric spatial representations, which, respectively, represent the coding of spatial information in a relative manner by means of comparisons among entities in space and the coding of spatial information in external coordinates by means of metric cues such as distance or length. It has been shown that at 7 months of age, infants spontaneously show categorical dichotomous discrimination of auditory space by differentiating objects within and beyond reach [57, 58] and by distinguishing spatial categories such as above vs. below and left vs. right [32, 63]. Early sensitivity to metric cues has been observed in 4.5–6.5 months old infants for the dimension of objects [64] and distance [36]. Nonetheless, methodological issues have been raised for the interpretation of such results since experimental paradigms typically used with infants employ observational measures of the infant's behavior that may reveal more low-level perceptual rather than conceptual representation. Indeed, it has been shown that at the age of 2 years, children are able to match objects by height when these objects are presented in containers of a fixed height, but not when they are presented without containers, indicating that toddlers make use of distance cues only when they can rely on relative cues [65]. A considerable improvement in the ability to code object size and location can be observed between the ages of 4 and 12 [40–42, 66], for example, in tasks that require to use a configuration of distal landmarks to infer object location [67]. This could be due to the development of a hierarchical coding system, which integrates metrics and categorical information [68]. Given the time course of spatial cognition development and the discrepancy between early and later acquisition of spatial skills, an interactionist approach has been proposed that acknowledges strong potentiality and tries to identify underlying mechanisms implicated in the transformation of early abilities into mature competence [69]. The underlying mechanisms responsible for the refinement of spontaneous spatial orientation skills might be found both in the biological and environmental experiences. Within the biological context, many improvements in spatial functioning have been associated with the maturation of specific brain regions such as the hippocampus. For instance, the maturation of the hippocampus-mediated ability to encode relations among multiple objects may determine an increase in the number of stimuli that children rely on during reorientation and navigation tasks [70]. Within the environmental context, experience involves interactions with objects in the physical world and learning conventional information about symbolic spatial representations, such as maps and models. Spatial competence is strictly dependent on experiential factors such as exploratory activities which are in turn related to the development of locomotor activities. For example, it has been suggested that the emergence of allocentric coding in the form of cue learning might derive from the onset of crawling around 8–9 months, while further locomotor experiences may facilitate place learning by stimulating children to observe and approach object arrays from different directions. Indeed, locomotion is not simply a maturational precursor to psychological changes, but it plays a crucial role in their genesis [71]. For example, crawling provides the infant with concrete experiences that may change his coding strategy, for example, permitting the infant to abandon an egocentric body-oriented localization of objects to one based on the use of environmental landmarks. Recent findings suggest that sighted children acquire spatial capabilities thanks to the reciprocal influence between visual perception and execution of movements [72]: children monitor the success of action through a sensory-motor feedback by matching expected and observed changes of visual information. Indeed, self-generated movements commonly help to perceive the space acoustically because they convey the proprioceptive sensation corresponding to the movement of the ears toward sound sources [73]. In other words, using the dichotomy between the body and its exterior, an individual acquires spatial competence through observation of the body's actions and the resulting sensory consequences: through self-generated movements, the nervous system learns sensorimotor contingencies [74], which reveal the spatial properties of the auditory space. Moreover, acting successfully entails affordances for action: since affordances change according to action capabilities and bodily characteristics, experiential factors are necessary especially during infancy when new skills are constantly appearing and bodily dimensions are changing rapidly [75].

These results suggest that early interaction between the visual input and other sensory and motor signals provides a powerful background to shape the development of spatial cognition in sighted children. But if vision is so important, how spatial development changes when the visual input is missing?

3. Development of spatial competence in the absence of vision

While the development of spatial cognition has been extensively studied in sighted individuals [50], less effort has been spent in understanding how the sense of space changes during development in children with visual impairment. Specifically, scientific research on the development of auditory localization skills in visually impaired children has provided contrasting results. For example, it has been shown that children with visual disabilities have an excellent spatial hearing, measured as the ability to discriminate differences in sound localization in the horizontal and vertical plane as well as the ability to reach or walk toward the sound source position [76]. On the contrary, several studies suggested that infants and children with severe congenital blindness have a developmental delay in sound localization abilities [23, 77–79] and motor responses to sound [80, 81]. For example, blind children do not reach for objects that produced sounds until the end of the first year, while sighted children start around 5 months [82]. Similarly, blind children show worse performances than sighted children in auditory bisection, minimum audible angle tasks [23], and audio depth tasks [78]. Other studies show mixed results, indicating that children with congenital visual disabilities show an initial neuromotor developmental delay but compensate for the lack of vision developing good manipulatory and walking skills thanks to the exploration of sounding objects in the environment [83]. Studies of proprioceptive localization of immediate and memorized targets have been used to compare the proprioceptive performance of sighted and blind individuals. For instance, it has been shown that early visual deprivation does not necessarily prevent the development of spatial representations in both early blind children [84] and adults [85]. Considering that spatial competence emerges gradually thanks to the reciprocal influence between visual perception and execution of movements [72], it is evident that visually impaired children not only lack the visual input necessary to establish the sensorimotor feedback that typically promotes spatial development, but also manifests a general delay in the acquisition of important locomotor and proprioceptive skills, which may cause them to accumulate much less spatial experience compared to their sighted peers [79, 86, 87]. It has long been known that the development of blind infants is delayed in self-initiated postures and locomotion [79, 88, 89]. While sighted children typically start to perform first individual actions and navigation from the first year of age, blind children without cognitive and motor impairments start to walk at about 30–32 months of age [90]. Moreover, from the first month of life, blind infants show delays in the vestibular and proprioceptive functions due to the lack of integration with the visual inputs typically provided during the development [91]. Finally, since visual feedback represents the most important incentive for actions and thus for the development of locomotion and mobility skills, the onset of several motor milestones (e.g., rolling, crawling, standing, and balancing) can be delayed in visually impaired infants [92, 93], suggesting that the visual feedback of the body is fundamental for the development of self-concept.

To perceive space, visually impaired children typically use hearing and touch. Despite the haptic sense provides essential information about the spatial layout of peripersonal space, such as the size, shape, position, and orientation of objects within reach, it typically conveys information only within the scope of the body. The case of hearing is particularly interesting because the auditory sense is not only the main channel for providing distal information but also it might be superior to all other sensory alternatives because it provides spatial information in both active and passive conditions and it does not necessarily involve direct contact with objects [94, 95]. At the same time, the use of hearing to perceive distal information might be particularly difficult for visually impaired children because in this case, they do not have any sensory feedback about sonorous objects in the far space. On the contrary, the haptic-proprioceptive system can provide accurate spatial data only within the scope of the body itself [96], and therefore a blind person must actively move in the environment to sequentially touch all the stimuli embedded in space. Several factors may contribute to increasing the difficulty in interpreting such contrasting results. For example, many studies on spatial hearing have been conducted within the framework of broader research on cognitive and motor skills development [87, 97] and reaching mixing the motor and the perceptual component of the observed behavior [83, 98]. In addition, different methodological approaches and stimuli have been used to assess similar aspects of auditory spatial perception: for instance, studies performed on visually impaired children under 3 years of age do not employ psychophysical procedures but they frequently use the sound of familiar voices or toys to gather information about auditory localization abilities in blind children [97]. In addition, in some cases, sighted and blind groups of children are not perfectly matched for age range and sometimes use also adults as comparison [76]. Finally, the difference between early and later loss of vision has not been often considered: many studies mix data from children with no visual experience with those of children with partial visual experience in the first period of life [76]. Instead, it has been demonstrated that the onset of blindness has a strong impact on spatial performance in adulthood: for example, late blind individuals who lost vision later in life after a normal visual experience during the first year of life perform equally or even better than sighted participants in several auditory spatial tasks (1, 50, 83, and 300). To summarize, although compensatory mechanisms for spatial perception have been demonstrated in blind adults, it is not clear whether an early visual impairment might delay the development of special auditory spatial skills. The development of spatial cognition is strictly related to the development of social cognition: the ability to independently navigate and orient ourselves in space facilitates engagement in social interactions. Indeed, a delay in the acquisition of language, motor or cognitive skills can have a direct impact on a child's social competence (106, 109, and 246). More recent works highlighted that preschool-age children with visual impairments often have difficulties engaging in positive social interactions, making their assimilation into preschool programs difficult. In fact, many do not display a full range of play behaviors [99–103] and spend more time engaging in solitary play interacting more with adults than with their sighted peers [81, 87, 89, 102–107]. Considering that the interaction among peers is essential for the development of cognitive, linguistic, social, and playing skills [108], the aforementioned delay in the acquisition of social competence in visually impaired children gives rise to feelings of frustration, rather than self-efficacy and independence which characterize the social experience of typical children. Indeed, the lack of visual information during early infancy often constitutes a risk for the development of the personality and emotional competence [89]. Nonetheless, when assessing social competence in visually impaired people, some other factors resulting from the loss of vision should be taken into account. For example, it has been shown that parenting style influences the socio-emotional development of sighted children [109–113] because parents represent the first influential setting that can produce appreciable differences in developmental outcomes in terms of psychological functions [114, 115]. Inconsistent, hostile and nonsensitive parenting behaviors have been associated with adjustment problems and social adversity during childhood [116, 117] and also with anxiety, depression, and other stress-related illnesses during adolescence [118, 119] and adulthood [120]. We speculate that a similar influence of parenting style holds also for blind children, especially because families of children with visual disabilities are more prone to experience various stressors such as concerns about the social acceptance of the child [121] and to face difficulties in initiating and sustaining social interactions [122], thus they might easily develop an overprotective behavior that negatively influences the social development of the visually impaired child. The negative effects of blindness on socio-emotional competence can be observed also in adulthood, with the impoverishment of the ability to perform everyday activities both in private settings like home and in public settings like workplace. Importantly, the decrease of functional abilities has been linked to the emergence of serious psychological problems in the blind population [123]. Indeed adults with visual impairments tend to feel more socially isolated and not properly supported compared to sighted individuals [123–126] and are at higher risk of developing depressive symptoms [105, 125, 127–131], principally because social competence depends on the ability to utilize visual cues [132]. Overall, several scientific findings suggest that visual impairments, especially if acquired later in life, can have profound consequences for the physical functioning, psychological well-being, and health service needs of older adults [133]. Consequently, early therapeutic interventions specifically focused on activities fostering the development of perceptual and motor abilities would improve the quality of life of children and adults with visual impairments. In the next section, we will present some tools developed to improve perceptual skills of visually impaired individuals and propose a new solution we recently developed for early intervention in visually impaired children.

4. Spatial tools for visually impaired children

The acquisition of spatial competence is typically a good indicator of the future ability to independently navigate in the environment and engage in positive social interaction with peers. While for sighted individuals, the visual feedback represents the most important incentive for actions and thus for the development of mobility and social skills, visually impaired individuals strongly rely on auditory and tactile landmarks to encode spatial and social information. Thus, the creation of technological devices to support visually impaired children in their spatial and social development would be a need. Nonetheless, despite the huge recent advancements in technological industry, most of the devices developed so far to address visually impaired population's needs are not widely accepted by adults and not easily adaptable to children [134].

As reported in the previous sections, visual impairments can determine spatial and social impairments during development. Technological support for the blind should fulfill two different but complementary tasks: the first is to substitute the absent sensory information (vision) with other sensory signals (audition and touch) for daily activities, and the second is to support the rehabilitation of impaired functions following sensory loss. This latter aspect is particularly important when the visual impairment occurs during the first year of life, because technological devices might represent an opportunity for children to develop perceptual and cognitive abilities by compensating for the sensory deprivation. Most of the technological supports developed to date have fulfilled mainly the first task, namely the substitution of vision with other modalities for everyday tasks such as object recognition.

Sensory substitution devices (SSDs) convert the stimuli, normally accessed through one sensory modality, into stimuli accessible to another sensory modality. Specifically, sensory substitution devices for visually impaired individuals aim at supplying the missing visual information with visual-to-tactile or visual-to-auditory conversion systems [135]. Typically, substitution systems based on visual-to-tactile conversion transforms images captured by a camera into tactile stimulations directed to users. From the first device developed in the mid-1960s by Bach-y-Rita (Tactile-Visual Sensory Substitution device or TVSS), that converts signals from a video camera into tactile stimulation applied to the back of the subject allowing for the recognition of lines and shapes [136], recent technological progress allowed the development of much smaller, portable, and wearable devices. For instance, wristbands, vests, belts, and shoes which allow hands-free interactions [137] and devices that can be placed on various body surfaces (e.g., fingers, wrist, head, abdomen, and feet) [138, 139]. Conversely, systems based on visual-to-auditory conversion transform the images captured by a camera into sounds transmitted to users via headphones. One of the most famous visual-to-auditory devices is the vOICe developed by Meijer [140] that associates height with pitch and brightness with loudness in a left-to-right scan of the visual image.

In our recent review, we listed the SSDs designed for visually impaired individuals by highlighting their main features and limitations for daily use [134]. In particular, we identified six main limitations that might determine low acceptance rate in adults and low adaptability in children:

- Invasiveness: SSDs can be physically invasive in the sense that in order to be used, they must be positioned on crucial body parts (e.g., ears or mouth), thus limiting perceptual functions in users or they must be transported (e.g., in backpacks), thus limiting users' navigation for weight and size;

- Extensive training: SSDs typically require long periods of training in order to be used because users need to learn how to interpret the output of the device, which is typically not immediate (e.g., sound loudness corresponds to pixel brightness in the vOICe [141]);

- High cognitive load: SSDs usually require high attentional resources, which makes it difficult for the user to focus on the main task they are performing when using the device;

- No clinical validation: SSDs frequently remain prototypes and do not reach the blind users market, principally because they are not validated on large sample patients through standardized clinical trials;

- Artificiality: SSDs are generally based on the idea that users can understand the properties of visual stimulus by listening (in the case of visual-to-auditory SSDs) or feeling (in the case of visual-to-tactile SSDs) a stimulus resulting from an artificial transformation code, missing an important aspect of the learning process, which is the association of action and perception.

Therefore, while sensory substitution devices have been shown to provide support for specific perceptual tasks in adults [142], they have never been tested in children principally because their use might too overwhelming for children. Nonetheless, technological development should be addressed especially to visually impaired children needs because cortical plasticity is maximal during the first year of life, therefore the benefit deriving from early interventions should be higher.

Moreover, technological development should lead to multimodal stimulation whose benefits have been repeatedly reported compared to unimodal stimulation [143–145], while most of the SSDs developed so far substitute the visual function with either the auditory or the tactile modality alone.

With this in mind, we developed a new device for visually impaired children (Audio Bracelet for Blind Interaction, ABBI, [146]), which is an audio bracelet that produces an auditory feedback of body movements when positioned on a main effector such as the wrist in order to provide a sensorimotor signal similar to that used by sighted children to construct a sense of space. Indeed, several reports indicate that sighted children typically acquire spatial competence by experiencing visuomotor correspondences [72]. In this sense, our device could be used to align the spatial understanding between one's own body and the external space through coupling auditory feedback with intentional motor actions. The audio movement created by the bracelet conveys spatial information and allows the blind user to build a representation of the movement in space in an intuitive and direct manner.

We validated the ABBI device with a clinical trial on an Italian sample of 44 visually impaired children aged 6–17 years old assigned to an experimental (ABBI training) or a control (classical training) rehabilitation condition. The experimental training group followed an intensive but entertaining rehabilitation for 12 weeks during which children performed ad-hoc developed audio-spatial exercises with the Audio Bracelet for Blind Interaction (ABBI). The clinical trial consisted of three sessions: pre-evaluation, training, and post-evaluation. Pre- and post-evaluation sessions lasted 60 min during which a battery of spatial and motor tests were performed [147]. The BSP (Blind Spatial Perception) battery comprised six tests: (1) auditory localization: the child listens to the sound produced by a set of loudspeakers positioned horizontally in front of him/her and localizes the sound source by pointing to it with a white cane; (2) auditory bisection: the child listens to a sequence of three sounds presented successively by a set of loudspeakers positioned horizontally in front of him/her and verbally reports whether the second sound is closer in space to the first or to the third one presented; (3) auditory distance: the child listens to two consecutive sounds produced by a set of loudspeakers positioned vertically in front of him/her in depth and verbally reports which of the two stimuli presented is closer in space to his/her own body; (4) auditory reaching: the child listens to a static sound positioned in far space and reaches the position of the sound by walking toward it; (5) proprioceptive reaching: the child repeats a movement trajectory after being presented with it by an external operator; (6) general mobility: the child walks straight on for three meters and then back to the starting position at his/her own pace. The training session lasted 12 weeks and children were assigned to the experimental training condition based on activities with the use of ABBI or to the classical training condition based on psychomotor lessons not necessarily involving sound localization activities. All children enrolled in the ABBI training group performed weekly training exercises with a trained rehabilitator for 45 min (9 h over 12 weeks) and weekly training sessions with a relative at home for 5 h (60 h over 12 weeks) for a total training period of 69 h. All training exercises were developed to train children' ability to recognize and localize sounds in space according to different levels of difficulty: (a) recognize and localize simple sound movements, such as a straight motion flow performed along the horizontal or sagittal planes in the front peri-personal space (first level); (b) recognize and localize complex sound movements, such as a motion flow performed randomly in space in the front peri-personal space, e.g., composite geometrical and nongeometrical figures (second level); (c) recognize and localize simple and complex sound movements in the back peri-personal space (third level); (d) recognize and localize simple and complex sound movements in the front and back in the extra-personal

	ABBI training	Control training	ABBI vs Control (p value)	ABBI Follow-up	ABBI vs ABBI Follow-up (p value)
	ΔA = T1 – T0, N= 18	ΔC = T1 – T0, N= 20	ΔA – ΔC	ΔA2 = T2 – T0, N= 10	ΔA – ΔA2
Auditory localization	2.80 (1.48) **	1.15 (0.78)	0.0001 ***	3.83 (2.22)	0.17
Auditory bisection	2.43 (2.12) ***	0.15 (0.66)	0.0005 **	3.18 (2.83)	0.11
Auditory distance	0.88 (2.41)	0.98 (1.66)	0.62	3.06 (1.93)	0.99
Auditory reaching	25.48 (12.12) ***	3.95 (12.19)	0.0005 **	17.12 (9.89)	0.17
Proprioceptive reaching	16.44 (10.40) ***	9.89 (7.18)	0.01 **	23.78 (17.92)	0.66
General mobility	3.53 (2.59) **	1.94 (0.95)	0.04 *	2.97 (2.78)	0.44

One year follow-up of the ABBI group (T2-T0). In order to evaluate the effects within groups, two-tailed t-tests assuming equal variances were performed between groups at baseline (T0) and post-training period (T1). Changes in the outcome measures were then calculated between baseline (T0) and post-training period (T1) in the ABBI training and classical training group (ΔA and ΔC), and between baseline (T0) and follow-up period (T2) in the ABBI training group (ΔA2). Data are presented as mean and standard deviation. The stars indicate the statistical significance of the corresponding t-test of the score difference ($p < 0.05$; **$p < 0.01$; ***$p < 0.001$). Table readapted from [148].*

Table 1.
Score difference (Δ) after 12 weeks training (T1-T0).

space (fourth level). The comparison of overall spatial performance before and after the training with a dedicated assessment battery indicated that the ABBI device is effective in improving spatial skills in an intuitive manner (see **Table 1** for a summary of results), confirming that in the case of blindness perceptual development can be enhanced with naturally associated auditory feedbacks to body movements [148]. Moreover, the validation of the ABBI device demonstrated that the early introduction of a tailored audio-motor training could potentially prevent spatial developmental delays in visually impaired children [149].

5. Conclusions

Visual experience is deemed to be fundamental for the acquisition of spatial competence; indeed, visually impaired children tend to manifest impairments in spatial and locomotor skills, causing a general developmental delay. The hearing sense can be boosted since an early age to foster compensatory mechanisms for the development of spatial perception, principally because compared to touch it can provide distal information [150]. There is evidence that multisensory training based on the action-perception link can improve spatial abilities in visually impaired children and prevent the risk of developmental delays and social exclusion [148, 149, 151].

Acknowledgements

We would like to thank all the children and parents for their willing participation in our studies and the Unit for Visually Impaired People (UVIP) members for their passionate work on visually impaired individuals.

Conflict of interest

The authors declare no conflict of interest.

Author details

Giulia Cappagli[1,2]* and Monica Gori[2]

1 Neurological Institute Foundation C. Mondino, Pavia, Italy

2 Italian Institute of Technology, Genova, Italy

*Address all correspondence to: giulia.cappagli@iit.it

References

[1] Thinus-Blanc C, Gaunet F. Representation of space in blind persons: Vision as a spatial sense? Psychological Bulletin. 1997;**121**(1):20

[2] Vasilyeva M, Lourenco SF. Spatial development. In: Lerner RM, Lamb ME, Freund AM, editors. The Handbook of Life-Span Development. Volume 1. Cognition, Biology, and Methods. Wiley; 2010. DOI: 10.1002/9780470880166.hlsd001020

[3] Pasqualotto A, Proulx MJ. The role of visual experience for the neural basis of spatial cognition. Neuroscience and Biobehavioral Reviews. 2012;**36**(4):1179-1187

[4] Foulke E. Perception, cognition and the mobility of blind pedestrians. In: Potegal M, editor. Spatial abilities: Development and physiological foundations. New York: Academic Press; 1982. pp. 55-76

[5] Millar S. Crossmodal and intersensory perception and the blind. In: Walk RD, Pick HL, editors. Intersensory Perception and Sensory Integration. Perception and Perceptual Development (A Critical Review Series). Boston, MA: Springer; 1981

[6] Zahorik P. Estimating sound source distance with and without vision. Optometry and Vision Science. 2001;**78**(5):270-275

[7] Pick HL, Warren DH, Hay JC. Sensory conflict in judgments of spatial direction. Perception & Psychophysics. 1969;**6**(4):203-205

[8] Flanagan JR, Beltzner MA. Independence of perceptual and sensorimotor predictions in the size–weight illusion. Nature Neuroscience. 2000;**3**(7):737

[9] Botvinick M, Cohen J. Rubber hands 'feel'touch that eyes see. Nature. 1998;**391**(6669):756

[10] Bertelson P, Aschersleben G. Temporal ventriloquism: Crossmodal interaction on the time dimension: 1. Evidence from auditory–visual temporal order judgment. International Journal of Psychophysiology. 2003;**50**(1-2):147-155

[11] Anderson PW, Zahorik P, editors. Auditory and Visual Distance Estimation. Proceedings of Meetings on Acoustics 161 ASA. Seattle, Washington; 2011;**12**(1):050004

[12] Alais D, Burr D. The ventriloquist effect results from near-optimal bimodal integration. Current Biology. 2004;**14**(3):257-262

[13] Heffner RS, Heffner HE. Hearing and sound localization in blind mole rats (*Spalax ehrenbergi*). Hearing Research. 1992;**62**(2):206-216

[14] King AJ. What happens to your hearing if you are born blind? Brain. 2014;**137**(1):6-8

[15] Knudsen EI, Brainard MS. Visual instruction of the neural map of auditory space in the developing optic tectum. Science. 1991;**253**(5015):85-87

[16] Knudsen EI, Knudsen PF. Vision guides the adjustment of auditory localization in young barn owls. Science. 1985;**230**(4725):545-548

[17] Withington-Wray D, Binns K, Keating M. The maturation of the superior collicular map of auditory space in the Guinea pig is disrupted by developmental visual deprivation. The European Journal of Neuroscience. 1990;**2**(8):682-692

[18] Wiesel TN, Hubel DH. Comparison of the effects of unilateral and bilateral

eye closure on cortical unit responses in kittens. Journal of Neurophysiology. 1965;**28**(6):1029-1040

[19] Withington D. The effect of binocular lid suture on auditory responses in the Guinea-pig superior colliculus. Neuroscience Letters. 1992;**136**(2):153-156

[20] Knudsen EI. Early blindness results in a degraded auditory map of space in the optic tectum of the barn owl. Proceedings of the National Academy of Sciences. 1988;**85**(16):6211-6214

[21] King AJ. Visual influences on auditory spatial learning. Philosophical Transactions of the Royal Society, B: Biological Sciences. 2008;**364**(1515):331-339

[22] King A, Carlile S. Changes induced in the representation of auditory space in the superior colliculus by rearing ferrets with binocular eyelid suture. Experimental Brain Research. 1993;**94**(3):444-455

[23] Vercillo T, Burr D, Gori M. Early visual deprivation severely compromises the auditory sense of space in congenitally blind children. Developmental Psychology. 2016;**52**(6):847

[24] Gori M, Sandini G, Martinoli C, Burr DC. Impairment of auditory spatial localization in congenitally blind human subjects. Brain. 2013;**137**(1):288-293

[25] Voss P. Auditory spatial perception without vision. Frontiers in Psychology. 2016;7:1960

[26] Piaget J, Inhelder B. La psychologie de l'enfant, coll.«Que sais-je?», no 369; 1967

[27] Inhelder B, Piaget J, Szeminska A. The Child's Conception of Geometry. New York: Basic Books; 1960

[28] Pick HL, Pick AD. A developmental and analytic study of the size-weight illusion. Journal of Experimental Child Psychology. 1967;**5**(3):362-371

[29] Spelke E, Lee SA, Izard V. Beyond core knowledge: Natural geometry. Cognitive Science. 2010;**34**(5):863-884

[30] Liben LS. Spatial development in childhood: Where are we now? In: Blackwell Handbook of Childhood Cognitive Development. Oxford: Blackwell Publishing; 2002. pp. 326-348

[31] Quinn PC, Cummins M, Kase J, Martin E, Weissman S. Development of categorical representations for above and below spatial relations in 3-to 7-month-old infants. Developmental Psychology. 1996;**32**(5):942

[32] Quinn PC. The categorization of above and below spatial relations by young infants. Child Development. 1994;**65**(1):58-69

[33] Baillargeon R, Spelke ES, Wasserman S. Object permanence in five-month-old infants. Cognition. 1985;**20**(3):191-208

[34] Baillargeon R. Object permanence in 3½-and 4½-month-old infants. Developmental Psychology. 1987;**23**(5):655

[35] Baillargeon R, DeVos J. Object permanence in young infants: Further evidence. Child Development. 1991;**62**(6):1227-1246

[36] Newcombe N, Huttenlocher J, Learmonth A. Infants' coding of location in continuous space. Infant Behavior & Development. 1999;**22**(4):483-510

[37] Lourenco SF, Huttenlocher J. The representation of geometric cues in infancy. Infancy. 2008;**13**(2):103-127

[38] Hund AM, Plumert JM. The stability and flexibility of spatial categories. Cognitive Psychology. 2005;**50**(1):1-44

[39] Spencer JP, Hund AM. Developmental continuity in the processes that underlie spatial recall. Cognitive Psychology. 2003;**47**(4):432-480

[40] Plumert JM, Hund AM. The development of memory for location: What role do spatial prototypes play? Child Development. 2001;**72**(2):370-384

[41] Sandberg EH, Huttenlocher J, Newcombe N. The development of hierarchical representation of two-dimensional space. Child Development. 1996;**67**(3):721-739

[42] Vasilyeva M, Duffy S, Huttenlocher J. Developmental changes in the use of absolute and relative information: The case of spatial extent. Journal of Cognition and Development. 2007;**8**(4):455-471

[43] van der Meer AL, Van der Weel F. Auditory guided arm and whole body movements in young infants. Advances in Sound localization. 2011:297-314

[44] Muir D, Field J. Newborn infants orient to sounds. Child Development. 1979:431-436

[45] Wertheimer M. Psychomotor coordination of auditory and visual space at birth. Science. 1961;**134**(3491):1692

[46] Ashmead DH, Hill EW, Talor CR. Obstacle perception by congenitally blind children. Perception & Psychophysics. 1989;**46**(5):425-433

[47] Morrongiello BA, Fenwick KD, Chance G. Crossmodal learning in newborn infants: Inferences about properties of auditory-visual events. Infant Behavior & Development. 1998;**21**(4):543-553

[48] Bower T, Dunkeld J, Wishart JG. Infant Perception of Visually Presented Objects. Science. 1979;**203**(4385):1137-1139

[49] Muir D, Hains S. The U-shaped developmental function for auditory localization. Journal of Cognition and Development. 2004;**5**(1):123-130

[50] Vasilyeva M, Lourenco SF. Development of spatial cognition. Wiley Interdisciplinary Reviews: Cognitive Science. 2012;**3**(3):349-362

[51] Piaget J, Inhelder B. Child's Conception of Space: Selected Works. New York, NY: Routledge; 2013

[52] Landau B, Spelke E. Geometric complexity and object search in infancy. Developmental Psychology. 1988;**24**(4):512

[53] Rieser JJ, Heiman ML. Spatial self-reference systems and shortest-route behavior in toddlers. Child Development. 1982:524-533

[54] Lew AR, Bremner JG, Lefkovitch LP. The development of relational landmark use in six-to twelve-month-old infants in a spatial orientation task. Child Development. 2000;**71**(5):1179-1190

[55] Newcombe N, Huttenlocher J, Drummey AB, Wiley JG. The development of spatial location coding: Place learning and dead reckoning in the second and third years. Cognitive Development. 1998;**13**(2):185-200

[56] Clifton RK. The development of spatial hearing in human infants. Developmental Psychoacoustics. 1992:135-157

[57] Clifton RK, Perris EE, Bullinger A. Infants' perception of auditory space. Developmental Psychology. 1991;**27**(2):187

[58] Litovsky RY, Clifton RK. Use of sound-pressure level in auditory distance discrimination by 6-month-old infants and adults. The Journal of the Acoustical Society of America. 1992;**92**(2):794-802

[59] Perris EE, Clifton RK. Reaching in the dark toward sound as a measure of auditory localization in infants. Infant Behavior & Development. 1988;**11**(4):473-491

[60] Hermer L, Spelke ES. A geometric process for spatial reorientation in young children. Nature. 1994;**370**(6484):57

[61] Hermer L, Spelke E. Modularity and development: The case of spatial reorientation. Cognition. 1996;**61**(3):195-232

[62] Nardini M, Jones P, Bedford R, Braddick O. Development of cue integration in human navigation. Current Biology. 2008;**18**(9):689-693

[63] Quinn PC, Adams A, Kennedy E, Shettler L, Wasnik A. Development of an abstract category representation for the spatial relation between in 6-to 10-month-old infants. Developmental Psychology. 2003;**39**(1):151

[64] Baillargeon R. Reasoning about the height and location of a hidden object in 4.5-and 6.5-month-old infants. Cognition. 1991;**38**(1):13-42

[65] Huttenlocher J, Duffy S, Levine S. Infants and toddlers discriminate amount: Are they measuring? Psychological Science. 2002;**13**(3):244-249

[66] Plumert JM, Hund AM, Recker KM. Organism-Environment Interaction in Spatial Development: Explaining Categorical Bias in Memory for Location. In: Plumert JM, Spencer JP, editors. The emerging spatial mind. New York, NY, US: Oxford University Press; 2007. pp. 25-52

[67] Leplow B, Lehnung M, Pohl J, Herzog A, Ferstl R, Mehdorn M. Navigational place learning in children and young adults as assessed with a standardized locomotor search task. British Journal of Psychology. 2003;**94**(3):299-317

[68] Newcombe NS. The nativist-empiricist controversy in the context of recent research on spatial and quantitative development. Psychological Science. 2002;**13**(5):395-401

[69] Newcombe NS, Huttenlocher J. Making Space: The Development of Spatial Representation and Reasoning. Cambridge, MA, US: The MIT Press; 2003

[70] Sutton JE, Joanisse MF, Newcombe NS. Spinning in the scanner: Neural correlates of virtual reorientation. Journal of Experimental Psychology. Learning, Memory, and Cognition. 2010;**36**(5)

[71] Uchiyama I, Anderson DI, Campos JJ, Witherington D, Frankel CB, Lejeune L, et al. Locomotor experience affects self and emotion. Developmental Psychology. 2008;**44**(5)

[72] Bremner AJ, Holmes NP, Spence C. Infants lost in (peripersonal) space? Trends in Cognitive Sciences. 2008;**12**(8):298-305

[73] Aytekin M, Moss CF, Simon JZ. A sensorimotor approach to sound localization. Neural Computation. 2008;**20**(3):603-635

[74] O'Regan JK, Noë A. A sensorimotor account of vision and visual consciousness. The Behavioral and Brain Sciences. 2001;**24**(5):939-973

[75] Adolph KE, Eppler MA, Gibson EJ. Crawling versus walking infants' perception of affordances for locomotion over sloping surfaces. Child Development. 1993;**64**(4):1158-1174

[76] Ashmead DH, Wall RS, Ebinger KA, Eaton SB, Snook-Hill MM, Yang X. Spatial hearing in children with visual disabilities. Perception. 1998;**27**(1):105-122

[77] Cappagli G, Gori M. Auditory spatial localization: Developmental delay in children with visual impairments. Research in Developmental Disabilities. 2016;**53**:391-398

[78] Cappagli G, Cocchi E, Gori M. Auditory and proprioceptive spatial impairments in blind children and adults. Developmental Science. 2017;**20**(3)

[79] Fraiberg S. Congenital sensory and motor deficits and ego formation. Annual of Psychoanalysis. 1977;**5**:169-194

[80] Fraiberg S, Siegel BL, Gibson R. The role of sound in the search behavior of a blind infant. The Psychoanalytic Study of the Child. 1966;**21**(1):327-357

[81] Adelson E, Fraiberg S. Gross motor development in infants blind from birth. Child Development. 1974:114-126

[82] Bayley N. Bayley Scales of Infant Development, Second Edition: Manual. San Antonio, TX: The Psychological; 1993

[83] Fazzi E, Signorini SG, Bomba M, Luparia A, Lanners J, Balottin U. Reach on sound: A key to object permanence in visually impaired children. Early Human Development. 2011;**87**(4):289-296

[84] Ittyerah M, Gaunet F, Rossetti Y. Pointing with the left and right hands in congenitally blind children. Brain and Cognition. 2007;**64**(2):170-183

[85] Gaunet F, Rossetti Y. Effects of visual deprivation on space representation: Immediate and delayed pointing toward memorised proprioceptive targets. Perception. 2006;**35**(1):107-124

[86] Landau B, Spelke E, Gleitman H. Spatial knowledge in a young blind child. Cognition. 1984;**16**(3):225-260

[87] Warren DH. Blindness and Early Childhood Development. New York, NY, US: American Foundation for the Blind; 1977

[88] Bigelow AE. Blind and sighted children's spatial knowledge of their home environments. International Journal of Behavioral Development. 1996;**19**(4):797-816

[89] Troster H, Hecker W, Brambring M. Longitudinal study of gross-motor development in blind infants and preschoolers. Early Child Development and Care. 1994;**104**(1):61-78

[90] Pérez-Pereira M, Conti-Ramsden G. Do blind children show autistic features. Autism and blindness: Research and reflections. 2005:99-127

[91] Prechtl HF, Cioni G, Einspieler C, Bos AF, Ferrari F. Role of vision on early motor development: Lessons from the blind. Developmental Medicine and Child Neurology. 2001;**43**(3):198-201

[92] Hallemans A, Ortibus E, Truijen S, Meire F. Development of independent locomotion in children with a severe visual impairment. Research in Developmental Disabilities. 2011;**32**(6):2069-2074

[93] Houwen S, Hartman E, Visscher C. Physical activity and motor skills in children with and without visual

impairments. Medicine and Science in Sports and Exercise. 2009;**41**(1):103-109

[94] Jacobson RD. Cognitive mapping without sight: Four preliminary studies of spatial learning. Journal of Environmental Psychology. 1998;**18**(3):289-305

[95] Wanet MC, Veraart C. Processing of auditory information by the blind in spatial localization tasks. Perception & Psychophysics. 1985;**38**(1):91-96

[96] Ungar S. Cognitive mapping without visual experience. In: Kitchin R, Freundschuh S, editors. Cognitive Mapping: Past Present and Future. London: Routledge; 2000

[97] Hüg MX, Arias C, Tommasini FC, Ramos OA. Auditory localization and precedence effect: An exploratory study in infants and toddlers with visual impairment and normal vision. Research in Developmental Disabilities. 2014;**35**(9):2015-2025

[98] Bigelow AE. Development of the use of sound in the search behavior of infants. Developmental Psychology. 1983;**19**(3)

[99] GuralnickMJ,ConnorRT,HammondM, Gottman JM, Kinnish K. Immediate effects of mainstreamed settings on the social interactions and social integration of preschool children. AJMR-American Journal on Mental Retardation. 1996;**100**(4):359-377

[100] Guralnick MJ, Gottman JM, Hammond MA. Effects of social setting on the friendship formation of young children differing in developmental status. Journal of Applied Developmental Psychology. 1996;**17**(4):625-651

[101] McConnell SR, Odom SL. A multimeasure performance-based assessment of social competence in young children with disabilities. Topics in Early Childhood Special Education. 1999;**19**(2):67-74

[102] Rettig M. The play of young children with visual impairments: Characteristics and interventions. Journal of Visual Impairment & Blindness. 1994;**88**(5):410-420

[103] Sacks S, Kekelis L, Gaylord-Ross R. The Development of Social Skills by Blind and Visually Impaired Students: Exploratory Studies and Strategies. New York, NY, US: American Foundation for the Blind; 1992

[104] Andersen ES, Dunlea A, Kekelis LS. Blind children's language: Resolving some differences. Journal of Child Language. 1984;**11**(3):645-664

[105] Parsons S. Function of play in low vision children: II. Emerging patterns of behavior. Journal of Visual Impairment & Blindness. 1986;**80**(6):777-784

[106] Schneekloth LH. Play environments for visually impaired children. Journal of Visual Impairment & Blindness. 1989;**83**(4):196-201

[107] Skellenger AC, Hill EW. Effects of a shared teacher-child play intervention on the play skills of three young children who are blind. Journal of Visual Impairment & Blindness. 1994;**88**(5):433-445

[108] Hartup WW. Social relationships and their developmental significance. The American Psychologist. 1989;**44**(2):120

[109] Booth CL. Predicting social adjustment in middle childhood: The role of preschool attachment security and maternal style. Social Development. 1994;**3**(3):189-204

[110] Harker CM, Ibanez LV, Nguyen TP, Messinger DS, Stone WL. The effect of parenting style on social smiling in infants at high and low risk for ASD. Journal of

Autism and Developmental Disorders. 2016;**46**(7):2399-2407

[111] Kaufmann D, Gesten E, Santa Lucia RC, Salcedo O, Rendina-Gobioff G, Gadd R. The relationship between parenting style and children's adjustment: The parents' perspective. Journal of Child and Family Studies. 2000;**9**(2):231-245

[112] Kochanska G, Coy KC, Tjebkes TL, Husarek SJ. Individual differences in emotionality in infancy. Child Development. 1998;**69**(2):375-390

[113] Landry SH, Smith KE, Swank PR, Assel MA, Vellet S. Does early responsive parenting have a special importance for children's development or is consistency across early childhood necessary? Developmental Psychology. 2001;**37**(3):387

[114] Bronfenbrenner U, Ceci SJ. Nature-nuture reconceptualized in developmental perspective: A bioecological model. Psychological Review. 1994;**101**(4):568

[115] Lomanowska A, Boivin M, Hertzman C, Fleming AS. Parenting begets parenting: A neurobiological perspective on early adversity and the transmission of parenting styles across generations. Neuroscience. 2017;**342**:120-139

[116] Lyons-RuthK,RepacholiB,McLeodS, SilvaE.Disorganizedattachmentbehavior in infancy: Short-term stability, maternal and infant correlates, and risk-related subtypes. Development and Psychopathology. 1991;**3**(4):377-396

[117] Wakschlag LS, Hans SL. Relation of maternal responsiveness during infancy to the development of behavior problems in high-risk youths. Developmental Psychology. 1999;**35**(2):569

[118] Key JM. Perceptions of poor maternal care are associated with adolescent depression. Journal of Affective Disorders. 1995;**34**(2):95-100

[119] Martin G, Bergen HA, Roeger L, Allison S. Depression in young adolescents: Investigations using 2 and 3 factor versions of the parental bonding instrument. The Journal of Nervous and Mental Disease. 2004;**192**(10):650-657

[120] Enns M, Cox B, Clara I. Parental bonding and adult psychopathology: Results from the US National Comorbidity Survey. Psychological Medicine. 2002;**32**(6):997-1008

[121] Leyser Y, Heinze A, Kapperman G. Stress and adaptation in families of children with visual disabilities. Families in Society. 1996;**77**(4):240-249

[122] Moore V, McConachie H. Communication between blind and severely visually impaired children and their parents. The British Journal of Developmental Psychology. 1994;**12**(4):491-502

[123] Foxall MJ, Barron CR, Von Dollen K, Jones PA, Shull KA. Predictors of loneliness in low vision adults. Western Journal of Nursing Research. 1992;**14**(1):86-99

[124] Emerson D. Facing loss of vision-the response of adults to visual impairment. Journal of Visual Impairment & Blindness. 1981;**75**(2):41-45

[125] Evans JR, Fletcher AE, Wormald RP. Depression and anxiety in visually impaired older people. Ophthalmology. 2007;**114**(2):283-288

[126] Fitzgerald RG. Reactions to blindness: An exploratory study of adults with recent loss of sight. Archives of General Psychiatry. 1970;**22**(4):370-379

[127] Burmedi D, Becker S, Heyl V, Wahl H-W, Himmelsbach I. Emotional and social consequences of age-related low

vision. Visual Impairment Research. 2002;**4**(1):47-71

[128] Burmedi D, Becker S, Heyl V, Wahl H-W, Himmelsbach I. Behavioral consequences of age-related low vision. Visual Impairment Research. 2002;**4**(1):15-45

[129] Nyman SR, Gosney MA, Victor CR. Emotional well-being in people with sight loss: Lessons from the grey literature. British Journal of Visual Impairment. 2010;**28**(3):175-203

[130] Nyman SR, Dibb B, Victor CR, Gosney MA. Emotional well-being and adjustment to vision loss in later life: A meta-synthesis of qualitative studies. Disability and Rehabilitation. 2012;**34**(12):971-981

[131] O'Donnell C. The greatest generation meets its greatest challenge: Vision loss and depression in older adults. Journal of Visual Impairment and Blindness. 2005;**99**(4):197-208

[132] Van Hasselt VB. Social adaptation in the blind. Clinical Psychology Review. 1983;**3**(1):87-102

[133] Horowitz A. The prevalence and consequences of vision impairment in later life. Topics in Geriatric Rehabilitation. 2004;**20**(3):185-195

[134] Gori M, Cappagli G, Tonelli A, Baud-Bovy G, Finocchietti S. Devices for visually impaired people: High technological devices with low user acceptance and no adaptability for children. Neuroscience and Biobehavioral Reviews. 2016;**69**:79-88

[135] Proulx MJ, Harder A. Sensory substitution. Visual-to-auditory sensory substitution devices for the blind. Dutch Journal of Ergonomics/Tijdschrift voor Ergonomie. 2008;**33**:20-22

[136] Bach-y-Rita P, Collins CC, Saunders FA, White B, Scadden L. Vision substitution by tactile image projection. Nature. 1969;**221**(5184):963

[137] Velázquez R. Wearable assistive devices for the blind. In: Wearable and Autonomous Biomedical Devices and Systems for Smart Environment. Berlin, Heidelberg: Springer-Verlag; 2010;**75**:331.349

[138] Kaczmarek KA. The tongue display unit (TDU) for electrotactile spatiotemporal pattern presentation. Scientia Iranica. 2011;**18**(6):1476-1485

[139] Bach-y-Rita P, Kaczmarek KA, Tyler ME, Garcia-Lara J. Form perception with a 49-point electrotactile stimulus array on the tongue: A technical note. Journal of Rehabilitation Research and Development. 1998;**35**:427-430

[140] Meijer PB. An experimental system for auditory image representations. IEEE Transactions on Biomedical Engineering. 1992;**39**(2):112-121

[141] Striem-Amit E, Cohen L, Dehaene S, Amedi A. Reading with sounds: Sensory substitution selectively activates the visual word form area in the blind. Neuron. 2012;**76**(3):640-652

[142] Maidenbaum S, Abboud S, Amedi A. Sensory substitution: Closing the gap between basic research and widespread practical visual rehabilitation. Neuroscience and Biobehavioral Reviews. 2014;**41**:3-15

[143] Bremner AJ, Spence C. Unimodal experience constrains while multisensory experiences enrich cognitive construction. The Behavioral and Brain Sciences. 2008;**31**(3):335-336

[144] Lewkowicz DJ. Perception of dynamic and static audiovisual sequences in 3-and 4-month-old infants. Child Development. 2008;**79**(5):1538-1554

[145] Shams L, Seitz AR. Benefits of multisensory learning. Trends in Cognitive Sciences. 2008;**12**(11):411-417

[146] Porquis LB, Finocchietti S, Zini G, Cappagli G, Gori M, Baud-Bovy G, editors. ABBI: A wearable device for improving spatial cognition in visually-impaired children. In: 2017 IEEE Biomedical Circuits and Systems Conference (BioCAS). Turin: IEEE; 2017. pp. 1-4

[147] Finocchietti S, Cappagli G, Giammari G, Cocchi E, Gori M. Test–retest reliability of BSP, a battery of tests for assessing spatial cognition in visually impaired children. PLoS One. 2019;**14**(4):e0212006

[148] Cappagli G, Finocchietti S, Cocchi E, Giammari G, Zumiani R, Cuppone AV, et al. Audio motor training improves mobility and spatial cognition in visually impaired children. Scientific Reports. 2019;**9**(1):3303

[149] Cappagli G, Finocchietti S, Baud-Bovy G, Cocchi E, Gori M. Multisensory rehabilitation training improves spatial perception in totally but not partially visually deprived children. Frontiers in Integrative Neuroscience. 2017;**11**:29

[150] Ungar S, Blades M, Spencer C. Can a tactile map facilitate learning of related information by blind and visually impaired people? A test of the conjoint retention hypothesis. In: Anderson M, Meyer B, Olivier P, editors. Diagrammatic Representation and Reasoning. Heidelberg: Springer Verlag; 2002

[151] Cappagli G, Finocchietti S, Baud-Bovy G, Badino L, D'Ausilio A, Cocchi E, et al. Assessing social competence in visually impaired people and proposing an interventional program in visually impaired children. IEEE Transactions on Cognitive and Developmental Systems. 2018;**10**(4):929-935

Chapter 16

Sensory Substitution for Visual Impairments: A Technological Review

Md Masum Billah, Zulkhairi Mohd Yusof, Kushsairy Kadir and Abdul Malik Mohd Ali

Abstract

This work shows the study of the people who are deprived of a sensory modality that affects brain organization and cognition. By studying, the blind or visual impaired helps learn about how sensory experience in each sense is required for specific brain systems to develop, and how the technologies help in plasticity change in their absence. The sensory-motor deprivation model serves to assess the roles of critical developmental periods, compensatory cross-modal plasticity, and sensory-independent (a-modal) processes in the human brain. Sensory substitution enables a new era for blind people. Therefore, this research will commit a complete review on the sensory substitution for visual impairments.

Keywords: blindness, visual technology, impairments, technology, eye-sight

1. Introduction

Visual weaknesses and visual impairment are practically basic wonders for the individuals who truly need help from others to navigate starting with one spot then onto the next. This gathering of individuals is denied of their ordinary life because of their visual issues. Despite the fact that a great deal of looks into have been done and some are proceeding for the improvement of assistive frameworks for this gathering which is totally unusable that can be acknowledged when practically 98% of visually impaired and outwardly debilitated individuals are totally relying upon the white stick as it were. Be that as it may, some are for the most part observed with the pooches in western nations for outside development, however despite everything it thinks about some peril while crossing the street and finding the method for course. Lab-scale models and couple of items for blinds are not finished enough for the visually impaired without the white stick or the help from others, so blinds cannot move alone while the advances are accessible. In this manner, another innovation which can be known as a tangible substitution as opposed to utilizing the assistive framework may assist the visually impaired individuals with moving alone with no other help.

2. Damage of visual sensory

2.1 Methods for recovery

Reclamation of tangible contribution in outwardly debilitated utilizing photographic inserts seems, by all accounts, to be an alluring option in contrast to tactile substitution gadgets, as they give a feeling of "genuine" vision, visual qualia (when contrasted with giving just visual data of vision). Gadgets dependent on different methodologies was demonstrated few encouraging outcomes, the visually impaired clients can, somewhat, use visual phosphenes produced by a portion of these gadgets to encounter important visual percepts. Be that as it may, in spite of the fact that they are at the forefront of medicinal, mechanical and logical advances, there are as yet a few noteworthy issues as of now keeping these methodologies from ending up evident clinical arrangements. As a matter of first importance, their intrusive nature makes them inclined to dangers identified with surgeries, for example, aggravation, drain, and expanded to deadness. Additionally, retinal prostheses are not material for populaces to visually impaired, as they require the presence of leftover practical retinal ganglion cells and visual tracts, while different visual impairment etiologies bring about their damage or nonattendance. Furthermore, these strategies are costly: the single sort of retinal embed which has as of late obtained in 2013 the principal FDA endorsement for constant implantation, Second Sight's Argus II, which is currently the main business visual embed, is accessible at a costly expenses.

Subsequently, the sight substitution (currently ending up economically accessible past starter clinical preliminaries) do not yet give locate that looks like characteristic achievement specifically creating a really valuable and utilitarian vision, at moderate expenses still cannot seem to become to ideally end up accessible later on and empower the treatment of more extensive etiologies.

2.2 Gadgets for visual sensory replacement

The elective way to deal with sight replacement to the visually impaired is tangible exchange. Tactile replacement alludes change qualities tangible methodology upgrades other methodology. It is conceivable to supplant vision by contact or tryout, tryout or vestibular faculties by contact, and so forth. On account of visual deficiency, SSDs speak to a non-intrusive recovery approach in which visual data is caught by an outer gadget, for example, a camcorder and conveyed to the visually impaired by means of a human-machine interface as sound-related or material information. Braille was developed for composing spearheaded made ready to present day using speck code. Be that as it may, Braille can work for material changed disconnected from printed visual letters to Braille specks and cannot be utilized for internet perusing of customary letters. As of late other perusing substitutions have been created for internet perusing, for example, the Optacon (a print-totactual-picture gadget concocted for perusing emblazoned in different variants of committed content to-discourse motors. Notwithstanding these perusing helps, a lot of exertion has been put resources into creating gadgets planned for improving the portability of the visually impaired. The white stick used to precisely test for hindrances speaks to the least complex, most normally utilized gadget. Both the Braille framework and the stick arrangements, which were immediately adjusted by visually impaired clients, propose that now and again the easiest arrangement may be the one that is the most broadly utilized. Be that as it may, as of late further developed partners of the stick have turned out to be accessible, for example, electronic travel helps intended to be utilized alongside the white stick so as to broaden the separation for ecological review and subsequently increment speed and proficiency of movement.

As opposed to these gadgets which are commonly intended for a restricted reason and are fruitful in supplanting just certain practical parts of vision, increasingly advanced procedures that supplant vision through material or sound-related data have been created in the course of the most recent couple of decades. The first focused on methodology to replacement of eye sight, because of the effortlessness and simplicity of changing visual into material sign which are both portrayed by two axes portrayals as shown in **Figure 1** [1].

Albeit amazingly extraordinary, both sound-related and material SSDs can conceivably be helpful for the visually impaired (however observe insights concerning their impediments in the following area; primarily the requirement for unequivocal preparing, the potential intrusion of sound-related sources of info and the low transient goals) [2–5]. Late tests demonstrate that blindfolded located people, and sometimes even the visually impaired can figure out how to translate the transmitted data and use it in a few basic visual undertakings, particularly in the wake of preparing or delayed utilization of the gadget [6].

2.3 Challenges in sight restoration

Current sight rebuilding endeavors, regardless of whether through intrusive or non-obtrusive strategies, still face a few difficulties to be appropriate to the general outwardly impeded populace.

These might be isolated to two primary highlights:

- Passing on data with adequate handy visual goals, or sharpness.

- Empowering visual useful handling of consistently complex scenes and undertakings

- Despite the fact that the two may appear to be to some degree compatible, they originate from altogether places.

Besides, at present the most progressive adaptation of visual inserts, retinal prostheses, are actually constrained to giving a restricted field of view because of issues in making inward embeds to fit the anatomical structure of the retina [7].

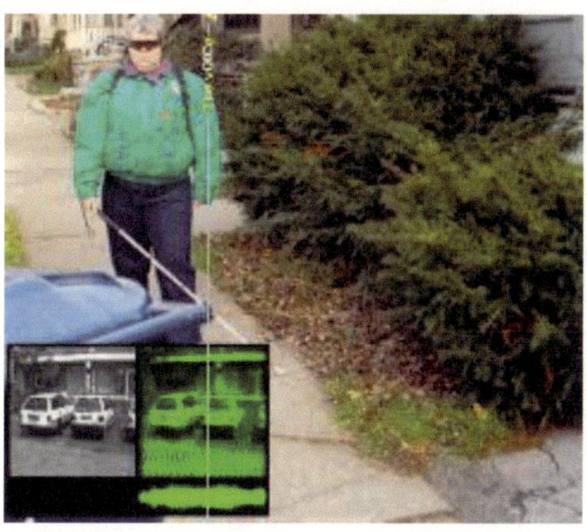

Figure 1.
Gadget for future sensory substitution [1].

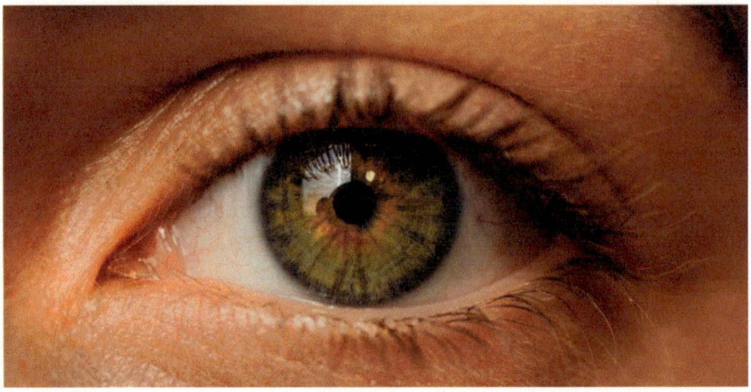

Figure 2.
Eye sight complication.

Maybe additional significantly, subsequent sharpness become less compare to anticipated given the number of pixels, on grounds that the interpretation from specialized goals to utilitarian keenness is exceptionally perplexing as shown in **Figure 2**.

The issue of recommended usage of gadget is portrayed outcomes. The gadget gives from the earlier the most noteworthy hypothetical goals, hence a main possibility for visual restoration. Its principle detriments lie in the multifaceted nature of the generally low fleeting goals. In spite of the fact that the SSD change standards are moderately basic, deciphering pictures requires unequivocal and very broad preparing, which was not in presence at the beginning of my exploration. As a major aspect of the examination venture, I built up a focused on preparing convention in "figuring out how to see" utilizing the system. The subsequent issue, which will be nitty gritty in the following segment, has to do with cerebrum association, pliancy and neurorehabilitation, which is increasingly mind boggling, and relates to our comprehension of mind work [8, 9].

3. Visual rehabilitation features

Although additional creating to recovery procedures is as yet a huge innovative test, tactile rebuilding endeavors just transmitting the sight data, whichever by means of different by providing vision through the characteristic visual framework to the mind. As it were, when initially acquainted with the cerebrum of an inherently visually impaired individual, the visual data is futile on the grounds that that individual does not have any past involvement on which such data can be deciphered. Besides, the mind of such people may do not have a working visual framework for translating the recently presented data and giving it useful significance. Indeed, even on account of non-innately daze who have had some past visual experience, one cannot expect that re-acquainting visual data with their minds will naturally result in completely refined visual observation, since their "visual" cerebrum areas may now be incorporated into other, non-visual cerebrum systems [10]. This exercise rises up out of the moderately fruitful restoration of hard of hearing and auditorily weakened people utilizing cochlear inserts, which additionally requires express educating for individuals to figure out how to create new relationship among sounds and their sources. Besides, such recovery is joined and empowered by relating versatility in the sound-related cortex to react to the recently conveyed information. **Figure 3** shows the clinical visual rehabilitation process generally practiced in the rehabilitation center.

DOI: http://dx.doi.org/10.5772/intechopen.89147

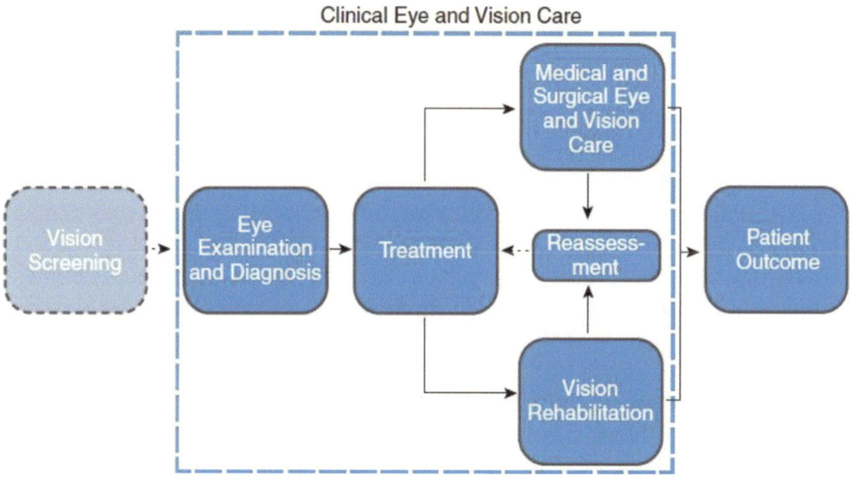

Figure 3.
Clinical visual rehabilitation process.

In reality, a few early endeavors at careful sight reclamation for visual information may likewise not get the job done if there should be an occurrence of vision [11–13]. The patients in these investigations indicated significant trouble in perceiving common articles and conditions, even after an extensive stretch of viewing preparing. This was particularly valid for 'ventral stream capacities', for example, shape and structure acknowledgment, figure ground isolation, profundity, size, and so forth. These visual disabilities remained so intense that in some announced cases the in fact "outwardly reestablished" individual retreated to living in useful self-characterized visual deficiency with no capacity to use the visual information now accessible to them. This is genuine notwithstanding for individuals who have lost their sight at more seasoned ages: an ongoing late-beginning visually impaired sight reclamation quiet whose sight was lost at 17 years old and reestablished 51 years after the fact additionally indicated real shortfalls in visual discernment. This demonstrates enabling the visual data to enter the mind through a practical retina does not ensure or empower full or characteristic visual discernment. Subsequently, accomplishing full useful tactile rebuilding might be conceivable on the off chance that we consider the specificities of intellectual and neural working of the tangible disabled, a subject which will be exhibited straightaway [14].

3.1 Damage significances

Once endeavoring for comprehend psyches and cerebrums of people damage a tangible methodology, an imperative take data of the numerous variables that influence the association cognitively. These are joined from our hereditary auras and the cerebrum's common formative way, diverted relying upon natural variables and explicit individual encounters and exercises, and through progressively novel psychological difficulties and requests forced by nonstandard tangible sources of info. In particular, so as to accomplish the equivalent useful level in their regular daily existence, the individuals who experience the ill effects of tactile misfortune need to create procedures which empower them to extricate data to accomplish their objectives from elective sources to make up for their visual impairment. Such alterations are intervened through rebuilding in other tactile or higher-request psychological capacities (for instance over the top utilization of memory systems, see subtleties underneath). Accordingly, unique psychological requests lead to various individual encounters and exercises, which thusly advance a specific example of plastic rearrangement inside the sensory system.

Moreover, it is imperative to remember that different subpopulations of people experiencing visual misfortune and varying in etiology or beginning of tangible misfortune contrast in their potential for versatility. The early beginning of tangible misfortune experienced in inborn visual impairment triggers the most sensational instances of versatility and empowers broad mind rebuilding which makes up for the shortfalls, producing a strikingly unexpected useful system in comparison to the one seen in ordinarily located people or people who have supported cerebrum or fringe wounds sometime down the road. Inborn or early-beginning visual deficiency influences huge bits of the mind, particularly when coming about because of fringe harm (for example broken retina or the tactile tracts), which do not harm the mind itself, however rather retain portions of the cerebrum from their common information, leaving it basically jobless. The visually impaired do not deteriorate. Or maybe, they experience broad versatility coming about in altogether changed neural responsiveness just as utilitarian contribution in non-visual psychological capacities. Critical, albeit normally less broad plastic changes, likewise happen in populaces experiencing non-inherent tactile misfortune. The neuroplasticity is clear normal mind actuation in the visually impaired when contrasted and that of the located, just as in its social appearances, e.g., tactile explicit psychological aptitudes, which are all essential to the capacity to reestablish locate sometime down the road.

The main proof for the broad rearrangement experienced by the cerebrums of the inherently visually impaired can be found in the revealed upgraded tangible and psychological capacities of such people which make up for their tactile shortages. Daze people need to make up for their absence of vision, the methodology which ordinarily enables one to "comprehend what is the place by looking and is perfect for giving simultaneous data to one another, attracting consideration regarding pertinent outside signs and incredibly encouraging spatial coding. In spite of the fact that the visually impaired cannot secure data for item limitation and acknowledgment by looking, despite everything they need this data to explore to find and perceive the articles around them for instance. Accordingly, they need to get this data through option, tangible or other, methodologies. For example, as right on time as the age of the Mishnah that was realized that visually impaired people had better memory capacities looked at. Thus, it has been demonstrated that the visually impaired have predominant material and sound-related discernment capacities: for example, they can all the more likely separate between little material dabs or sound-related spatial areas than the located, and even to more readily distinguish smells. In any case, the visually impaired do not generally perform better on such undertakings, proposing that ideal advancement of certain parts of tactile handling in the unaffected modalities may rely upon, or possibly advantage from, simultaneous visual info. Moreover, when looking at changed populaces of the visually impaired, it turns out to be evident that the recognized advantages in some sound-related and material undertakings depend, as it were, on the age at sight misfortune [15].

In particular, these points of interest are frequently, yet not constantly, constrained to the innately and early-beginning visually impaired, though the exhibition of the late blinded will in general take after that of the located, reflecting contrasts in the measurement of visual experience between these populaces. Notwithstanding, there is likewise proof showing that compensatory benefits additionally happen in the late visually impaired, in which case they might be interceded by various neurophysiological components as point by point in the following areas. Critically, albeit delayed involvement with a diminished number of accessible tactile modalities prompts such advantages, these do not show up naturally. For instance, it has been demonstrated that visually impaired youngsters have huge troubles with certain assignments, particularly those which expect reference to outside signals, getting bearings and spatial relations between items. Such undertakings are trying for the visually impaired, as they have bargained spatial portrayals and depend for the most part on self-reference and development groupings. Therefore, the visually impaired have issues perceiving possibly valuable data expected to play out these sorts of assignments and do not have the advantages which could emerge from all the while accessible vision. For instance, simultaneous visual info can encourage acknowledgment and learning of accommodating sound-related or somatosensory highlights given that the presence of excess or covering data from more than one methodology is by and large connected with controlling consideration and improved learning [16]. In any case, such acknowledgment of valuable signals or the alignment of sound-related and material space is in the end conceivable even without vision, as it might be accomplished utilizing various prompts, for instance those originating from self-movement. Significantly, despite the fact that it might require moderately extensive preparing to arrive at a phase where the missing tangible information is swapped and made up for by comparable data from different modalities, spatial portrayals which are at long last created based on haptic and sound-related contribution of the visually impaired appear to be equal to the outwardly based ones in the located. Generally speaking, the discoveries demonstrate that the visually impaired, when they figure out how to manage the accessible tangible modalities, can indicate equivalent or unrivaled execution in numerous errands when contrasted with the located. This preferred position can even be undermined by the nearness of visual data, as demonstrated by second rate execution of the somewhat visually impaired. In this manner, the accessible proof will in general counter the thought that tangible misfortune prompts general maladjustment and brokenness in capacities outside the missing methodology. An incredible opposite, this general-misfortune theory ought to be relinquished for the option, compensatory speculation which recommends that tactile misfortune prompts the unrivaled improvement of the rest of the faculties [17].

These interesting compensatory capacities are the aftereffect of plastic changes in the cerebrums of the visually impaired. Over the most recent couple of decades, neural connects of revealed weakness actuated changes in psychological capacities and procedures have been altogether contemplated, giving an abundance of data with respect to the cerebrum's capacities to change. Studies researching neural handling of innately dazzle people, just as creature models of these conditions, demonstrate that the cerebrum is equipped for vigorous versatility reflected in significantly adjusted working of whole mind systems. Significant proof relating to the modified intellectual handling and the practical status of the occipital cortex in the visually impaired stems from electrophysiological contemplates which have researched non-visual tangible elements of the visually impaired. These yielded outcomes demonstrating shorter latencies for occasion related possibilities (ERP) in sound-related and somatosensory assignments in the visually impaired as opposed to the located, proposing increasingly effective handling in these undertakings. In the visually impaired, huge numbers of these progressions begin to happen inside days following the beginning of visual impairment and in this manner influence the intrinsically visually impaired as well as the late visually impaired, who likewise show critical revamping in the occipital cortex in spite of the fact that to a lesser degree. For instance, late-beginning visually impaired individuals show enactment in their essential visual cortex for language recognition.

This versatility, particularly in the early-beginning visually impaired, may go about as a twofold edged sword. From one viewpoint, it enables the visually impaired adapt to better to visual impairment by supporting compensatory capacities, and yet it may meddle with sight rebuilding endeavors by exasperating the first elements of the visual cortex, as will be itemized in the following segment.

3.2 Developmental periods of sensory loss

When talking about various kinds of neuroplastic changes and potential instruments fundamental them, and the unfavorable consequences for the regularly creating visual framework with regards to visual restoration, underline that these shift altogether rely upon the age at beginning of visual deficiency, just as its span. These distinctions mirror a few factors: the cerebrum's capability to change at various times of advancement, the measure of involvement with visual or sound-related preparing preceding tangible misfortune and the measure of training with the rest of the faculties or some unique material. The most significant of these components mirrors the way that the general potential for any type of plastic changes differs gigantically over the life expectancy. In spite of the fact that the cerebrum holds some capacity to change all through life, it is by and large accepted and tentatively supported that the sensory system is most plastic during its advancement, both on account of ordinary improvement and following mind damage [18]. The creating cerebrum is an exceedingly unique framework which experiences a few unmistakable stages from cell development to the fast development and ensuing end of un-utilized neural connections before at long last going into an increasingly steady stage following adolescence. The utilitarian task of individual cerebrum locales which happens during this time is vitally reliant on synaptic improvement which incorporates extreme changes that frequently occur in spurts. In the visual cortex, during the primary year after birth, the quantity of neurotransmitters develops hugely and is accordingly downsized to the grown-up level around the age of 11 through broad abatements in synaptic and spine thickness, dendritic length or even the quantity of neurons. This procedure is basically controlled by understanding and neural action: neurotransmitters which are utilized are fortified while those which are not strengthened or effectively utilized are killed. Synaptic improvement is exceptionally subject to rivalry between approaching data sources, the absence of which can bring about a diminished degree of synaptic correction and perseverance of repetitive associations in adulthood. This procedure of synaptic pruning speaks to a genuinely ceaseless and expanded tuning of neural circuits and can be diverged from different sorts of changes which happen at exceptionally short timescales. During such times of strengthened and improvement of sensory loss, a huge operational procedure was required for recovery. Along these lines, wounds influencing various phases of advancement, notwithstanding when they happen at a generally comparable ages, may trigger unmistakable examples of compensatory neuroplastic changes and lead to various degrees of recuperation. In particular, early investigations of recuperation after visual misfortune in creature recommended that vision is especially delicate to getting regular contribution during early advancement, and that visual hardship notwithstanding for brief terms, yet at an early formative beginning, may irreversibly harm the capacity to typically see vision at more seasoned ages. Instances of waterfall evacuation in outwardly disabled youngsters bolster these discoveries. For instance, youngsters brought into the world with thick respective waterfalls and afterward treated during the primary year of life later by and large create typical vision, and are not debilitated at either low level visual capacities and abnormal state capacities. Since these abilities surpass those present during childbirth in the outwardly ordinary youngster, the typical presentation of waterfall inversion patients likely suggests that the neural circuits fundamental these capacities can recoup totally from a brief time of prior visual hardship. In any case, if the waterfalls are not expelled early enough, the waterfall inversion patients may later experience the ill effects of decreased visual keenness and hindrances abnormal state capacities, for example, diminished visual gathering capacities and hindered face preparing doubt even after early youth, visual data is significant for the crystallization of visual associations long after the finish of pruning, however the deficiencies created from short visual hardship starting at early immaturity for instance are progressively moderate [16–18].

In this way, visual hardship, particularly if showing from the get-go throughout everyday life, can devastatingly affect the capacity to process vision. Additionally, the capacity of the cerebrum to adjust, or the potential for neuroplasticity after adolescence is viewed as much lower than in youth. Moreover, the pliancy found in adulthood will in general outcome from various neurophysiological systems, which may not get the job done to help visual recovery. For instance, the vigorous, transient pliancy saw in blindfolding for a few days may emerge from the enlistment of officially existing, however ordinarily unused, hindered or conceal pathways which become accessible once the source or explanation behind such covering is evacuated. Along these lines, a few types of grown-up pliancy do not reflect that portrayed by the production of new availability designs. In neurotic states, wounds, or late tangible misfortune, versatility might be blended. Fast changes mirroring the exposing of existing associations happening in the primary stage advance and may empower resulting moderate, yet increasingly perpetual basic changes.

3.3 Visual cortex in the brain

Another factor worth considering in this regard is the huge intricacy of the visual preparing led in the cerebrum, and its imperative fundamental neural structures. The regularly created visual framework is a complex neural engineering of parallel and interweaved handling, with a perplexing division-of-work in which various areas have practical experience in the preparing of various visual highlights, errands and even articles. For instance, the visual cortex is included two handling streams. The ventral occipital-fleeting pathway has been connected with visual handling of structure, object character and shading. Its partner is viewed as the dorsal occipital-parietal "where/how" pathway, or the "dorsal stream", which examines visuo-spatial data about article area and takes an interest in visuo-engine arranging and outwardly guided development. It has been more than once demonstrated that in typically located individuals who have endured a sore in one of these alleged neural modules or notwithstanding preparing streams, the impression of items handled in this district might be seriously impeded [19]. For instance, the twofold separation between the preparing of the two streams has been altogether approved by investigations of confined sores independently influencing visual item personality acknowledgment (visual agnosia) and article visuo-engine spatial control, and an injury or deafferentation of the VWFA may bring about alexia, or procured dyslexia.

The anatomical reason for this division has additionally been contemplated, and shows a mind boggling example of base up availability, starting with the essential visual cortex and making two parallel (however not totally free) anatomical network streams, one of which leads dorsally, through the back parietal cortex towards the premotor cortex, accordingly making a characteristic "way" towards arrangement for movement and spatial handling, while different leads through zone V4, which is specific for the shading and size of visual, to inferotemporal territories containing complex visual article portrayals, and up to the prefrontal cortex. Thus, the various leveled handling of the low-level highlights of the states of letters, their further sequencing to words and after that to progressively extract semantic portrayals additionally shows in an anatomical preparing pathway. This hard-wired bottom up availability example makes a solid limitation towards the age of these streams and districts within the sight of typical visual contribution during improvement. In any case, the production of two separate visual streams, or that of independent area specific locales inside the streams, and their utilitarian selectivity may not be so trifling without visual info, which denies the visual cortex of its regular information, particularly given the distinctive powerlessness to versatility over the life expectancy. Since these streams and locales have been demonstrated to be basic for the best possible preparing of item shapes, areas just as better evaluation highlights, for example, content (as confirm by the previously mentioned injury contemplates), it is conceivable to ask whether visual acknowledgment can happen at all without building up the full degree of the complex visual cortex design.

Every one of the components nitty gritty so far show the requesting provokes that still should be handled by sight rebuilding endeavors. In the event that the visually impaired cerebrum has experienced broad changes, and the inherently visually impaired mind might be considerably more definitely modified since it did not get the visual data sources guiding its ordinary advancement in the first place, how might we anticipate that the visually impaired should figure out how to see vision?

4. Auditory sensory substitution

Sound-related SSDs can offer, in any event hypothetically, incredibly high goals. While one such gadget utilized in research and with an end goal to restore the visually impaired has a maximal hypothetical goal of just 124 pixels can on a fundamental level create a lot higher goals, up to 25,344 pixels. Nonetheless, its real practical visual sharpness has never been tried as far as we could possibly know, and particularly not in a visually impaired clients bunch methodically. It is consequently critical to decide the most ideal visual sharpness that can be accomplished by visually impaired people utilizing such a sound-related SSD, so as to comprehend the potential estimation of these gadgets [20, 21]. Besides, as basic formative periods for view of common for confinement the medicinal methods for sight rebuilding (for instance, a few uncommon records of sight reclamation in adulthood brought about just incompletely useful vision, likely because of such restrictions; it is fascinating to decide whether early-beginning and intrinsically dazzle grown-ups can figure out how to see fine "visual" subtleties after numerous long stretches of visual deficiency utilizing SSDs.

4.1 Sounds: sensory substitution

A few investigations have indicated enlistment of visually impaired for different assignments that copy the visual errands of similar districts in the located. This

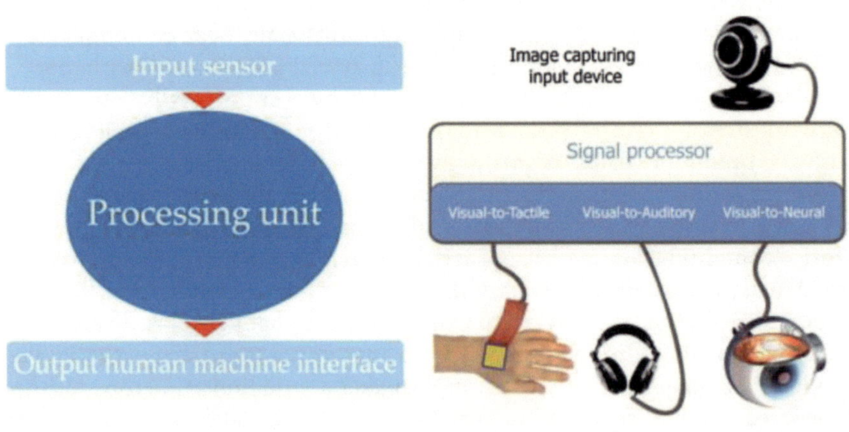

Figure 4.
Auditory sensory substitution concepts.

incorporates enlistment of the material improvements through a perusing task. Notwithstanding, few examinations have indicated selectivity to one errand over another and less yet have researched the presence in the visually impaired of a basic component of the ventral visual cortex, to be specific, its local selectivity for perceptual classes that despite the fact that our SSD change rations the state of the letters, it is impossible that a particular low-level tangible shape handling emulating vision drives the initiation or selectivity saw in our outcomes, since the physical measurements on which it is based contrast incredibly from those portraying both visual and material as shown in **Figure 4**. In particular, visual highlights that have been proposed to drive the selectivity for letters, for example, high-recurrence vision.

5. Conclusion

This work shows the study of the people who's are deprived of a sensory modality that affects brain organization and cognition. By studying, the blind or visual impaired helps learn about how sensory experience in each sense is required for specific brain systems to develop, and how the technologies help in plasticity change in their absence. The sensory-motor deprivation model serves to assess the roles of critical developmental periods, compensatory cross-modal plasticity and sensory-independent (a-modal) processes in the human brain. Therefore, this research will commit a complete review on the sensory substitution for visual impairments.

Acknowledgements

The authors would like to thank Universiti Kuala Lumpur British Malaysian Institute for generous support to complete this research.

Conflict of interest

The authors declare no conflict of interest.

Author details

Md Masum Billah, Zulkhairi Mohd Yusof*, Kushsairy Kadir and Abdul Malik Mohd Ali
Universiti Kuala Lumpur British Malaysian Institute (UniKL BMI), Kuala Lumpur, Malaysia

*Address all correspondence to: zulkhairi@unikl.edu.my

References

[1] Maidenbaum S, Abboud S, Amedi A. Sensory substitution: Closing the gap between basic research and widespread practical visual rehabilitation. Neuroscience & Biobehavioral Reviews. 2014;**41**:3-15

[2] Schinazi VR, Thrash T, Chebat DR. Spatial navigation by congenitally blind individuals. WIREs Cognitive Science. 2016;**7**(1):37-58. http://dx.doi.org/10.1002/wcs.1375

[3] Maidenbaum S, Hanassy S, Abboud S, Buchs G, Chebat DR, Levy-Tzedek S, et al. The "EyeCane", a new electronic travel aid for the blind: Technology, behavior & swift learning. Restorative Neurology and Neuroscience. 2014;**32**(6):813-824

[4] Proulx MJ, Ptito M, Amedi A. Multisensory integration, sensory substitution and visual rehabilitation. Neuroscience and Biobehavioral Reviews. 2014;**41**:1-2

[5] Kristjánsson Á, Moldoveanu A, Jóhannesson ÓI, Balan O, Spagnol S, Valgeirsdóttir VV, et al. Designing sensory-substitution devices: Principles, pitfalls and potential 1. Restorative Neurology and Neuroscience. 2016;**34**(5):769-787

[6] Dundon NM, Bertini C, Làdavas E, Sabel BA, Gall C. Visual rehabilitation: Visual scanning, multisensory stimulation and vision restoration trainings. Frontiers in Behavioral Neuroscience. 2015;**9**:192

[7] N Sahni J, Angi M, Irigoyen C, Semeraro F, R Romano M, Parmeggiani F. Therapeutic challenges to retinitis pigmentosa: From neuroprotection to gene therapy. Current Genomics. 2011;**12**(4):276-284

[8] Goetz GA, Mandel Y, Manivanh R, Palanker DV, Čižmár T. Holographic display system for restoration of sight to the blind. Journal of Neural Engineering. 2013;**10**(5):056021

[9] Goetz GA, Palanker DV. Electronic approaches to restoration of sight. Reports on Progress in Physics. 2016;**79**(9):096701

[10] Kruegle HA, Blumenthal A. Inventors; Allen Vision Systems Inc, assignee. Low vision rehabilitation system. United States patent US 5,777,715. 1998

[11] Visser ES, Visser R, van Lier HJ, Otten HM. Modern scleral lenses part I: Clinical features. Eye & Contact Lens. 2007;**33**(1):13-20

[12] Tao Y, Hu H. Building a visual tracking system for home-based rehabilitation. In: Proc. of the 9th Chinese Automation and Computing Society Conf. In the UK. Vol. 20. 2003. pp. 343-448

[13] Ordikhani-Seyedlar M, Sorensen HB,Kjaer TW, Siebner HR, Puthusserypady S. SSVEP-modulation by covert and overt attention: Novel features for BCI in attention neuro-rehabilitation. In: 2014 36th Annual International Conference of the IEEE Engineering in Medicine and Biology Society. IEEE; 2014. pp. 5462-5465

[14] Capelle C, Trullemans C, Arno P, Veraart C. A real-time experimental prototype for enhancement of vision rehabilitation using auditory substitution. IEEE Transactions on Biomedical Engineering. 1998;**45**(10):1279-1293

[15] Collignon O, Voss P, Lassonde M, Lepore F. Cross-modal plasticity for the spatial processing of sounds in visually deprived subjects. Experimental Brain Research. 2009;**192**(3):343

[16] King AJ. Visual influences on auditory spatial learning.

Philosophical Transactions of the Royal Society, B: Biological Sciences. 2008;**364**(1515):331-339

[17] Gori M, Sandini G, Martinoli C, Burr DC. Impairment of auditory spatial localization in congenitally blind human subjects. Brain. 2013;**137**(1):288-293

[18] Kooijman AC. Rehabilitation of visual impairments in patients with brain damage. In: Low Vision: Research and New Developments in Rehabilitation. IOS Press; 1994:**11**:287

[19] Cohen H, Kane-Wineland M, Miller LV, Hatfield CL. Occupation and visual/vestibular interaction in vestibular rehabilitation. Otolaryngology–Head and Neck Surgery. 1995;**112**(4):526-532

[20] Smiddy WE, Hamburg TR, Kracher GP, Gottsch JD, Stark WJ. Contact lenses for visual rehabilitation after corneal laceration repair. Ophthalmology. 1989;**96**(3):293-298

[21] Serdarevic ON, Renard GJ, Pouliquen Y. Randomized clinical trial comparing astigmatism and visual rehabilitation after penetrating keratoplasty with and without intraoperative suture adjustment. Ophthalmology. 1994;**101**(6):990-999

Chapter 17

Audio Cortical Processing in Blind Individuals

Monica Gori, Maria Bianca Amadeo, Giulio Sandini and Claudio Campus

Abstract

This chapter focuses on the cortical processing of auditory spatial information in blindness. Research has demonstrated enhanced auditory processing in blind individuals, suggesting they compensate for lacking vision with greater sensitivity in other senses. A few years ago, we demonstrated severely impaired auditory precision in congenitally blind individuals when performing an auditory spatial metric task: participants' thresholds for spatially bisecting three consecutive, spatially distributed sound sources were seriously compromised. Here we describe psychophysical and neural correlates of this deficit, and we show that the deficit disappears if blind individuals are presented with coherent spatio-temporal cues (short space associated with short time and vice versa). Instead, when the audio information presents incoherent spatio-temporal cues (short space associated with long time and vice versa), sighted individuals are unaffected by the perturbation while blind individuals are strongly attracted to the temporal cue. These results suggest that blind participants use temporal cues to make audio spatial estimations and that the visual cortex seems to have a functional role in these perceptual tasks. In the present chapter, we illustrate our hypothesis, suggesting that the lack of vision may drive construction of multisensory cortical network coding space based on temporal instead of spatial coordinates.

Keywords: blindness, visual cortex, space, time, neural plasticity

1. Introduction: the development of space representation

The development of a multisensory space representation of the environment is crucial for humans to interact with objects and each other. Different sensory modalities represent space using varying reference systems: vision relies on retinotopic coordinates, audition on head-centered coordinates, and touch on body-centered ones. To perceive a multisensory world, human brains must combine the spatial information arriving from all the sensory modalities into a coherent representation. The visual modality seems to have a crucial role in this important step, and specifically in the process of developing an integrated multisensory representation of the environment. If vision is so important, then an obvious question arises: what happens to space representation when the visual input is missing? Studies of animals suggest that the lack of vision in the first period of life alters the development of space representation. For example, auditory spatial maps of juvenile barn owls change after visual adaptation with prismatic spectacles [1]. Likewise, total visual deprivation in young ferrets is associated with the development of disordered auditory spatial maps [2]. Similar transitory effects occur in humans. In a number of studies, auditory space representation altered after short periods of adaptation to non-aligned auditory and visual stimuli [3, 4]. In agreement with this idea, research shows the representation of the auditory space is dominated by visual experience among young children [5]. Taken together, these results support not only the idea that vision is important for developing auditory space representation, but also that its absence may interfere with such development.

2. Space representation and blindness

Since blindness represents a unique condition to investigate the role of the visual modality in the development of space representation, many researchers have investigated this topic. However, contradictory results have been found. Lack of visual experience is associated with an enhancement of auditory (e.g., [6–11]) and tactile modalities [12] in blind compared with sighted individuals according to some studies. Results show that early blind subjects have enhanced skills in auditory pitch discrimination [13], localization of peripheral sounds in the horizontal plane [7, 10, 11], and ability to form spatial topographical maps underlying simple auditory localization [14, 15]. In particular, Lessard et al. [10] investigated the three-dimensional spatial mapping in early blind individuals by considering monaural and binaural listening conditions. Authors observed that early blind subjects show equal or better accuracy compared to sighted subjects when localizing single sounds. Moreover, they observed that early blind people could correctly localize sounds monaurally compared to sighted participants. Neurophysiological results indicate a clear response of the occipital cortex of blind individuals to auditory stimuli (e.g., [8, 16–19]), revealing even topographic organization [20–24]. The absence of visual input also drives anatomical changes in the auditory cortex (e.g., [25, 26]). On the other side, other studies in humans and animals show that lack of vision is associated with spatial deficits. For example, studies show that blindness affects one's ability to estimate the absolute distance of auditory cues [27–29], audio metric tasks [30, 31], auditory distance discrimination, and proprioceptive reproduction [32]. Research has also demonstrated poorer skills of blind compared to sighted people for localization of sounds along the mid-sagittal plane [11].

These results suggest that the mechanisms that subtend the development of space representation remain unclear. They also support that the role of the visual modality in space representation varies based on spatial properties, producing in some cases enhanced or impaired skills in blind individuals. The mechanisms behind this require clarification.

3. Audio metric impairment in blind individuals

Another exception of the enhanced skills of blind individuals in space representation is the ability to perform an audio spatial bisection task [30]. Contrary to previous works studying pitch and timbre discrimination [13, 33], or localization of single sounds in space [7, 10], the bisection task requires estimation and comparison of different locations in space. While sighted children of 6 years of age can perform it [5], our study found that blind individuals were strongly impaired in this task. The results were in agreement with previous findings of our group showing that, during development, the visual modality dominates the multisensory spatial percept in audio-visual conditions of the bisection task, suggesting that the visual input might be crucial for the development of audio spatial bisection skills [5]. During the task, participants sat 180 cm from the center of a bank of 23 speakers and perceived three sounds: the first speaker (on the left) and the last speaker (on the right) delivered the first and the third sounds, respectively. The second sound came from an intermediate speaker between the first and the last one (see **Figure 1**). Participants verbally reported whether the second sound was closer to the first (i.e., left) or to the last (i.e., right) sound.

While sighted individuals succeeded at the task, with responses varying systematically as a function of speaker position (a standard deviation of 4.3°), blind individuals provided almost random responses. However, the same deficit was absent for other tasks, such as the minimal audible angle task in which participants were asked to evaluate which sound was from the left in a sequence of two sounds (this result is in agreement with previous studies [10]). The deficit we reported for the bisection task was far larger than the perceptual enhancements that have been reported before, and it was highly consistent among blind individuals. **Figure 2** reports the individual thresholds for the minimum audible angle against individual thresholds for the bisection task: the thresholds of blind individuals are over the equality line. While the study observed no difference between groups for the minimum audible angle (t test, $p = 0.21$), groups significantly differed for the bisection thresholds (Wilcoxon signed ranks test, $p < 0.01$; bootstrap sign-test: $p < 10^{-5}$). We performed other tests we do not report here so as to show the specificity of the deficit and its independency from the kind of sound used (e.g., the pointing task; for more details, see [30]). We also performed a temporal version of the bisection task, in which the participants performed the same task in the temporal domain. Participants had to report if the second sound was closer to the first or to the last in time. In this task, no deficit emerged, suggesting that the deficit was not due to a general/aspecific impairment, to task incomprehension, or to attention and memory problems associated with task difficulty.

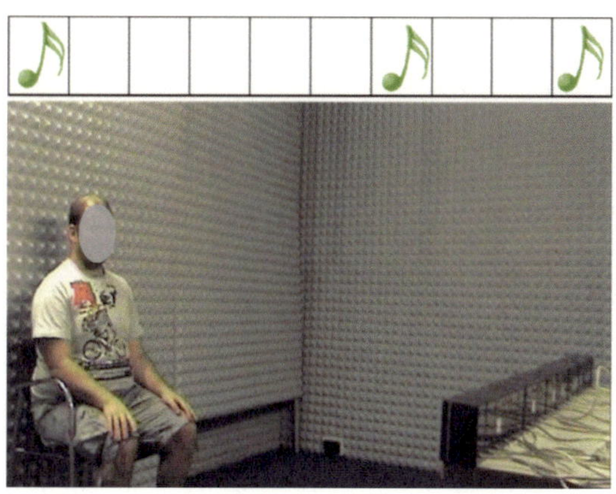

Figure 1.
Description of the spatial bisection task. Participants were aligned with the central speaker (i.e., 0°) and listened to a sequence of three sounds. The first and the third sound were delivered from the first speaker on the left (i.e., −25°) and the last speaker on the right (i.e., +25°) respectively, whereas the second sound derived from an intermediate speaker between the first and the last one (i.e., between −25° and +25°). Participants were asked whether the second sound was closer to the first (i.e., left, −25°) or the last (i.e., right, +25°) sound. Upper panel reports an exemplar trial in which the second sound is closer to the last (i.e., right) sound.

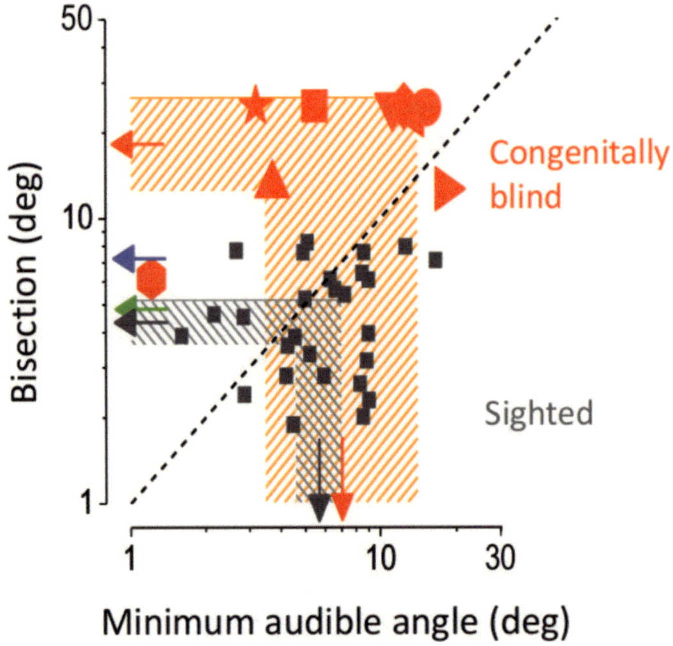

Figure 2.
Individual data, plotting bisection thresholds against minimal audible angle. Arrows at the margin show the geometric means of each group as well as the shaded areas of 95% confidence intervals. The blue and green arrows show the average thresholds for 7- and 10-year-old children, respectively (taken from a previous study) [5]. The dashed diagonal line is the equality line: while the thresholds of sighted subjects are scattered around this line, all except one non-sighted subject are above it. Indeed, the only non-sighted subject with bisection threshold that falls within the control range had a threshold for minimal audible angle that was six times lower than the mean of the controls, meaning the subject's data point sits well above the bisection line. With permission from Gori et al. [30].

4. Cortical processing of space and blindness

Scientific evidence suggests that the auditory and somatosensory systems colonize the visual cortex of congenitally blind individuals to a certain extent (e.g., [16, 34]). For example, studies that were performed with fMRI [35–38] and event-related potentials (ERPs [39, 40]) show that the visual cortex shows a strong and reliable response to sound presented alone. Tomasello et al. [41] have recently proposed a neurocomputational model to explain the visual cortex recruitment during language processing in congenitally blind individuals. For what concerns space representation, Collignon and colleagues [42] compared the brain activity of early blind and sighted individuals during a spatial and pitch task using the same stimuli for both. Authors observed that the processing of sounds recruited the occipital cortex, and the spatial processing of audio spatial stimuli also activated the dorsal occipital stream involved in visuospatial/motion processing in sighted individuals. They concluded that some regions of the right dorsal occipital stream specialize toward processing spatial information without the necessity of visual experience. Not only are visual areas activated during auditory tasks, but also localization abilities of blind subjects are strongly associated with the magnitude of visual cortex activity [8, 43, 44]. For example, early blind people localize sounds more accurately than those who are sighted under monaural conditions [10]. Their activation in right-hemisphere striate and ventral extrastriate areas correlates with the performance in a pointing task to monaurally presented sounds [8]. These results suggest that the enhancement of some auditory skills of blind individuals may reflect in the recruitment of the visual cortex. From this arises the question: what about the impaired skills, such as in the case of the bisection task? If the visual information is important for the development of audio space bisection [45], as we reported in the previous section, then we may expect the visual cortex of sighted and not of blind individuals [30] should be recruited for this audio processing. We recently used EEG to measure activation of the occipital cortex of sighted and blind individuals during the audio bisection task [45, 46]. **Figure 3** illustrates the scalp maps elicited by the second sound of the spatial bisection task when it was delivered from the left (i.e., −4.5°, see left panel) and the right side (i.e., +4.5°, see right panel) in the 50- to 90-ms time window after sound onset, for sighted (**Figure 3A**) and blind participants (**Figure 3B**). In the case of both groups, two strong positivities emerged: one involving central areas and one involving parieto-occipital areas. However, the latter positivity showed a specific contralateral pattern during the spatial bisection task that was only in sighted subjects (**Figure 3A**). In early blind participants (**Figure 3B**), the parieto-occipital response was strongly attenuated and not contralateral to the sound spatial position.

To provide evidence that the early contralateral component that we observed over the occipital scalp actually involved generators in occipital areas, we performed comparisons between groups at the source level (**Figure 4**). Results suggest that sighted subjects showed a stronger occipital and temporal activation contralateral to the physical sound position, while early blind subjects exhibited reduced activation in contralateral cortical areas and an increased activation in ipsilateral cortical areas.

In early blind individuals, the laterality was absent, which means that early visual experience mediates development of this contralateral early occipital response. The data suggest that visual modality plays a key role in the development of an early occipital response that is specific for space perception and auditory stimuli. In sighted subjects, the acoustic recruitment of the visual brain may be necessary to build a spatial metric of the environment using high resolution and flexibility that only the visual brain is capable of implementing. Lack of vision

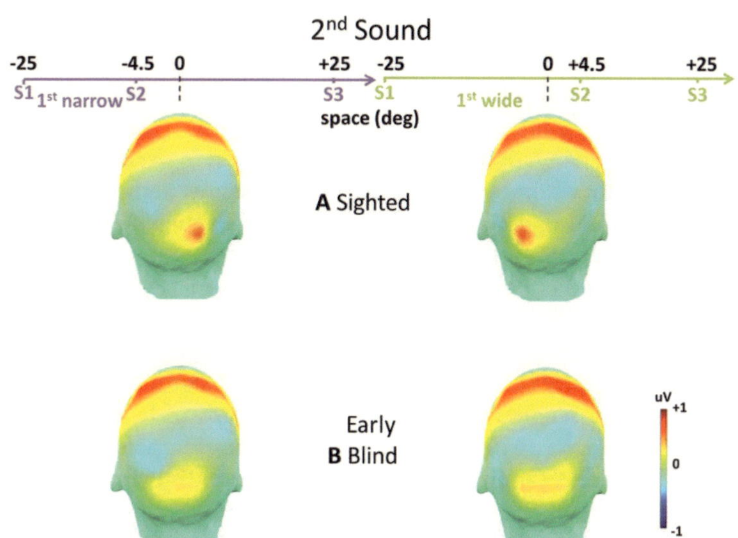

Figure 3.
Scalp maps of the mean ERP amplitude in the selected time window (50–90 ms) after the second sound of the spatial bisection task, for sighted (A) and blind (B) groups. Left and right panels of the figure report the conditions in which S2 was presented from either −4.5° (i.e., narrow first distance) or + 4.5° (i.e., wide first distance), respectively, and independently of timing (±250 ms). With permission from Campus et al. [46].

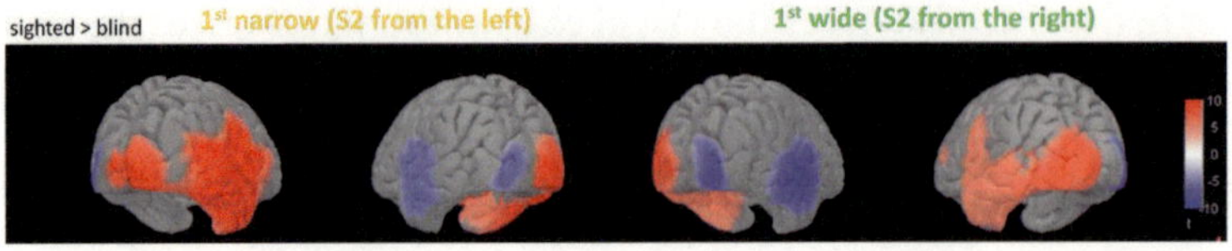

Figure 4.
Average source activity within the selected time window (50–90 ms) compared between sighted and blind subjects. Left and right panels of the figure report the conditions in which S2 was presented from either the left (i.e., −4.5°, narrow first distance) or the right side (i.e., +4.5°, wide first distance), respectively. We report results of paired two tailed t *tests with the scale in terms of t-statistic. We also display significant values of t statistic: reddish and bluish colors indicate stronger activations in sighted and early blind subjects, respectively, while intensity indicates magnitude of t (i.e., strength of difference). Only t values corresponding to* $p < 0.0001$ *after FDR correction appear. Adapted with permission from Campus et al. [46].*

seems to impact the development of this processing and underlying neural circuits, thereby impairing understanding of Euclidean relationships, such as those involved in solving a spatial bisection task. These findings agree with our previous behavioral results [30], at the same time revealing that the neural correlates of the audio space bisection deficit reported in blind individuals might correspond to reduction of early occipital contralateral activation. We speculate that cortical activation underlying the C1 ERP component (usually elicited by visual stimuli) plays a fundamental role in the construction of metrics in the spatial domain independently of the involved sensory modality. Moreover, the construction of spatial metrics may depend on visual experience.

5. Blindness duration and cortical reorganization

The lack of vision seems to interfere with the development of space representation, so an interesting question is: what happens when the subject loses visual input later in life? Late blindness is a condition worthy of investigation concerning this issue because spatial hearing of late blind subjects is shaped by unique combination of visual calibration in childhood and prolonged blindness in adulthood. As well as for early blind individuals, research on late blind individuals shows contrasting results at both the behavioral and cortical levels. For example, scientific evidence shows that, late blind individuals are better compared to sighted people in using spectral cues when they localize sound position in peripheral regions [47, 48]. Similar to early blind participants, they also show auditory and tactile recruitment of occipital regions [49–51]. Voss and colleagues [43] investigated the effect of blindness on brain activity by using positron emission tomography (PET) during one binaural and one monaural sound source discrimination task (SSDT) in early and late-onset blind individuals. In their study, Voss et al. observed that no difference was present between groups for the binaural task. Contrarily, during the monaural condition, early blind individuals performed significantly better than all the other groups (in agreement with the behavioral study of Lessard and colleagues [10]). Late blind subjects are more similar to sighted individuals concerning other skills too, such as absolute auditory distance estimation [27], locational judgments after a perspective change in small-scale space [52], audio shape recognition and navigation tasks [53]. In a recent study from our group [54], late blind individuals were involved to allow the study to investigate how blindness duration (BD) affects auditory spatial bisection skills and neural correlates. In late blind individuals, we replicated the same behavioral and EEG experiment previously performed among early blind people (see section above, [46]). We observed that the early (50–90 ms) ERP response, previously observed in sighted [45] and not in early

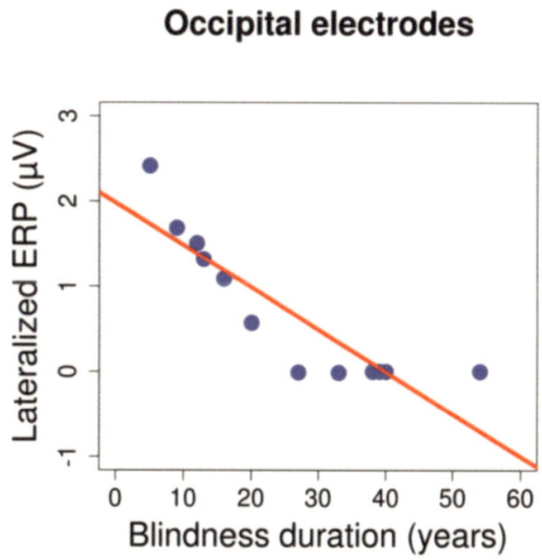

Figure 5.
Results of linear regression analyses in late blind individuals. Years of blindness duration (BD) negatively correlate with lateralized (i.e., contralateral-ipsilateral to S2 position) ERP amplitude in a 50- to 90-ms time window after S2 for the spatial bisection task. With permission from Amadeo et al. [54].

blind [46] individuals, is dependent on the amount of time spent without vision (i.e., BD, [54]). In particular, we observed that a shorter period of blindness links to stronger contralateral activation in the visual cortex (see **Figure 5**) and better performance during spatial bisection tasks. Contrarily, we observed non-lateralized visual activation and lower performance in individuals who had experienced a longer period of blindness.

Time spent without vision seems to gradually impact neural circuits underlying the construction of space representation in late blind participants. On the one hand, duration of blindness directly impacts both neural and behavioral correlates of late blind individuals during auditory spatial processing similarity between neural circuits and competences of late blind individuals with short blindness duration and, confirming there is indeed a key relationship between visual deprivation and auditory spatial abilities in humans. On the other hand, the sighted people suggest that an early visual experience is necessary and sufficient to fully develop neural areas involved in complex representations of space. These results agree with previous works in animals showing visual information during the first years of life is essential toward calibrating auditory space representation in the brain [5, 30, 31, 53, 55].

6. Time to infer space in blindness

Almost 100 years ago, Piaget [56] stated that the temporal metric is strictly related to spatial metric development: "Space is a still of time, while time is space in motion" [57]. What Piaget did not discuss is the role of different sensory modalities in this link. Visual experience is important for the development of spatial metric representations, such as for bisecting sounds. Starting from Piaget's idea, one might hypothesize that when vision is unavailable, such as in the case of blindness, temporal representation of events can set spatial representation. Indeed, while early and late blind individuals with long blindness duration show strong deficits in terms of spatial bisection tasks, they show performance and cortical activations similar to sighted individuals in the time domain, such as in a temporal bisection task [45]. In support of this hypothesis, we recently tested and verified that space representation of blind individuals is strongly influenced by the temporal representation of events [58]. We performed different versions of the spatial bisection task in sighted and blind individuals, in which we presented spatial and temporal independent, coherent, and conflicting information (**Figure 6** top panel). Similar to the original version of the bisection task [30], in one condition the temporal delay between the three sounds was always the same, and only spatial cues were relevant to compute the task (i.e., Equal bisection, **Figure 6A** top panel). In other conditions instead, we presented a spatio-temporal coherent or conflicting information. For example, in the coherent bisection, a longer spatial distance between the first and the second sound was associated with a longer temporal delay between the two sounds, and the reverse was the case for shorter distances (see **Figure 6B** top panel). In the opposite bisection, a longer spatial distance between the first and the second sound was associated with a shorter temporal delay between the two sounds, and the reverse for shorter distances (see **Figure 6C** top panel). Thanks to these two manipulations, it was possible to disentangle the role of spatial and temporal cues when it comes to the audio spatial bisection task. Our results show that these manipulations modified the performance of blind but not sighted participants. Indeed, in blind individuals, the spatial bisection deficit observed in the original version of the task disappeared when the study presented coherent temporal and spatial cues, and it increased in the conflicting condition. **Figure 6** (lower panels) plots the proportion of answer "second sound closer to the third sound" as a function of the position of the second sound for one blind (in red) and one age-matched sighted individual (in gray). In the equal bisection condition, we observed the same deficit observed previously [30], with random responses and no psychometric function for the blind subject. Interestingly, in the

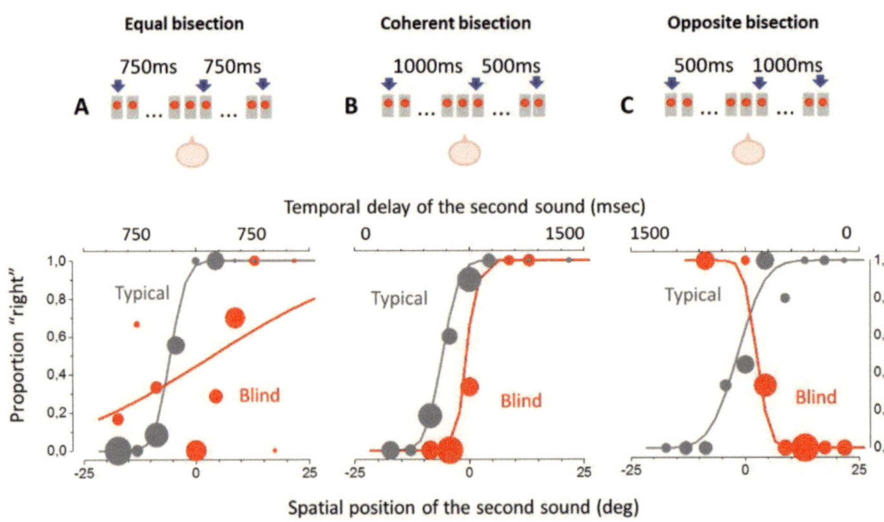

Figure 6.
Bisection tasks: coherent and conflicting manipulations of space and time. Results of the three conditions of the spatial bisection task for a typical blind participant (red symbols) and a typical sighted control (gray symbols). Subjects sat in front of an array of 23 speakers, which are illustrated by the sketches. (A) Equal spatial bisection. Top: the time interval between the first and the second sound (750 ms) was equal to the time interval between the second and the third sound. Bottom: proportion of trials judged "closer to the right sound source" plotted against the speaker position for the second sound. The size of the dots is proportional to trial number at that position. We fitted both sets of data with the Gaussian error function. (B) Coherent spatial bisection. Top: spatial distances and temporal intervals between the three sounds were directly proportional (e.g., long spatial distance and long temporal interval). Bottom: same as for (A). (C) Opposite spatial bisection. Top: spatial distances and temporal intervals between the three sounds were inversely proportional (e.g., long spatial distance and short temporal interval). Bottom: same as for (A) and (B). With permission from Gori et al. [58].

coherent bisection condition, the deficit disappeared and there was similar performance between the sighted and blind participants. More interestingly, in the opposite bisection condition (**Figure 6C**), while there was no effect of the manipulation that was evident in the sighted individual, in the blind individual, the response was inverted (i.e., the psychometric function was reversed and presented in the opposite direction than expected).

Performance of blind individuals reveals a strong temporal dominance for the spatial bisection task, suggesting that temporal cue is attracting the spatial auditory response [58]. A possible explanation is that, while the retinotopic organization of the visual cortex may support the reorganization underlying some enhanced audio spatial skills in blindness (such as the sound localization ability), it may be insufficient to guarantee the development of more complex spatial skills, such as those required for the audio spatial bisection task. Our results about the role of time in space representation suggest that temporal information can act as an alternative cue for reorganizing space representation subtending some more complex spatial abilities.

7. Space, time, and speed

How can temporal information support space processing in blindness? It might be that, for some complex spatial representations, the visual system calibrates the auditory sense of space by processing the speed of the stimuli. Neurons that process speed information have been demonstrated for the visual modality in the visual cortex [59]. These neurons could be responsible for processing information during spatial bisection tasks.

In typical conditions, it may be that the visual system facilitates transfer of audio processing from a temporal to a spatial coordinate system. Indeed, audition is the most reliable sense to represent time information, and vision is the most reliable sense to represent space information. The mediator between auditory time and visual space could be velocity processing, which may represent a channel of communication between the two sensory systems. **Figure 7** reports a graphical description of how vision and audition may collaborate to estimate space and time starting from the speed properties of an object. Concerning space estimation in sighted individuals, given the higher weight of vision, it is independent of the temporal coordinates of the stimulus for both coherent (**Figure 7A**) and conflicting (**Figure 7B**) situations. On the other hand, when the visual information is unavailable, the spatial counterpart seems unable to develop and blind individuals seem to rely only on temporal coordinates to infer metric spatial information. One might then speculate that when the visual network is impaired, blind individuals internalize a statistical prior (i.e., a prior on the constant velocity of stimuli) derived from environmental statistics. This drives them to infer space from time. This idea is in agreement with the Imputed Velocity Theory [60], which asserts that humans intuitively attribute constant velocity to a single object moving through space over time. If we assume that blind individuals assume a prior of constant velocity of objects in space, they can use this information to extract space cues using time cues. This strategy would help blind people to overcome metric problems by using unimpaired temporal maps to decode spatial metrics. This may also facilitate their interaction with others (**Figure 7** left). This mechanism would be adaptive for blind individuals as it allows them to process spatial information correctly at the auditory level based on its temporal representation. On the other side, this mechanism could be maladaptive when conflicting spatial and temporal information is provided, as blind individuals can be deceived by the temporal

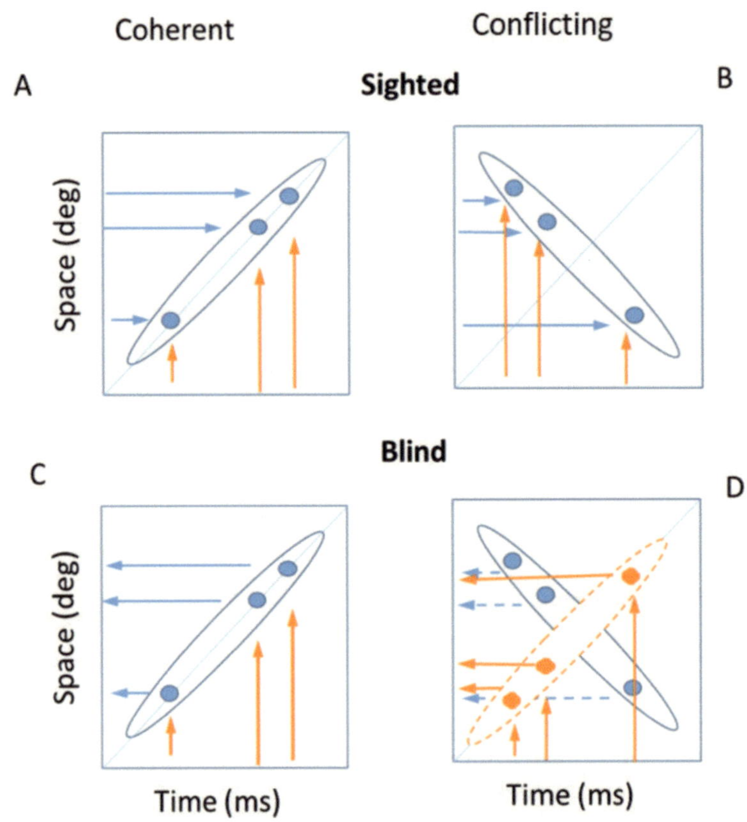

Figure 7.
Graphical model of our theory. In sighted individuals, spatial estimation is independent of the temporal cue of the stimulus for both coherent (A) and conflicting (B) information. Blind individuals infer spatial information using temporal coordinates of the stimulus assuming constant velocity. When spatial-temporal coherent stimuli are present, the spatial estimation can be successfully extracted by the temporal cue (C). On the other hand, when conflicting spatial-temporal information (D) is provided, the temporal cue is wrongly used to drive the spatial sound position assuming constant velocity.

cue in the spatial evaluation, perceiving an illusory spatial position of the sound based on its temporal coordinates (**Figure** 7 right).

These findings support the cross-sensory calibration theory [5, 61], suggesting that visual information is necessary for normal development of auditory sense of space. In children younger than 12 years of age, there is visual dominance over audition in spatial bisection, and an auditory dominance over vision in temporal bisection [5]. The cross-sensory calibration of the visual system for the spatial bisection explains why blind subjects show a specific temporal response to the spatial bisection task, while also showing different processing to solve Euclidean, metric, relationships. We can speculate that these processes could be mediated in sighted but not in blind people by pathways involving the superior colliculus [30, 55, 62]. The present study adds new evidence, showing other possible interactions during development among sensory modalities, as well as spatial and temporal domains.

8. Conclusion

A lack of vision hampers strategies and neural circuits underlying complex spatial metrics, driving to multisensory interactions that bring to code space based on temporal instead of spatial coordinates. These findings open new opportunities for developing sensory substitution devices and rehabilitation technologies for blind people, where spatial and temporal cues could be simultaneously manipulated to convey richer information.

Acknowledgements

The authors acknowledge the contribution of David Burr and Concetta Morrone in helping to shape the line of research that forms the basis of this chapter, including their continuous support and their participation in some of the experiments reported.

Conflict of interest

The authors declare no conflicts of interest.

Author details

Monica Gori[1*], Maria Bianca Amadeo[1,2], Giulio Sandini[3] and Claudio Campus[1]

1 Unit for Visually Impaired People, Italian Institute of Technology, Genova, Italy

2 Department of Informatics, Bioengineering, Robotics and Systems Engineering, Università degli Studi di Genova, Genova, Italy

3 Robotics, Brain and Cognitive Sciences Department, Italian Institute of Technology, Genova, Italy

*Address all correspondence to: monica.gori@iit.it

References

[1] Knudsen EI. Capacity for plasticity in the adult owl auditory system expanded by juvenile experience. Science. 1998;**279**(5356):1531-1533

[2] King AJ, Carlile S. Changes induced in the representation of auditory space in the superior colliculus by rearing ferrets with binocular eyelid suture. Experimental Brain Research. 1993;**94**(3):444-455

[3] Recanzone GH. Rapidly induced auditory plasticity: The ventriloquism aftereffect. Proceedings of the National Academy of Sciences of the United States of America. 1998;**95**(3):869-875

[4] Zwiers MP, Van Opstal AJ, Paige GD. Plasticity in human sound localization induced by compressed spatial vision. Nature Neuroscience. 2003;**6**(2):175-181

[5] Gori M, Sandini G, Burr D. Development of visuo-auditory integration in space and time. Frontiers in Integrative Neuroscience. 2012;**6**:77

[6] King AJ, Parsons CH. Improved auditory spatial acuity in visually deprived ferrets. The European Journal of Neuroscience. 1999;**11**(11):3945-3956

[7] Roder B, Teder-Salejarvi W, Sterr A, Rosler F, Hillyard SA, Neville HJ. Improved auditory spatial tuning in blind humans. Nature. 1999;**400**(6740):162-166

[8] Gougoux F, Zatorre RJ, Lassonde M, Voss P, Lepore F. A functional neuroimaging study of sound localization: Visual cortex activity predicts performance in early-blind individuals. PLoS Biology. 2005;**3**(2):e27

[9] Lewald J. Vertical sound localization in blind humans. Neuropsychologia. 2002;**40**(12):1868-1872

[10] Lessard N, Pare M, Lepore F, Lassonde M. Early-blind human subjects localize sound sources better than sighted subjects. Nature. 1998;**395**(6699):278-280

[11] Zwiers MP, Van Opstal AJ, Cruysberg JR. A spatial hearing deficit in early-blind humans. The Journal of Neuroscience. 2001;**21**(9):RC142: 1-RC142: 5

[12] Goldreich D, Kanics IM. Tactile acuity is enhanced in blindness. The Journal of Neuroscience. 2003;**23**(8):3439-3445

[13] Gougoux F, Lepore F, Lassonde M, Voss P, Zatorre RJ, Belin P. Neuropsychology: Pitch discrimination in the early blind. Nature. 2004;**430**(6997):309

[14] Tinti C, Adenzato M, Tamietto M, Cornoldi C. Visual experience is not necessary for efficient survey spatial cognition: Evidence from blindness. Quarterly Journal of Experimental Psychology. 2006;**59**(7):1306-1328

[15] Fortin M, Voss P, Lord C, Lassonde M, Pruessner J, Saint-Amour D, et al. Wayfinding in the blind: Larger hippocampal volume and supranormal spatial navigation. Brain. 2008;**131**(Pt 11):2995-3005

[16] Weeks R, Horwitz B, Aziz-Sultan A, Tian B, Wessinger CM, Cohen LG, et al. A positron emission tomographic study of auditory localization in the congenitally blind. The Journal of Neuroscience. 2000;**20**(7):2664-2672

[17] Poirier C, Collignon O, Devolder AG, Renier L, Vanlierde A, Tranduy D, et al. Specific activation of the V5 brain area by auditory motion processing: An fMRI study. Brain Research. Cognitive Brain Research. 2005;**25**(3):650-658

[18] Renier L, De Volder AG. Cognitive and brain mechanisms in sensory

substitution of vision: A contribution to the study of human perception. Journal of Integrative Neuroscience. 2005;**4**(4):489-503

[19] Striem-Amit E, Amedi A. Visual cortex extrastriate body-selective area activation in congenitally blind people "seeing" by using sounds. Current Biology. 2014;**24**(6):687-692

[20] Voss P, Zatorre RJ. Organization and reorganization of sensory-deprived cortex. Current Biology. 2012;**22**(5):R168-R173

[21] Collignon O, Voss P, Lassonde M, Lepore F. Cross-modal plasticity for the spatial processing of sounds in visually deprived subjects. Experimental Brain Research. 2009;**192**(3):343-358

[22] Rauschecker JP. Developmental plasticity and memory. Behavioural Brain Research. 1995;**66**(1-2):7-12

[23] Collignon O, Charbonneau G, Peters F, Nassim M, Lassonde M, Lepore F, et al. Reduced multisensory facilitation in persons with autism. Cortex. 2013;**49**(6):1704-1710

[24] Collignon O, Champoux F, Voss P, Lepore F. Sensory rehabilitation in the plastic brain. Progress in Brain Research. 2011;**191**:211-231

[25] Korte M, Rauschecker JP. Auditory spatial tuning of cortical neurons is sharpened in cats with early blindness. Journal of Neurophysiology. 1993;**70**(4):1717-1721

[26] Elbert T, Sterr A, Rockstroh B, Pantev C, Muller MM, Taub E. Expansion of the tonotopic area in the auditory cortex of the blind. The Journal of Neuroscience. 2002;**22**(22):9941-9944

[27] Wanet MC, Veraart C. Processing of auditory information by the blind in spatial localization tasks. Perception & Psychophysics. 1985;**38**(1):91-96

[28] Kolarik AJ, Cirstea S, Pardhan S. Evidence for enhanced discrimination of virtual auditory distance among blind listeners using level and direct-to-reverberant cues. Experimental Brain Research. 2013;**224**(4):623-633

[29] Kolarik AJ, Pardhan S, Cirstea S, Moore BC. Auditory spatial representations of the world are compressed in blind humans. Experimental Brain Research. 2017;**235**(2):597-606

[30] Gori M, Sandini G, Martinoli C, Burr DC. Impairment of auditory spatial localization in congenitally blind human subjects. Brain. 2014;**137**(Pt 1): 288-293

[31] Finocchietti S, Cappagli G, Gori M. Encoding audio motion: Spatial impairment in early blind individuals. Frontiers in Psychology. 2015;**6**:1357

[32] Cappagli G, Finocchietti S, Cocchi E, Gori M. The impact of early visual deprivation on spatial hearing: A comparison between totally and partially visually deprived children. Frontiers in Psychology. 2017;**8**:467

[33] Doucet ME, Guillemot JP, Lassonde M, Gagne JP, Leclerc C, Lepore F. Blind subjects process auditory spectral cues more efficiently than sighted individuals. Experimental Brain Research. 2005;**160**(2):194-202

[34] Sadato N, Pascual-Leone A, Grafman J, Ibanez V, Deiber MP, Dold G, et al. Activation of the primary visual cortex by Braille reading in blind subjects. Nature. 1996;**380**(6574):526-528

[35] Amedi A, Stern WM, Camprodon JA, Bermpohl F, Merabet L, Rotman S, et al. Shape conveyed by visual-to-auditory sensory substitution activates the lateral occipital complex. Nature Neuroscience. 2007;**10**(6):687-689

[36] Lane C, Kanjlia S, Omaki A, Bedny M. "Visual" cortex of congenitally blind adults responds to syntactic movement. The Journal of Neuroscience. 2015;**35**(37):12859-12868

[37] Bedny M, Pascual-Leone A, Dodell-Feder D, Fedorenko E, Saxe R. Language processing in the occipital cortex of congenitally blind adults. Proceedings of the National Academy of Sciences of the United States of America. 2011;**108**(11):4429-4434

[38] Roder B, Stock O, Bien S, Neville H, Rosler F. Speech processing activates visual cortex in congenitally blind humans. The European Journal of Neuroscience. 2002;**16**(5):930-936

[39] Kujala T, Alho K, Kekoni J, Hamalainen H, Reinikainen K, Salonen O, et al. Auditory and somatosensory event-related brain potentials in early blind humans. Experimental Brain Research. 1995;**104**(3):519-526

[40] Focker J, Best A, Holig C, Roder B. The superiority in voice processing of the blind arises from neural plasticity at sensory processing stages. Neuropsychologia. 2012;**50**(8):2056-2067

[41] Tomasello R, Wennekers T, Garagnani M, Pulvermuller F. Visual cortex recruitment during language processing in blind individuals is explained by Hebbian learning. Scientific Reports. 2019;**9**(1):3579

[42] Collignon O, Vandewalle G, Voss P, Albouy G, Charbonneau G, Lassonde M, et al. Functional specialization for auditory-spatial processing in the occipital cortex of congenitally blind humans. Proceedings of the National Academy of Sciences of the United States of America. 2011;**108**(11):4435-4440

[43] Voss P, Gougoux F, Zatorre RJ, Lassonde M, Lepore F. Differential occipital responses in early- and late-blind individuals during a sound-source discrimination task. NeuroImage. 2008;**40**(2):746-758

[44] Voss P, Lepore F, Gougoux F, Zatorre RJ. Relevance of spectral cues for auditory spatial processing in the occipital cortex of the blind. Frontiers in Psychology. 2011;**2**:48

[45] Campus C, Sandini G, Concetta Morrone M, Gori M. Spatial localization of sound elicits early responses from occipital visual cortex in humans. Scientific Reports. 2017;**7**(1):10415

[46] Campus C, Sandini G, Amadeo MB, Gori M. Stronger responses in the visual cortex of sighted compared to blind individuals during auditory space representation. Scientific Reports. 2019;**9**(1):1935

[47] Voss P, Lassonde M, Gougoux F, Fortin M, Guillemot JP, Lepore F. Early- and late-onset blind individuals show supra-normal auditory abilities in far-space. Current Biology. 2004;**14**(19):1734-1738

[48] Fieger A, Roder B, Teder-Salejarvi W, Hillyard SA, Neville HJ. Auditory spatial tuning in late-onset blindness in humans. Journal of Cognitive Neuroscience. 2006;**18**(2):149-157

[49] Buchel C, Price C, Frackowiak RS, Friston K. Different activation patterns in the visual cortex of late and congenitally blind subjects. Brain. 1998;**121**(Pt 3):409-419

[50] Voss P, Gougoux F, Lassonde M, Zatorre RJ, Lepore F. A positron emission tomography study during auditory localization by late-onset blind individuals. NeuroReport. 2006;**17**(4):383-388

[51] Burton H, McLaren DG. Visual cortex activation in late-onset, Braille naive blind individuals: An fMRI study during semantic and phonological tasks with heard words. Neuroscience Letters. 2006;**392**(1-2):38-42

[52] Lehtinen-Railo S, Juurmaa J. Effect of visual experience on locational judgements after perspective change in small-scale space. Scandinavian Journal of Psychology. 1994;**35**(2):175-183

[53] Gori M, Cappagli G, Baud-Bovy G, Finocchietti S. Shape perception and navigation in blind adults. Frontiers in Psychology. 2017;**8**:10

[54] Amadeo MB, Campus C, Gori M. Impact of years of blindness on neural circuits underlying auditory spatial representation. NeuroImage. 2019;**191**:140-149

[55] King AJ. What happens to your hearing if you are born blind? Brain. 2014;**137**(Pt 1):6-8

[56] Piaget J, Inhelder B. The Psychology of the Child. New York: Basic Books; 1962

[57] Piaget J. The Child's Conception of Time. New York, NY: Ballantine Books; 1927

[58] Gori M, Amadeo MB, Campus C. Temporal cues influence space estimations in visually impaired individuals. iScience. 2018;**6**:319-326

[59] Liu J, Newsome WT. Functional organization of speed tuned neurons in visual area MT. Journal of Neurophysiology. 2003;**89**(1):246-256

[60] Huang YL, Jones B. On the interdependence of temporal and spatial judgments. Perception & Psychophysics. 1982;**32**(1):7-14

[61] Gori M. Multisensory integration and calibration in children and adults with and without sensory and motor disabilities. Multisensory Research. 2015;**28**(1-2):71-99

[62] King AJ, Hutchings ME, Moore DR, Blakemore C. Developmental plasticity in the visual and auditory representations in the mammalian superior colliculus. Nature. 1988;**332**(6159):73-76

Chapter 18

The Application of Geographic Information Systems to Support Wayfinding for People with Visual Impairments or Blindness

Susanne Zimmermann-Janschitz

Abstract

People with visual impairments or legal blindness are relying on differing, comprehensive information utilized for their individual mobility. Increasing the personal mobility of people with disabilities and thereby achieving a self-determined life are major steps toward a more inclusive society. Research and applications on mobility issues of people with visual impairments or blindness mainly focus on technical applications or assistive orientation and navigation devices, and less work is covering the individual needs, e.g., regarding the information required for wayfinding. Moreover, active participation of people with disabilities in research and development is still limited. ways2see offers a new online application to support individual mobility in context of pre-trip planning for people with visual impairments or blindness based on a Geographic Information System (GIS). Obstacles, barriers, landmarks, orientation hints, and directions for wayfinding are generated by user profiles. The underlying network for GIS analysis is designed as pedestrian network. This individually coded network approach integrates sidewalks and different types of crossings and implements various orientation and navigation attributes. ways2see integrates three research realms: firstly, implementing a participative and transdisciplinary research design; secondly, integrating personalized information aligned with the individual user needs; and thirdly, presenting result of GIS analysis through an accessible designed user interface.

Keywords: geographic information systems, GIS, disabilities, visual impairments, blindness, mobility, orientation, navigation, wayfinding, network analysis

1. Introduction: why another orientation and navigation tool?

Geographic information science is a well-established approach in the context of navigation, wayfinding, and orientation—as long as the focus is given to motorized vehicles, e.g., Google, OpenStreetMap, etc. With rising importance of sustainability issues during the last decades, alternative modes of transportation gained interest, and geographic information systems (GISs) were progressively used, also for analyzing cycling and walking behavior [1, 2]. A GIS is an analytical tool to manage, store, analyze, and visualize spatial information. Simplified it can be seen as a digital map including a database to access and investigate spatial relations.

Narrowing down wayfinding and orientation to pedestrians and especially to persons with disabilities, up to now research is still at the beginning. However, demographic changes, the rising demand for (social) sustainability, and therefore strategies of equity and inclusion to generate diversity and to overcome barriers in Western societies force geography to provide (spatial) answers for the elderly and people with disabilities.

The need for autonomous and independent mobility underlines the demand of people with disabilities and the elderly for social equity and their full participation in society and in societal life [3, 4]. Contrary to these requirements, the design and development of urban space, the lack of offers in (public) transport infrastructure and information, and barriers in the built environment and above all in the mindset of civil society still exclude people with disabilities. Particularly exposed are people with visual impairments or legal blindness; they consequently experience a reduced mobility in their daily life. This can be underpinned by some statistical figures, e.g., more than 50% of persons with visual impairments in Austria perceive themselves as moderate up to severely mobility impaired [5].

Existing GIS applications to increase the mobility of people with disabilities can be categorized upon various parameters; among others one key element is the type of disability [6]. GIS approaches for persons physically restricted in their mobility like wheelchair users, persons with crutches, parents with strollers, or elderly people show a wide variety in theoretical discussions as well as in practical implementations, mostly focusing on accessibility issues [7–11]. Solutions to support independent mobility for persons who are visually impaired or blind often remain either on a theoretical level or as project ideas, as special solutions or prototypes. Concerning their spatial extent, they are typically valid for a limited space like university campuses or small districts of cities; others require cost-intensive devices that are sometimes yet difficult to manage [12, 13].

However, people with visual impairments or blindness can benefit from the possibilities to plan and prepare their activities in space, as long as the supporting tools fulfill a number of requirements. Tools have to provide information about accessibility of facilities and the built environment and additionally have care for accessibility of information through a manageable and easy-to-operate user interface and an appropriate description of route directions.

The paper presents the theoretical background of a "GIS4all" and, in particular, the results of the project "ways2see," which implements the theory for people with visual impairments or blindness. GIS4all is a framework, which intends to conceptualize the scope of action for the application of an inclusive, trans-, and interdisciplinary GIS providing answers for spatial information, orientation, and navigation issues of people with and without disabilities. Since persons with visual impairments or blindness require complex and alternative spatial information for wayfinding, the focus of the application project "ways2see" was given to this user group.

The design and product development of the assistive tool ways2see are supporting orientation and navigation as pre-trip planning instrument for people with visual impairments or blindness. ways2see provides information on facilities as well as routing information adapted to the needs of the target group, which will support them or assist persons in preparing ways in so far unknown environments. The goal of ways2see is twofold. (1) The design and presentation of information for the target group include special cartography on the one hand and on the other hand, an applicable web-user interface at the front end which is capable for screen readers. (2) The individual selection and description of routes presented by the tool are comparable to the description used by orientation and mobility (O&M) trainers, including hints and landmarks for orientation, warning of obstacles, and simultaneously avoiding barriers in the routing.

The underlying network for pedestrian routing was developed using ArcGIS Desktop and Server, and the application ways2see is based on ArcGIS Web AppBuilder. The development embodies a participative and iterative process, following the motto of inclusion, "nothing about us without us," not only with the goal to produce an assistive tool for the target group but also to raise awareness in society for the topics of disability and inclusion.

2. Theoretical background

The origins of tools intended to increase the mobility of people with visual impairments or blindness can be seen in tactile maps, reaching back hundreds of years [14]. With the evolvement of information and communication technologies (ICT) in the mid of the last century, electronic and assistive tools gained importance [13]. Since then, various approaches, using wearable devices (e.g., electronic white canes) and sight replacing aids up to robotic help, have been developed and evaluated from various scientific backgrounds (e.g., see [15, 16]). Geographic information systems as integrative part of mobility solutions do not play an important role in these reviews; sometimes they are even not mentioned. One reason for this can be seen in the mapping part of the software, since (digital) maps—regardless on which device they are presented—barely meet the needs of visually impaired users.

Although showing a bottleneck with maps, GISs offer main advantages: the possibility to address spatial relationships as well as processes and present spatial analytical results. Based on the spatial and therefore geographical perception, GIS applications for mobility issues of people with visual impairments or blindness can be split into four main scopes: (1) the field of application or use, (2) the spatial environment, (3) the information and navigation aspects, and (4) the presentation and communication of information and/or the analytical results. The following discussion reflects the literature mainly since 2010, and a detailed description of approaches before is given in [16, 17].

(1) An overall classification of the applications is dealing with the category and purpose of usage. This reflects on the one hand the application fields like tourism purposes, emergency management or planning, and decision support tools [18–22]. On the other hand, the purpose of the trip can be split up upon the use in form of pre-trip planning or on-trip planning. Pre-trip applications show a focus in web applications and discuss various accessibility aspects of maps (user-oriented content, design, and functionalities), the design of the interface, and the degree of interactivity as well as the communication to the users [22–24]. With the availability of GPS, on-trip applications gained interest. They are mainly used for navigation and routing in different surroundings, using various devices (smartphones, wearable and portable assistive technology, etc.). Additionally, they give special interest to critical situations along the routes, e.g., intersections or obstacles [25–28].

(2) Taking a closer look at the spatial environment, the orientation and navigation support give emphasis either on indoor settings [29, 30], outdoor navigation [31–33], or a combination of both [34]. Golledge et al. [35] elaborated one of the basic approaches, discussing the spatial context of mobility for people with visual impairments or blindness. Since different technologies have to be integrated to define the position of the person along a route on-trip, a combination with different technologies (RFID, Bluetooth, DGPS, etc.), regarding the surrounding where the

navigation takes place, is involved, including tracking functionalities to determine the accurate and current position [26, 31, 36].

(3) Analyzing the information and data necessary for navigation purposes, three different core elements to enhance the process are crucial. Landmarks or navigation hints are added to improve wayfinding and the descriptions of directions [37–40]. Obstacle detection helps to increase "safe" orientation and navigation in unknown areas [21, 41, 42]. Additionally, a special focus is given to critical locations or areas along routes. Especially intersections need a more detailed description, respectively, and a different navigation process [28, 43, 44]. Finally, the integration of pedestrian paths is critically important to be able to distinguish between left- and right-hand side of a street [45].

(4) The bottleneck of GIS for people with visual impairments or blindness was already identified in the mapping part. Therefore, the presentation of information and transfer to the users has to include adopted visual elements [46–48] as well as audio and/or haptic assistive devices [33, 49–52]. This important front-end part of mobility assisting electronic devices leads to a second component of accessibility issues. Next to the accessibility of the urban environment, which can be indicated as first issue, the assistive tools themselves have to be accessible, including web accessibility. This means the operability of the software similar to the accessibility of the presented information, e.g., as maps have to be provided with special/universal design and extended/substituted with haptic and/or acoustic information.

The discussion of recent work on increasing individual mobility of persons with visual impairments or blindness finally results in a list of challenges, which are addressed in ways2see and are tackled in this paper:

- Availability and density of detailed spatial data
- Data about critical areas, e.g., intersections and crossings
- Lack of data about pedestrian path network
- Possibility to personalize information, e.g., directions
- Accuracy of positioning during the navigation process (in- and outdoor)

Roentgen et al. [39] summarized in their review that "The limited accuracy of the turn instructions and the 'roughness' of the information provided were regarded as insufficient." [37] conclude furthermore "Therefore there is a requirement to not only improve the availability and accessibility of graphical information but also to provide more context sensitive information (e.g. via profiles and points of interest) as geographical data is of little use on its own for understanding the environment, and the relationship between the individual and their surroundings."

3. Methods

The structure of the methods corresponds with the results and discussion (Section 4).

3.1 Fundamentals of ways2see in a framing model GIS4all

The project ways2see is embedded in a wider context with an overall goal and general idea: to design and implement a GIS4all, a GIS which presents spatial information to all persons with (and without) disabilities, regardless of the type of

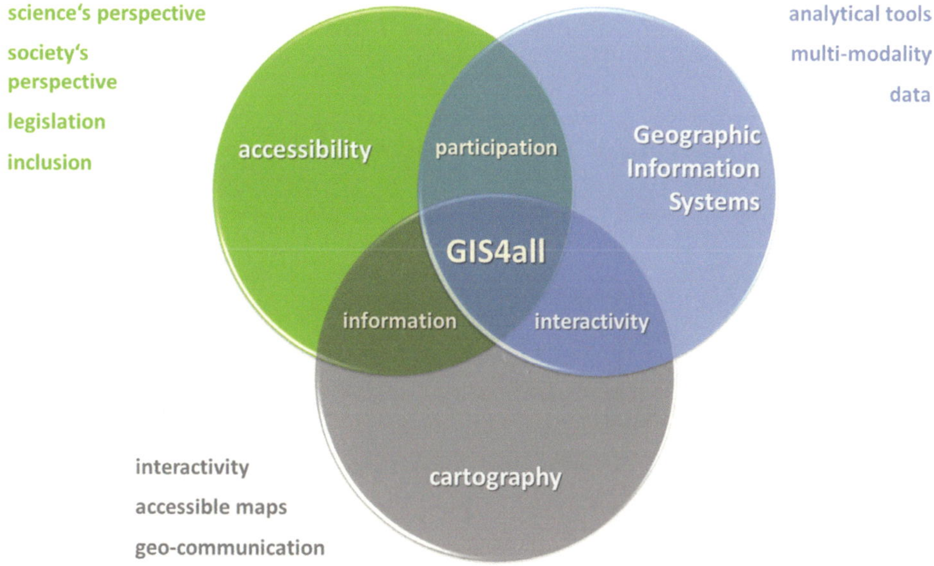

Figure 1.
Three pillars of GIS4all.

their disability. The intention of this inclusive approach is firstly to conceptualize a theoretical framework for GIS and secondly to transfer the scientific results into practice by designing a marketable product, namely, ways2see (https://www.barrierefrei.uni-graz.at/ways2see).

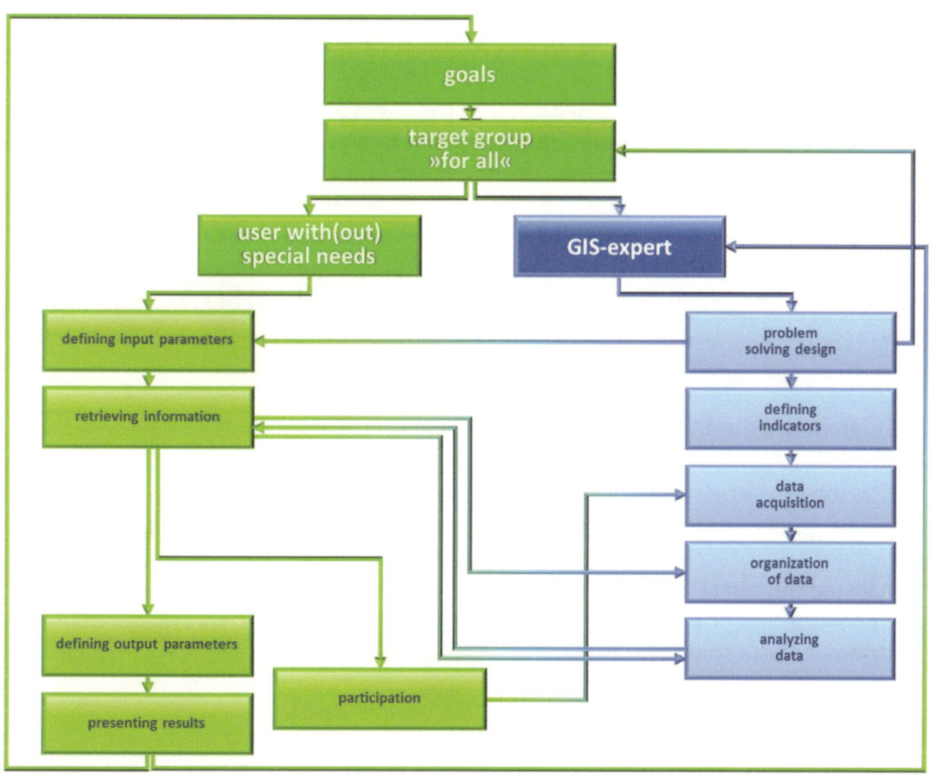

Figure 2.
Conceptual model of GIS4all.

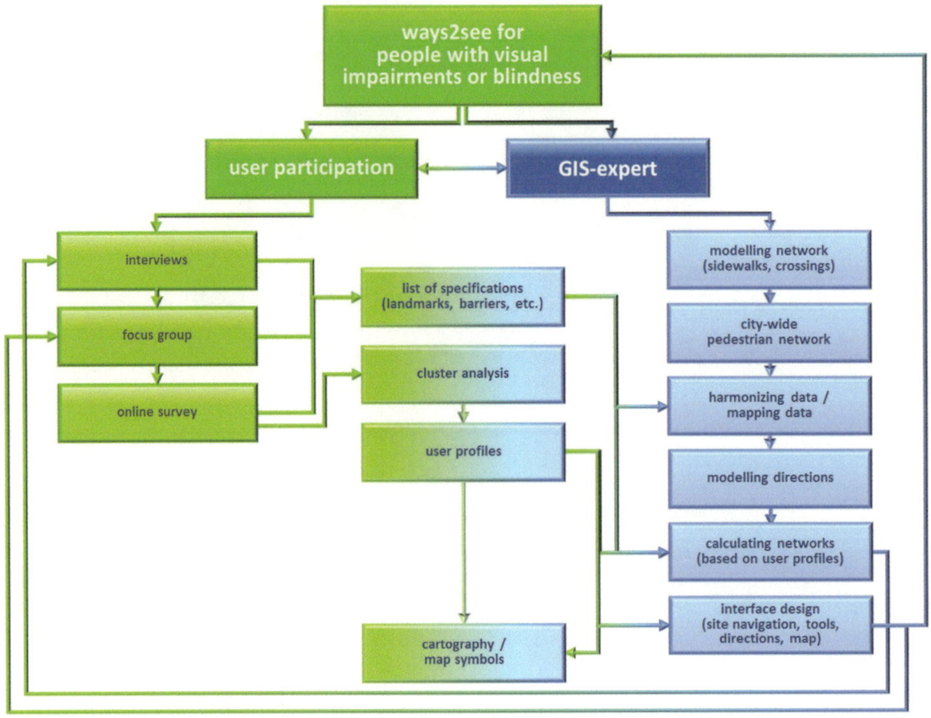

Figure 3.
Applied methods and generated results in ways2see.

The framing model GIS4all results from a theoretical discussion, including three main disciplines: disability studies, cartography, and GIS [17]. **Figure 1** illustrates these three pillars along with topics significant for the GIS4all model.

The literature review resulted in a construction kit made up of detailed building bricks for implementation. **Figure 2** shows the conceptual model of GIS4all, which also works as system model and GIS model. The overall intention of GIS4all is to present information to people with (and without) disabilities through an online platform toward four strategies: the information can be retrieved (1) using easy language, (2) is supported with a sign language avatar, and (3) is including needs for people with physical impairments as well as (4) people with visual impairments or blindness. The model illustrates the process design and will be transferred to ways2see (Section 4.2, **Figure 3**) narrowing down the concept "for all" to people with visual impairments or blindness.

3.2 Inclusion: together toward new ways

The integration of prospective users in the development and design process of ways2see, based on the motto "nothing about us without us," is following a trans-disciplinary procedure with iterative interactions with the target group, people with visual impairments and blindness. Special and thorough interest is given to the active integration of persons with visual impairments or blindness and participative processes, conducting the following methods:

- Guided interviews with orientation and mobility trainers

- In-depth interviews with users from the target group

- Focus group work with participants of the target group, O&M trainers, and educational staff

- Design workshops with participants of the target group, O&M trainers, and educational staff

- A nationwide online survey with people with visual impairments or blindness

The results of the online survey were analyzed with descriptive and exploratory statistical analyses. A hierarchical cluster analysis, intended to highlight unknown structures within the data, is used to identify inherent information in the data about the specific needs of the target group. The cluster analysis was conducted in IBM SPSS Statistics 23, using Ward's algorithm with squared Euclidean distance, and resulted in five clusters as user profiles (Section 4.2).

Clarke et al. [53] indicate a need for careful consideration of involving users, due to the various and different needs of the target group. Additionally, participation raises the chance for acceptance and a wider use of the final product. Martin et al. [54] stated that especially communication tools and screen readers are more likely to be abandoned compared to, e.g., tools to assist in daily living, if not reflected carefully and making the target group aware before ready for the market.

Following the inclusive approach of ways2see with the integration of people with visual impairments or blindness into the development and evaluation process, further workshops with the target group, discussions, and a comprehensive testing of the prototype were conducted. The integration process can be defined as iterative and mutually supportive and beneficial for both sides—the prospective users and the project team.

3.3 Pedestrians, not motorized vehicles: a network for people with visual impairments or blindness

As stated before, most navigation systems use street centerlines as a basis for their routing algorithm. Since this lacks precision for wayfinding for people with visual impairment or blindness, a network based on sidewalks was generated using zonal information. Along with the sidewalk-based network oriented toward the needs of pedestrians, additional technical or GIS-oriented challenges of ways2see were addressed through the following methodological approaches:

- Automated data processing and implementation through scripts, extended with data collected through fieldwork

- Definition of network attributes to serve the different needs

- Design of a user-oriented interface, based on user profiles, including application design as well as cartographic design

- Implementation of ways2see as a marketable product

Spatial analyses are executed in ArcGIS Desktop 10.4, the GIS functionalities are using ArcGIS Server 10.3 capabilities, and the implementation is using the Developer Edition of ArcGIS Web AppBuilder.

3.4 Accessibility through the user interface and map design

The interface design starts off with a focus toward compatibility with the most commonly used screen readers and Internet browsers, retrieved from the project online survey and the information presented by the [55]. Parallel to compatibility issues, the design has to include the possibility to deploy different contrasts and colors to the users, following the individual needs.

The user interface of ways2see is designed using the Developer Edition of ArcGIS Web AppBuilder. The two analytical tools—wayfinding and orientation as well as looking for point of interest (POI) in the surrounding—are implemented using pre-defined widgets in the Web AppBuilder, adapted through coding. Establishing ways2see on a project server using ArcGIS Server 10.3 allows full adaption of the map to the project needs as well as integrating the concept of vector tiles, which provides a faster map access.

3.5 Quality attracts users

To assure the quality of ways2see, to increase the probability of use, and to inform the user group of the availability of ways2see, three strategies finally need to be mentioned. Next to the participative development process, prospective users conducted comprehensive testing using the prototype. Prior to this, ways2see passed extensive testing by the project team. Quality assurance was additionally provided through an external evaluation of the project after implementing the prototype. Since the evaluator shows next to his GIS skills special expertise in cartography, the final product also benefits regarding map design and definition of user-oriented map symbols.

4. The way to a marketable tool: ways2see results and discussion

4.1 Study area: the dimension of a citywide project offers new challenges

The city of Graz with about 290,000 inhabitants and an area of 127 km^2 (49 mi^2) and 1200 kilometers (745 miles) of streets and path brings a new dimension into the design, development, and implementation of an O&M supporting tool. Especially the dimension of the city makes it necessary to compete with the amount of data—firstly regarding the acquisition of information and secondly due to the modeling and automatization of data, which has to be processed and updated on a regularly basis. The long history of the city, Graz received its city arms in 1245, can be seen in the structure of the city. A historic downtown area in combination with prospering suburban areas, mostly in the south and hilly and less populated spaces in the northeast, requires a model, which reflects various situations concerning sidewalks, intersections, or street crossings. Furthermore, the inner city as a UNESCO World Cultural Heritage with various historic sites bears hurdles toward the reduction of barriers and an inclusive urban planning.

4.2 User profiles for accessing personalized information

Guided interviews with four O&M trainers and two persons from the project cooperation partner Odilien-Institute were conducted to estimate the need for the application ways2see. The results served as basis for a focus group work, with the goal to get a more detailed view on information and data needed for ways-2see. The group consisted of 31 people, including 16 people with blindness.

In terms of gender, the group was split into around one-third female and two-third male participants.

The results of the theoretical and methodological discussion, the focus group work, and the expert interviews build the background for an online survey intended to reach a wider audience and to broaden the perspectives. One constraint associated with the online questionnaire is that predominantly persons with visual impairments or blindness, which are able to handle a computer or are supported by an assistive person, can provide answers. Another limitation is given with the way the audience is addressed. The target group is contacted through federations of people with visual impairments or blindness, where persons register on an optional basis, since there is no organization in Austria, where all persons of the target group are recorded. Despite this, the answers provided by the target group offer a classification of needs of people with visual impairments or blindness regarding their mobility in daily life.

A list of specifications, including points of interest, landmarks, orientation hints, dangerous spots, and movement barriers, is compiled from the guided and in-depth interviews, the focus group work, and the online survey. The list of specifications was generated from a feasibility study, dealing with the availability and possibility of automated data integration. The result is indicating the limits of ways2see from a technical perspective on the one hand and the limitation regarding data acquisition on the other hand. For example, it is neither possible to implement movable obstacles like bicycles parked on sidewalks into the system nor to map the citywide lowering of sidewalks for driveways. This is also contrasting the idea of integrating freely available data or automated data acquisition for ways2see when ensuring quality as well as timeliness of data.

The nationwide survey shows a response rate of 11%. 1000 people were contacted in the online survey, which is a comparably small portion of 318,000 persons with visual impairments or blindness (thereof 3000 blind) in Austria [56]. The reasons for this are stated in Section 3.2—one reason is that people with visual impairments or blindness cannot be addressed through a central institution and a second reason is that the survey was conducted online.

The cluster analysis, based on the results of the online survey, presents five clusters in the heterogeneous group of people of visual impairments and blindness:

- Cluster 1: Accompanied
- Cluster 2: Elderly blind
- Cluster 3: Independent adults
- Cluster 4: Tech-savvy, age 20–40
- Cluster 5: Congenitally visually impaired, age under 20

A detailed description of the results of the cluster analysis is documented in [57]. These groups of prospective users work as initial point to deviate the user profiles, which are implemented in the network generation and user interface of ways2see. The following four profiles are implemented in ways2see, evaluated in focus group work and in a design workshop with persons of the target group:

- Short routes preferred, regardless of infrastructure of crossings.
- Tactile pavement and accessible pedestrian signals preferred.

- Avoid crossings without tactile pavement and accessible pedestrian signals, and show all orientation hints.

- Choose individual settings.

Figure 3 illustrates the methodological approaches combined with the essential results of the design and development of ways2see. It is reflecting and applying the conceptual model of GIS4all given in Section 3.1 for the target group of people with visual impairments or blindness (**Figure 2**).

4.3 A new pedestrian network for the city of Graz and new routing information for the target group

As stated in the theoretical background, the generation of a pedestrian network based on sidewalks is critically important, since people with visual impairments or blindness need to distinguish between the left-hand side and right-hand side of a street. Most of the available navigation tools use centerlines of streets as basic network information—even for pedestrian routing. Consequently, this leads to a coarse representation of directions, since they are based either using terminology involved in car navigation and/or imprecise guidance. Persons with sight are still able to navigate following these directions, since they rely on landmarks like street names, signs, etc. People with visual impairments or blindness need more specific, additional information, for example, where they are walking along (a wall, a fence, etc.), the distinction and location of "safe" crossings, landmarks that are ascertainable with the white cane, or barriers and objects which bear a danger.

Another challenge is that pedestrian networks are commonly not available in city data and their generation is cost- and time-intensive. ways2see uses a semiautomatic generation of the pedestrian network based on the centerlines of sidewalks. The attempt to use the methodology of [58], who developed a standardized procedure to generate sidewalks based on fixed distances from the street centerlines, failed due to varying street width and a lack of availability of this information in the data. Neis and Zielstra [59] used OpenStreetMap as data source for network generation, likewise offering limited level of detail and too general for the target group. The deduction of sidewalk centerlines for ways2see is using the zoning map, which indicates traffic zones including the street, the sidewalks and parking areas, etc. In combination with street centerlines of the Graph Integration Platform [60], a freely available dataset of the open government data, sidewalks were calculated and integrated, using ArcGIS scripts. The advantage of this approach is the potential to transfer the model to other cities/regions. The model achieves an accuracy level of 86%. Although only 14% of line segments are left to be inspected, the whole city was reviewed in fieldwork. This decision was taken to get sidewalk information at the best quality, since some particular information cannot be derived from other data sources.

The generation of the pedestrian network includes modeling intersections and crossings. A considerable portion of the target group relies on crossings equipped with accessible pedestrian signals, which has to be documented in the modeling process. In case of inexistence of crosswalks and (accessible) pedestrian signals, intersections without infrastructure were modeled by using scripting to avoid long detours. This situation is found predominantly in the suburban parts of the city with single-home setting.

The sidewalk-oriented pedestrian network works as basis but requires additional attributes for the orientation and navigation of people with visual impairments or blindness. A major challenge turned out in adding directional linear-based information to the network. The information, what kind of objects a person is moving along as well as where (linear) objects are located, e.g., house walls, fences, etc., is an important element of orientation and navigation information for the target group. Especially linear-based information is missing in existing tools. The possibility to include this kind of information in the direction settings is not provided in the network generation of ArcGIS. Additionally, the complexity of data cannot be represented in the standard network model. The network allows the combination of orientation features along the road like surface, availability of sidewalks, and use of sidewalks as well as landmarks and barriers to calculate the route, but not their display in the directions, which are provided to the user for wayfinding. Challenges identified with assigning necessary data to the network are encountered with new strategies to include this information through the adoption of the background xml files and direction settings. To produce a clear result without redundant information, the directions have to be post-processed before presenting to the user.

The final result is a citywide network, representing the centerlines of sidewalks, including crossings as unsecured crossings, crosswalks with and without pedestrian signals, and crossings using accessible pedestrian signals (**Figure 4**). A modeling process realized with scripts and Python makes this important step transferable to other regions.

The attributes of the pedestrian network are representing the requirements of the target group and are based on the list of specification (Section 4.2). The attributes, which are detailing the navigation information, are:

- Directional representation of objects along the sidewalk
- Availability, type, and surface of sidewalks
- Landmarks, obstacles, and barriers

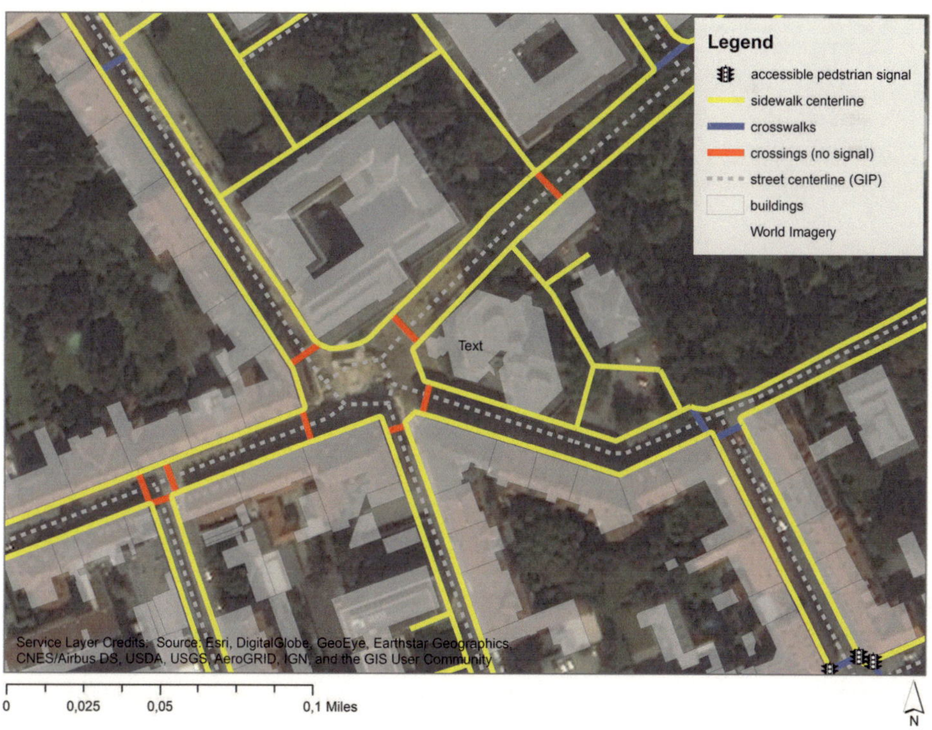

Figure 4.
Basic elements of the pedestrian network, city of Graz.

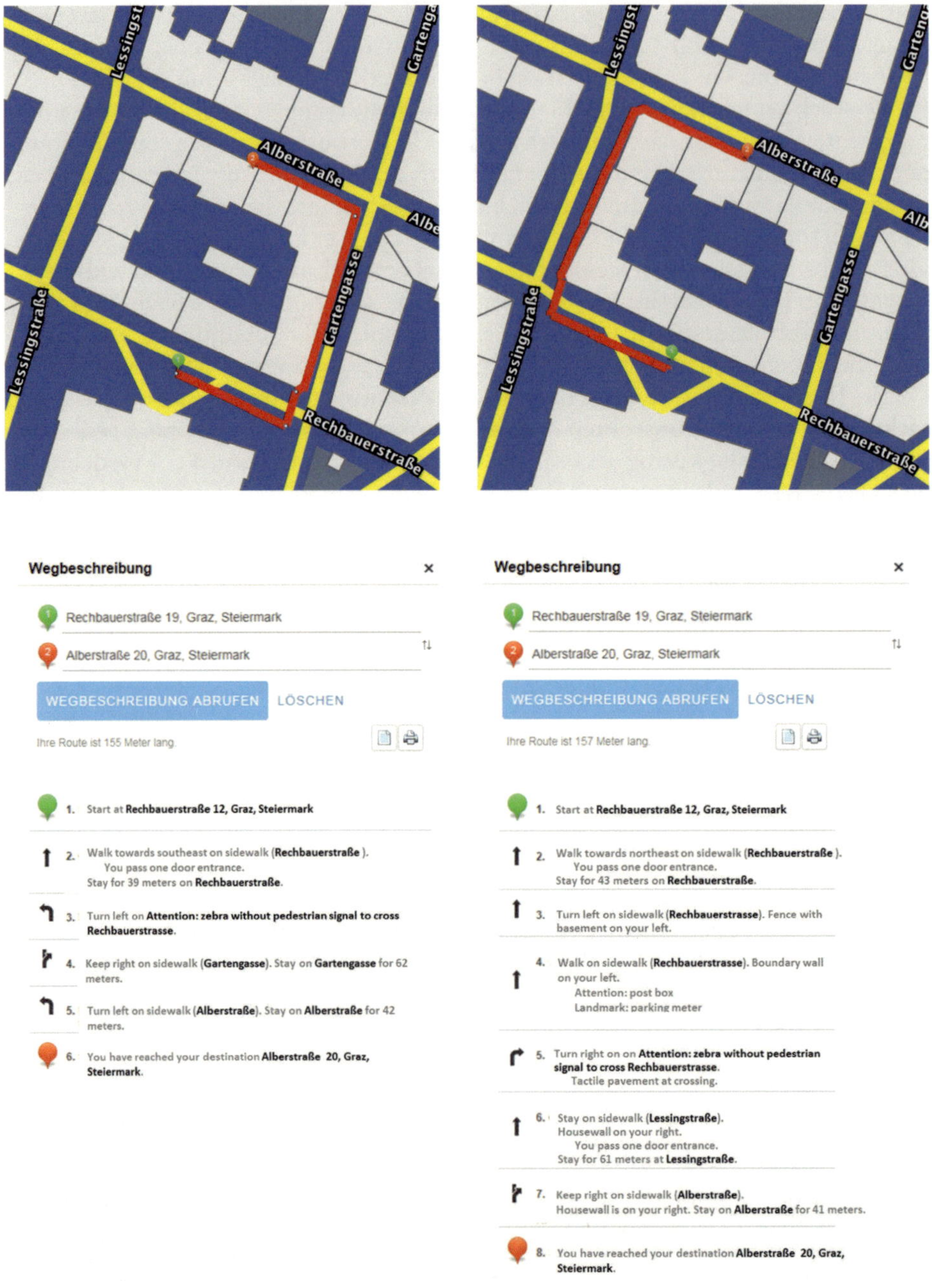
Lessingstraße
Gartengasse
Albe
Albe
Alberstraße
Rechbauerstraße
Wegbeschreibung
Rechbauerstraße 19, Graz, Steiermark
Alberstraße 20, Graz, Steiermark
WEGBESCHREIBUNG ABRUFEN
LÖSCHEN
Ihre Route ist 155 Meter lang.
1. Start at Rechbauerstraße 12, Graz, Steiermark
2. Walk towards southeast on sidewalk (Rechbauerstraße).
You pass one door entrance.
Stay for 39 meters on Rechbauerstraße.
3. Turn left on Attention: zebra without pedestrian signal to cross Rechbauerstrasse.
4. Keep right on sidewalk (Gartengasse). Stay on Gartengasse for 62 meters.
5. Turn left on sidewalk (Alberstraße). Stay on Alberstraße for 42 meters.
6. You have reached your destination Alberstraße 20, Graz, Steiermark.
Wegbeschreibung
Rechbauerstraße 19, Graz, Steiermark
Alberstraße 20, Graz, Steiermark
WEGBESCHREIBUNG ABRUFEN
LÖSCHEN
Ihre Route ist 157 Meter lang.
1. Start at Rechbauerstraße 12, Graz, Steiermark
2. Walk towards northeast on sidewalk (Rechbauerstraße).
You pass one door entrance.
Stay for 43 meters on Rechbauerstraße.
3. Turn left on sidewalk (Rechbauerstrasse). Fence with basement on your left.
4. Walk on sidewalk (Rechbauerstrasse). Boundary wall on your left.
Attention: post box
Landmark: parking meter
5. Turn right on on Attention: zebra without pedestrian signal to cross Rechbauerstrasse.
Tactile pavement at crossing.
6. Stay on sidewalk (Lessingstraße).
Housewall on your right.
You pass one door entrance.
Stay for 61 meters at Lessingstraße.
7. Keep right on sidewalk (Alberstraße).
Housewall is on your right. Stay on Alberstraße for 41 meters.
8. You have reached your destination Alberstraße 20, Graz, Steiermark.

Figure 5.
Example of routes based on two different profiles. Left, short routes preferred; right, show all orientation hints.

Based on the user profiles given in Section 4.2, these attributes are differently combined and weighted in the network. This is resulting in differing routing results and directions presented to the users, based on the selected profile.

Figure 5 exemplarily shows the main components of two different descriptions of directions. The user profile "short routes preferred" needs less orientation hints. The profile "avoid crossings without tactile pavement and accessible pedestrian signals, show all orientation hints" uses a detailed description of the route and avoids "unsecured" crossings.

4.4 Design of the user interface: new ways to see

The user interface of ways2see is concise, easy to use, self-explanatory, and accessible. It is integrating the user profiles resulting from the cluster analysis (Section 3.2). ways2see as an Internet-based application is all-time available.

The interface is using a straightforward navigation strategy, with the following steps:

- Welcome and introduction of the tool including links to a glossary and help
- Decision for the user profile to be used (**Figure 6a**)
- Decision, what to do:
    1. Retrieving directions between two addresses or retrieving directions between current position and an address (**Figure 6b**)
    2. Searching for POIs and retrieving directions to a selected POI (**Figure 6c**)
- Presentation of the result:
    1. Detailed directions for wayfinding (according to the selected user profile) (**Figure 7**)
    2. Map visualizing the route as well as POI (**Figure 7**)
    3. Text-based list of addresses of POI
- Option to export the information for "offline" or analogue use

On the first view, the map-focused design of Web AppBuilder seems to be a contrary to the goal of accessibility. However, the concise and minimal design with a comprehensive task menu offers the possibility to adapt the interface toward the needs of accessibility and compatibility with screen reader software. Therefore, a pre-defined template is adjusted through removing needless functionalities and adding text labels to menu elements. Text labels support on the one hand visibility and identification of menu buttons with the screen reader; on the other hand, they are selectable with the keyboard. Next to the keyboard first strategy, the interface is navigable with mouse and touchscreens. The user interface has the advantage of an automated arrangement of buttons and tools depending on the used end device (computer screen, tablet, smartphone). As indicated with the straightforward strategy, the buttons are offered consecutively step by step. Consequently, a button is offered only, if necessary selections, e.g., choosing the user profile, have already been made. The decision of searching for a POI or selecting a wayfinding process can only be done after defining the user profile.

Finally, the map, which is split up into a base map and additional layers presenting target group-oriented information, has to be briefly discussed. The base map shows the basic city structures including street centerlines, green areas, rivers, and buildings, following the idea of [61], who developed a base map for Austria. Additional layers will integrate cartography for visually impaired users. As stated in Section 3.3, special interest is given to the directions, since this is the most essential result for users not able to read the map due to their limited sight. Directions have to

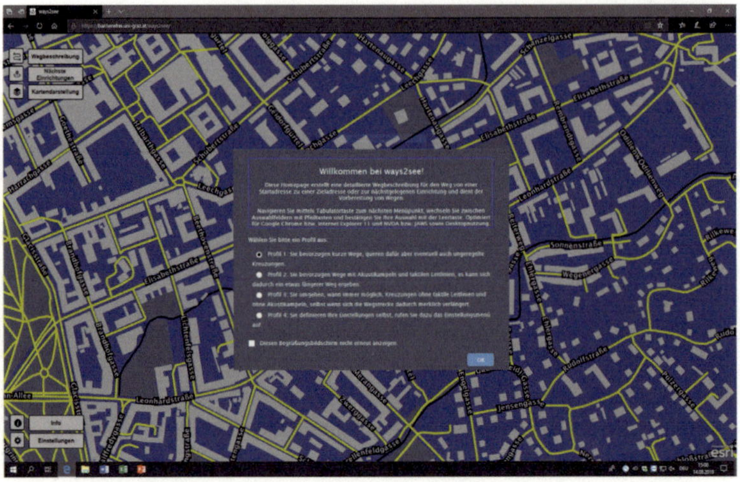

(a)

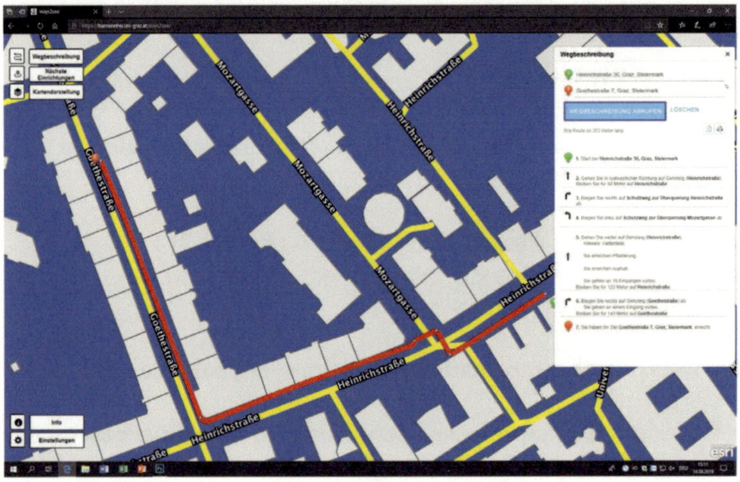

(b)

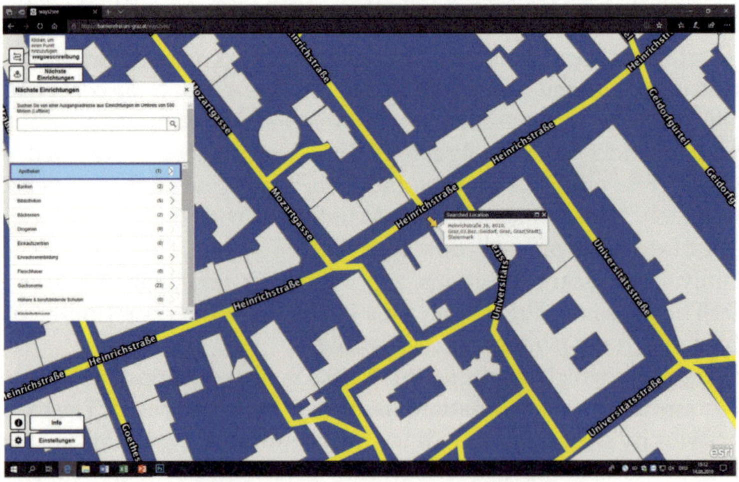

(c)

Figure 6.
(a) Welcome screen of ways2see offering basic information and selection of user profile. (b) Wayfinding between two addresses. (c) Search for facilities in the surrounding area.

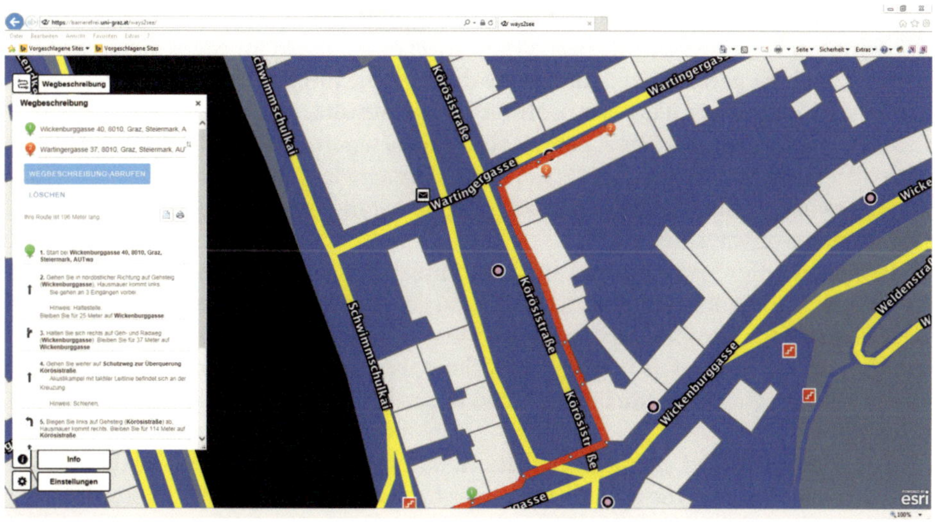

Figure 7.
Map with directions based on a selected user profile.

be readable with screen readers and can be exported—either to be used for adding further, personalized information or to be used on-trip. Routes, obstacles, barriers, and landmarks as well as points of interest are displayed using special designed map symbols. Furthermore, the performance of different browsers was tested regarding the implementation of personal settings (size and color schemes,) and the design of the user interface was adopted toward the most common browsers. However, the map component is challenging, since every browser handles the presentation of the map differently. At this point, it has to be mentioned that ways2see was developed for the screen readers NVDA and JAWS 16.0.

As restriction has to be indicated, outdated software might not offer compatibility and/or present optimized map result. As participatory part of ways2see initially, the integration of data provided by users (crowdsourcing) was conceived (cp. **Figure 2**). Although this is still on the project agenda, the technical realization opens up a completely new dimension due to the necessity to review and georeference the information as well as to think about the validity of data and user registration issues.

5. Conclusion

People with disabilities and their (spatial) needs are still at the edge—in society as well as in geography/science. To allow people moving away from this fringe, an essential step can be made by increasing the personal and individual mobility. Mobility means independency, e.g., from assisting persons, is enhancing quality of life, and finally is widening the individual (spatial) scope, which potentially leads to more interrelation and inclusion in society.

ways2see offers a new tool to people with visual impairments or blindness, which increases the personal mobility by supporting orientation and wayfinding for pre-trip planning. The user interface of ways2see is designed toward the needs of the target group and offers the possibility of personalization through different user profiles. The results of pre-trip planning are (1) information about facilities in the surrounding and/or (2) personalized directions for wayfinding toward these facilities or defined addresses. As a difference to existing tools, the results show (3) an extensive number of attributes presented as orientation and navigation hints along routes, (4) a user profile based indication of obstacles for the avoidance of barriers, and (5) personalized directions through the integration of this information in the routing analysis. The user profile-oriented results can be provided through GIS analysis on an expert level behind the scenes, where spatial data is analyzed with different network settings. Special focus hereby is given to the definition of the basic network, using sidewalks and adapting the standard network settings to the requirements of ways2see.

Parallel to offer user-oriented and customizable information as routes and route directions, the results are presented to the target group in an accessible way by specific interface design, map layout, and map symbols. The Internet platform itself and the list of addresses as POI and directions are available with and are suitable for screen readers. ways2see can be described as accessible tool providing information about accessibility.

The combination of spatial information; its analysis with geographic technologies, namely, GIS; and the application toward a marginalized group underpins the potential of geography in disability studies by a clear positioning of the competence for spatial approaches. ways2see is the result of a participative process, integrating persons with visual impairments or blindness through iterative steps into the development process. Different strategies were elaborated and are used to meet the needs of the target group. Inter- and transdisciplinarity is guaranteed through the partner network and allows the development of a marketable product.

In a future perspective, ways2see not only provides spatial information as orientation and navigation information but shows the potential to work as supporting tool in urban development and planning processes and can help to reduce barriers in the urban environments and—furthermore—in our minds. It is also intended as one way to raise awareness in society and herewith to promote social sustainability and inclusion.

Acknowledgements

ways2see is funded by the Austrian Research Promotion Agency (FFG). Special thanks are given to the project team. SynerGIS Informationssysteme GmbH is responsible for the coding, and Odilien-Institute—Society for People with Visual Impairment or Blindness is providing applied knowledge and expertise. The Department of Geography and Regional Science, University of Graz, is the scientific leader of the project.

The author would like to express special thanks to Sebastian Drexel, Antonia Dückelmann, Simon Landauer, Bettina Mandl and Jana Obermeier for their enthusiasm and personal commitment and their creative and innovative contributions to this project.

The author acknowledges the financial support of this publication by the University of Graz.

Author details

Susanne Zimmermann-Janschitz
Department of Geography and Regional Science, University of Graz, Graz, Austria

*Address all correspondence to: susanne.janschitz@uni-graz.at

References

[1] Carr LJ, Dunsiger SI, Marcus BH. Walk score™ as a global estimate of neighborhood walkability. American Journal of Preventive Medicine. 2010;**39**(5):460-463. DOI: 10.1016/j.amepre.2010.07.007

[2] Wuerzer T, Mason SG. Cycling willingness: Investigating distance as a dependent variable in cycling behavior among college students. Applied Geography. 2015;**60**:95-106. DOI: 10.1016/j.apgeog.2015.03.009

[3] Clarke P, Ailshire JA, Bader M, Morenoff JD, House JS. Mobility disability and the urban built environment. American Journal of Epidemiology. 2008;**168**(5):506-513. DOI: 10.1093/aje/kwn185

[4] Webber SC, Porter MM, Menec VH. Mobility in older adults: A comprehensive framework. The Gerontologist. 2010;**50**(4):443-450. DOI: 10.1093/geront/gnq013

[5] Sammer G, Uhlmann T, Unbehaun W, Millonig A, Mandl B, Dangschat J, et al. Identification of mobility-impaired persons and analysis of their travel behaviour and needs. Transportation Research Record: Journal of the Transportation Research Board. 2012;**2320**:46-54. DOI: 10.3141/2320-06

[6] Zimmermann-Janschitz S. Geographic information systems in the context of disabilities. Journal of Accessibility and Design for All (JACCESS). 2018;**8**(2):161-192. DOI: 10.17411/jacces.v8i2.171

[7] Beale L, Field K, Briggs D, Picton P, Matthews H. Mapping for wheelchair users: Route navigation in urban spaces. The Cartographic Journal. 2006;**43**(1):68-81

[8] Mobasheri A, Deister J, Dieterich H. Wheelmap: The wheelchair accessibility crowdsourcing platform. Open Geospatial Data, Software and Standards. 2017;**2**(1):27

[9] Sedlak P et al. Definition of contributions of geographic information systems for solving barrier-free environment issues. In: Proceedings of the 11th WSEAS International Conference on Applied Informatics and Communications, and Proceedings of the 4th WSEAS International Conference on Biomedical Electronics and Biomedical Informatics, and Proceedings of the International Conference on Computational Engineering in Systems Applications; 23-25 August 2011; Florence. Seven Point: WSEAS; 2011. pp. 198-203

[10] Svensson J. Accessibility in the urban environment for citizens with impairments: Using GIS to map and measure accessibility in Swedish cities. In: Proceedings of the 24th International Cartographic Conference (ICC); 15-21 November 2009; Santiago. International Cartographic Association; 2010. pp. 15-21

[11] Yairi IE, Igi S. Universal designed mobility support geographic information system for all pedestrians. Journal of the National Institute of Information and Communications Technology. 2007;**54**(3):135-145

[12] Lakde CK, Prasad PS. Review paper on navigation system for visually impaired people. International Journal of Advanced Research in Computer and Communication Engineering. 2015;**4**(1):2278-1021. DOI: DOI 10.17148/IJARCCE.2015.4134

[13] Roentgen U, Gelderblom G, Soede M, de Witte L. The impact of electronic mobility devices for persons who are visually impaired: A systematic review of effects and effectiveness. Journal of Visual Impairment and

Blindness. 2009;**103**(11):743-753. ISSN: 0145-482X

[14] Edman PK. Tactile Graphics. New York: American Foundation for the Blind; 1992

[15] Bhowmick A, Hazarika SM. An insight into assistive technology for the visually impaired and blind people: State-of-the-art and future trends. Journal on Multimodal User Interfaces. 2017;**11**(2):149-172. DOI: 10.1007/s12193-016-0235-6

[16] Cuturi LF, Aggius-Vella E, Campus C, Parmiggiani A, Gori M. From science to technology: Orientation and mobility in blind children and adults. Neuroscience and Biobehavioral Reviews. 2016;**71**:240-251. DOI: 10.1016/j.neubiorev.2016.08.019

[17] Janschitz S. Von Barrieren in unseren Köpfen und Karten ohne Grenzen. Geographische Informationssysteme im Diskurs der Barrierefreiheit—ein Widerspruch in sich oder unerkanntes Potenzial. [About Barriers in Our Minds and Maps without Borders. Geographic Information Systems in the Disability Discourse: Contradiction or Undiscovered Potential]. Vienna-Muenster: LIT-Verlag; 2012. 272 p

[18] Abe A, Maita N, Ooshida Y, Kano T. Proposal for a system based on the universal design approach for providing tourism information by linking RFID and GIS. In: Magyar G, Knapp G, Wojtkowski W, Wojtkowski WG, Zupancic J, editors. Advances in Information Systems Development. Boston, MA: Springer; 2007. pp. 247-258. DOI: 10.1007/978-0-387-70761-7_21

[19] Enders A, Brandt Z. Using geographic information system technology to improve emergency management and disaster response for people with disabilities. Journal of Disability Policy Studies. 2007;**17**(4):223-229

[20] Fernandes H, Conceicao N, Paredes H, Pereira A, Araujo P, Barroso J. Providing accessibility to blind people using GIS. Universal Access in the Information Society. 2012;**11**(4):399-407. DOI: 10.1007/s10209-011-0255-7

[21] Rice MT, Aburizaiza AO, Jacobson RD, Shore BM, Paez FI. Supporting accessibility for blind and vision-impaired people with a localized gazetteer and open source geotechnology. Transactions in GIS. 2012;**16**(2):177-190. DOI: 10.1111/j.1467-9671.2012.01318.x

[22] Fernandes H, Costa P, Filipe V, Paredes H, Barroso J. A review of assistive spatial orientation and navigation technologies for the visually impaired. Universal Access in the Information Society. 2019;**18**(1):155-168

[23] Petrie H, Johnson V, Strothotte T, Raab A, Fritz S, Michel R. MoBIC: Designing a travel aid for blind and elderly people. Journal of Navigation. 1996;**49**(01):45-52. DOI: 10.1017/S0373463300013084

[24] Zeng L, Weber G. Accessible Maps for the Visually Impaired. In: Proceedings of IFIP INTERACT 2011, Workshop on ADDW; 5-9 September 2011; Lisbon. Heidelberg: Springer; 2011. pp. 54-60

[25] Ahmetovic D, Manduchi R, Coughlan JM, Mascetti S. Mind your crossings: Mining GIS imagery for crosswalk localization. ACM Transactions on Accessible Computing (TACCESS). 2017;**9**(4):11

[26] Ivanov R. Real-time GPS track simplification algorithm for outdoor navigation of visually impaired. Journal of Network and Computer Applications.

2012;**35**(5):1559-1567. DOI: 10.1016/j.jnca.2012.02.002

[27] Mayerhofer B, Pressl B, Wieser M. ODILIA—A mobility concept for the visually impaired. In: International Conference on Computers for Handicapped Persons (ICCHP); 9-11 July 2008; Linz. Berlin-Heidelberg: Springer; 2008. pp. 1109-1116

[28] Liao CF. Using a smartphone application to support visually impaired pedestrians at signalized intersection crossings. Transportation Research Record: Journal of the Transportation Research Board. 2013;**2393**:12-20. DOI: 10.3141/2393-02

[29] Fernandes H, Filipe V, Costa P, Barroso J. Location based Services for the Blind Supported by RFID Technology. Procedia Computer Science. 2014;**27**:2-8. DOI: 10.1016/j.procs.2014.02.002

[30] Serrao M, Shahrabadi S, Moreno M, Jose JT, Rodrigues JI, Rodrigues JM, et al. Computer vision and GIS for the navigation of blind persons in buildings. Universal Access in the Information Society. 2015;**14**(1):67-80. DOI: 10.1007/s10209-013-0338-8

[31] Chen M, Lin H, Liu D, Zhang H, Yue S. An object-oriented data model built for blind navigation in outdoor space. Applied Geography. 2015;**60**:84-94. DOI: 10.1016/j.apgeog.2015.03.004

[32] Kammoun S, Mace MJM, Oriola B, Jouffrais C. Towards a geographic information system facilitating navigation of visually impaired users. In: 13th International Conference on Computers for Handicapped Persons (ICCHP); 11-13 July 2012; Linz. Berlin-Heidelberg: Springer; 2012. pp. 521-528. DOI: 10.1007/978-3-642-31534-3_77

[33] Velázquez R, Pissaloux E, Rodrigo P, Carrasco M, Giannoccaro N, Lay-Ekuakille A. An outdoor navigation system for blind pedestrians using GPS and tactile-foot feedback. Applied Sciences. 2018;**8**(4):578

[34] Karimi HA. Universal Navigation on Smartphones. New York: Springer US; 2011. DOI: 10.1007/978-1-4419-7741-0

[35] Golledge RG, Loomis JM, Klatzky RL, Flury A, Yang XL. Designing a personal guidance system to aid navigation without sight: Progress on the GIS component. International Journal of Geographical Information Systems. 1991;**5**(4):373-395. DOI: 10.1080/02693799108927864

[36] Brilhault A, Kammoun S, Gutierrez O, Truillet P, Jouffrais C. Fusion of artificial vision and GPS to improve blind pedestrian positioning. In: New Technologies, Mobility and Security (NTMS); 2011 4th IFIP International Conference on New Technologies, Mobility and Security; 7-10 February 2011; Paris. New York: IEEE; 2011. pp. 1-5. DOI: 10.1109/NTMS.2011.5721061

[37] Chandler E, Worsfold J. Understanding the requirements of geographical data for blind and partially sighted people to make journeys more independently. Applied Ergonomics. 2013;**44**(6):919-928. DOI: 10.1016/j.apergo.2013.03.030

[38] Laakso M, Sarjakoski T, Lehto L, Sarjakoski LT. An information model for pedestrian routing and navigation databases supporting universal accessibility. Cartographica. 2013;**48**(2):89-99. DOI: 10.3138/carto.48.2.1837

[39] Roentgen UR, Gelderblom GJ, de Witte LP. Users' evaluations of four electronic travel aids aimed at navigation for persons who are visually impaired. Journal of Visual Impairment and Blindness. 2011;**105**(10):612-623

[40] Serrao M, Rodrigues JM, du Buf JH. Navigation framework using visual landmarks and a GIS. Procedia Computer Science. 2014;**27**:28-37. DOI: 10.1016/j.procs.2014.02.005

[41] Bermeo A, Bravo M, Punin C, Ordoñez E, Huerta M. Obstacle detection system to improve mobility of people with visual impairment. In: IEEE ANDESCON; 22-24 August 2018; Cali. New York: IEEE; 2018. pp. 1-5

[42] Serna A, Marcotegui B. Urban accessibility diagnosis from mobile laser scanning data. ISPRS Journal of Photogrammetry and Remote Sensing. 2013;**84**:23-32. DOI: 10.1016/j.isprsjprs.2013.07.001

[43] Ahmetovic D, Manduchi R, Coughlan JM, Mascetti S. Zebra crossing spotter: Automatic population of spatial databases for increased safety of blind travelers. In: Proceedings of the 17th International ACM SIGACCESS Conference on Computers and Accessibility; 26-28 October 2015; Lisbon. New York: ACM; 2015. pp. 251-258

[44] Coughlan JM, Shen H. Crosswatch: A system for providing guidance to visually impaired travelers at traffic intersections. Journal of Assistive Technologies. 2013;**7**(2):131-142. DOI: 10.1108/17549451311328808

[45] Karimi HA, Kasemsuppakorn P. Pedestrian network map generation approaches and recommendation. International Journal of Geographical Information Science. 2013;**27**(5):947-962. DOI: 10.1080/13658816.2012.730148

[46] Brock A, Oriola B, Truillet P, Jouffrais C, Picard D. Map design for visually impaired people: Past, present, and future research. Médiation et Information. 2013;**36**:117-129

[47] Calle-Jimenez T, Lujan-Mora S. Web accessibility barriers in geographic maps. International Journal of Computer Theory and Engineering. 2016;**8**(1):167-174. DOI: 10.7763/IJCTE.2016.V8.1024

[48] Jenny B, Kelso NV. Color design for the color vision impaired. Cartographic Perspectives. 2007;**58**:61-67. DOI: 10.14714/CP58.270

[49] Morgan N, Saeed M. A comparative study of multimodal digital map interface designs for blind users. International Journal of Artificial Intelligence and Soft Computing. 2015;**5**(1):69-86. DOI: 10.1504/IJAISC.2015.067526

[50] O'Sullivan L, Picinali L, Gerino A, Cawthorne D. A prototype audio-tactile map system with an advanced auditory display. International Journal of Mobile Human Computer Interaction (IJMHCI). 2015;**7**(4):53-75. DOI: 10.4018/IJMHCI.2015100104

[51] Rodriguez-Sanchez MC, Moreno-Alvarez MA, Martin E, Borromeo S, Hernandez-Tamames JA. Accessible smartphones for blind users: A case study for a wayfinding system. Expert Systems with Applications. 2014;**41**(16):7210-7222. DOI: 10.1016/j.eswa.2014.05.031

[52] Wang Z, Li N, Li B. Fast and independent access to map directions for people who are blind. Interacting with Computers. 2012;**24**(2):91-106. DOI: 10.1016/j.intcom.2012.02.002

[53] Clarke Z, Judge S, Heron N, Langley J, Hosking I, Hawley MS. User involvement in the early development of assistive technology devices in Everyday Technology for Independence and Care. In: AAATE 2011; 31 August–1 September 2011; Maastricht. Assistive Technology Research Series. 2011;**29**:362-373. DOI: 10.3233/978-1-60750-814-4-362

[54] Martin JK, Martin LG, Stumbo NJ, Morrill JH. The impact of consumer

involvement on satisfaction with and use of assistive technology. Disability and Rehabilitation. Assistive Technology. 2011;**6**(3):225-242. DOI: 10.3109/17483107.2010.522685

[55] Center for Persons with Disabilities. WebAIM. Screen Reader User Survey #6 Results. Utah State University. 2017. Available from: http://webaim.org/projects/screenreadersurvey6/ [Accessed: 20 March 2017]

[56] Austria S. Menschen mit Beeinträchtigungen. Ergebnisse der Mikrozensus-Zusatzfragen 4. Quartal 2007. 2008. Available from: http://www.statistik.at/web_de/statistiken/gesundheit/gesundheitszustand/gesundheitliche_beeintraechtigungen/index.htm [Accessed: 27 October 2016]

[57] Zimmermann-Janschitz S, Mandl B, Dückelmann A. Clustering the mobility needs of persons with visual impairments or legal blindness. Transportation Research Record: Journal of the Transportation Research Board. 2017;**2650**(1):66-73. DOI: 10.3141/2650-08

[58] Ballester MG, Pérez MR, Stuiver HJ. Automatic pedestrian network generation. In: The 14th AGILE International Conference on Geographic Information Science; 18-21 April 2011; Utrecht. AGILE; 2011. Available from: https://agile-online.org/conference_paper/cds/agile_2011/contents/pdf/shortpapers/sp_116.pdf [Accessed: 20 March 2017]

[59] Neis P, Zielstra D. Generation of a tailored routing network for disabled people based on collaboratively collected geodata. Applied Geography. 2014;**47**:70-77. DOI: 10.1016/j.apgeog.2013.12.004

[60] Graph Integration Platform (GIP). 2016. Available from: http://www.gip.gv.at/home.html [Accessed: 13 January 2016]

[61] Schmidt M, Jörg W. basemap.at—Creating a harmonised web basemap for Austria. In: Jobst M, editor. Service-Oriented Mapping. Vienna: Jobstmedia Management Verlag; 2012. pp. 143-149

Chapter 19

Low-Vision Rehabilitation in Maculopathy

Giovanni Sato and Roberta Rizzo

Abstract

Maculopathy can have many causes: congenital, hereditary and acquired. The response of a maculopathy is the formation of a scotoma that can be relative or absolute with difficulty or impossibility to read, write and see the normal activities of daily life. The visually impaired person therefore has an insufficient level of visual ability to perform daily activities, work or leisure activities that are usual for individuals of the same age, sex and sociocultural status. A more or less serious low vision and a visual disability are thus created. The visually impaired person is able to use the eccentric visual residue in the preferential retinal network. With visual rehabilitation, a visual capacity lost by the patient is gained, developing eccentric fixation, giving the patient the awareness of his own possibilities to see and use the use of optical and electronic aids.

Keywords: maculopathy, low vision, rehabilitation, preferential retinal locus, neurovision training

1. Introduction

The most frequent maculopathy are age-related macular degeneration, myopic macular degeneration, diabetic edematous and exudative maculopathy, and hereditary macular dystrophy followed in order of frequency by Stargardt Disease, cone dystrophy, cone-rod dystrophy and Best disease. The ability requested from low-vision patients are in the first place to read again (90%) and then recognizing faces, writing, hand working, TV, theater and cinema watching, driving a car, inability to perform the standard daily working activity or hobby and relaxation, inability in the spatial orientation and mobility. The damage induced by AMD leads to a central absolute or relative scotoma of different shape and extension, with subsequent loss or reduction of the fine visual abilities like the reading process.

2. Low-vision rehabilitation in maculopathy: preferential retinal locus (PRL)

The low-vision patient with maculopathy of various origins can recover the visual ability with the presence of a little part of healthy retina called preferential retinal locus (PRL).

PRL is distant in varying degrees from the nonfunctioning fovea.

How to find and locate the PRL? In the presence of an absolute scotoma, the site and the extension of the scotoma must be precisely detected, and it has to be the preferential retinal locus (PRL) [1].

In 1982, Timberlake [1] used the scanning laser ophthalmoscopy (SLO) to do direct retinal perimetry. With SLO, he obtained a map with which the retinal locus was directly observable on a video of the fundus in patients with macular disease.

About the localization of PRL, Guez, Le Gargasson, Rigaudiere and O'Reagan (1993) reported that the PRL was located in 60% of the cases to the left of the visual field scotoma; Sunness et al. [2], Cummings and Rubin [3] in 63%; and Fletcher and Schuchard [4] in 34%. Trauzettel-Klosinski [5] found that in 50% of patients with Stargardt's juvenile maculopathy the eccentric fixation was located above the retinal lesion (below the visual scotoma).

Nilsson et al. [6, 7] studied 20 patients with age-related macular degeneration, an absolute central scotoma and a mean visual acuity of 0.04 (20/475) using scanning laser ophthalmoscopy (SLO) (**Figure 1**) that was used for microperimetry and determination of preferred retinal locus, localized in most patients to the left. Trying to read with a PRL to the left of the retinal lesion with the scotoma located in the direction of reading has been shown to be very disadvantageous. All 20 patients were trained to use a new PRL located above the macular atrophy, which is better for reading (corresponding to a location below the visual field scotoma)-first by reading the text under simultaneous fixation monitoring and instruction in the SLO and then by reading the printed text, using high magnification (mean 14.3×). With training (mean 5.2 h), it increased significantly ($p < 0.001$) the reading speed to 68.3 ± 19.4 words per min. Training of eccentric reading has thus proved to be very successful (**Figure 2**).

Nilsson test is a fundamental in low-vision rehabilitation: a large cross generated by the SLO with the center omitted to accommodate a large letter. The patient is asked to fixate on the center of the cross: the letter is invisible to the patient since it is located in the scotoma. The horizontal line is then moved upwards (or downwards) on the SLO screen step by step, and the patient is instructed to follow it until he can clearly identify the letter (**Figures 3** and **4**) [6].

The horizontal bar of the cross on the SLO screen is then elevated step by step, and the patient is told to follow the moving bar so as to fixate on the center of the cross at all times. This means that the projection of the bar on the retina gradually moves downwards together with the lesion until the projection of the letter on the retina finally becomes visible above the retinal lesion (below the visual field scotoma), as demonstrated in the figure. The horizontal bar moves in one direction on the SLO screen, viewed by the patient, and its projection on the retina in the

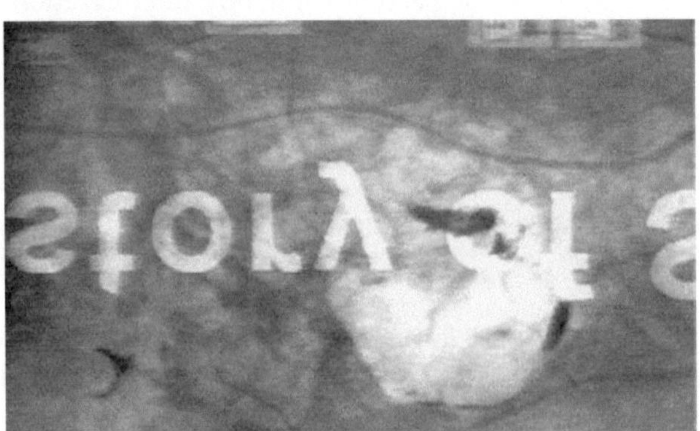

Figure 1.
Scanning laser ophthalmoscopy shows the site of PRL.

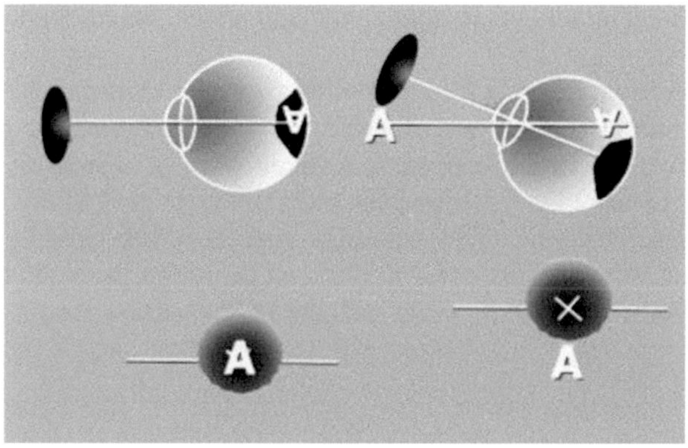

Figure 2.
In AMD with absolute scotoma, the central fixation places a letter in the foveal center, within the macular scar, corresponding to the visual field scotoma (left part of the figure). By looking upwards, moving the retinal lesion downwards and elevating the visual field scotoma, the letter is projected in the healthy retina above the lesion and seen below the scotoma (right part of the figure) [6].

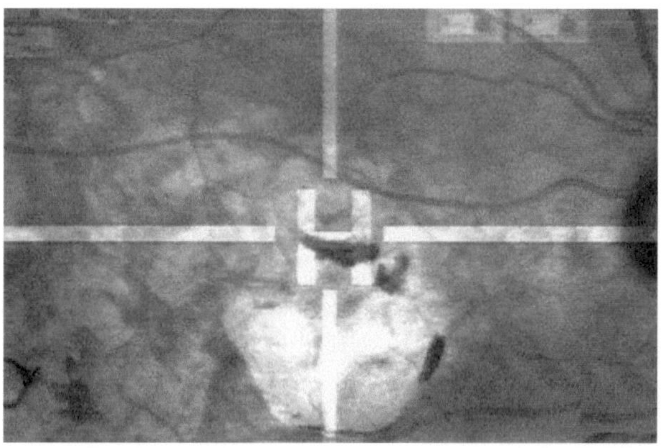

Figure 3.
A large cross is generated in the SLO screen, viewed by the patient: the center of the cross is omitted to accommodate a large-size letter. The patient is told to fixate the center of the cross but the letter placed in the center of the retinal lesion (visual field scotoma) is invisible to the patient.

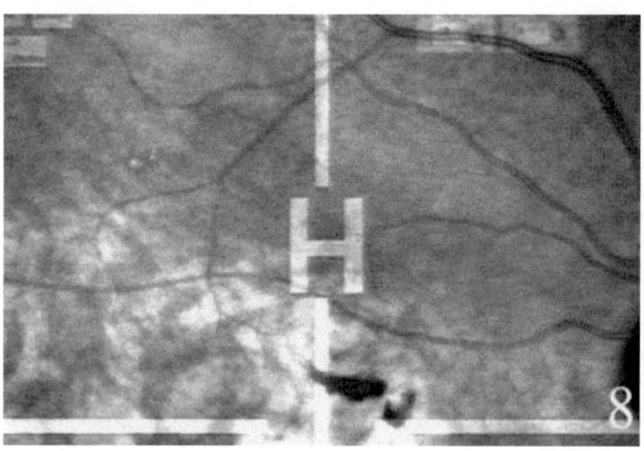

Figure 4.
Nilsson test.

opposite direction. The patient is repeatedly trained to find his new trained retinal locus (TRL).

After the training with SLO [6, 7], reading speed increased in 90% of the patients who accepted and learned eccentric viewing from an average of 9 words/min, which is far from fluent reading, to an average of 68 words/min.

Currently, SLO is not available and the tools to locate the PRL are represented by some type of microperimetry. There are also some low-tech test like Letter Scotometry and California Visual Field Test and Backman procedure [8, 9]. In the Age pre-microperimetry and after the end-age of SLO, the scotoma might be

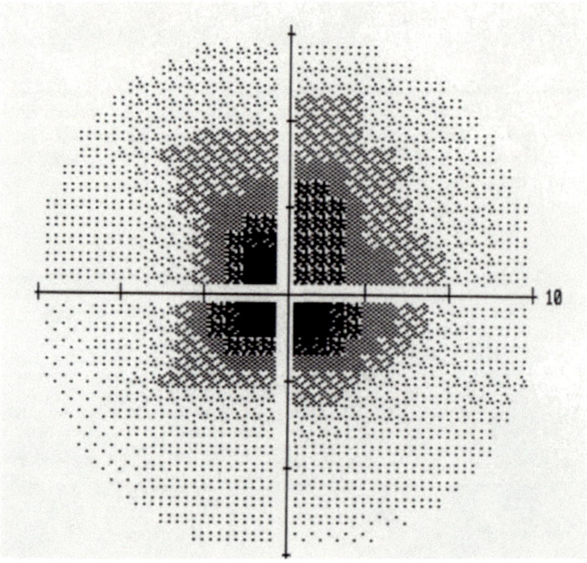

Figure 5.
Automatic computerized perimetry: absolute scotoma.

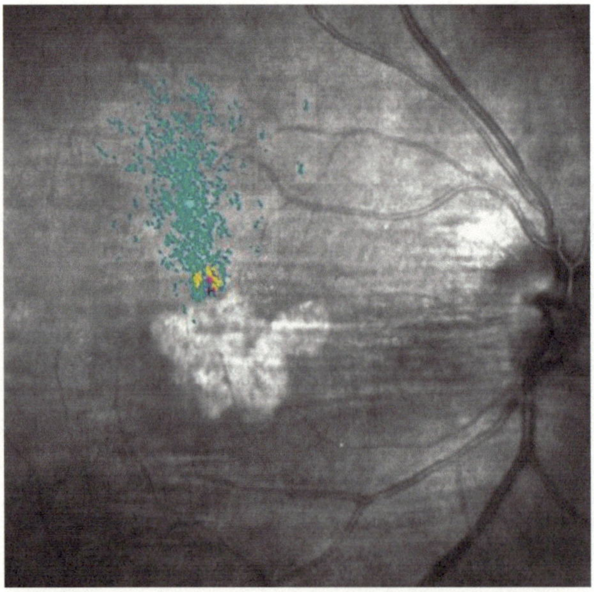

Figure 6.
Superior PRL in patients with loss of central vision in atrophic ARMD.

detected with Visual Field Test (Goldmann and automatic computerized perimetry) (**Figure 5**).

Microperimetry [10, 11] (MP) or fundus perimetry is a technology that allows the study of retinal sensitivity at different foveal and parafoveal areas as well as eye fixation and provides a direct correlation between anatomical and functional outcomes. Concerning ocular pathology, several studies have confirmed the usefulness of MP for evaluating and analyzing different retinal pathological conditions, such as age-related macular degeneration or glaucoma, and for analyzing the effect of different medical or surgical treatments for these conditions. MP has also been shown to be useful for visual training and rehabilitation using audiobiofeedback [11, 12].

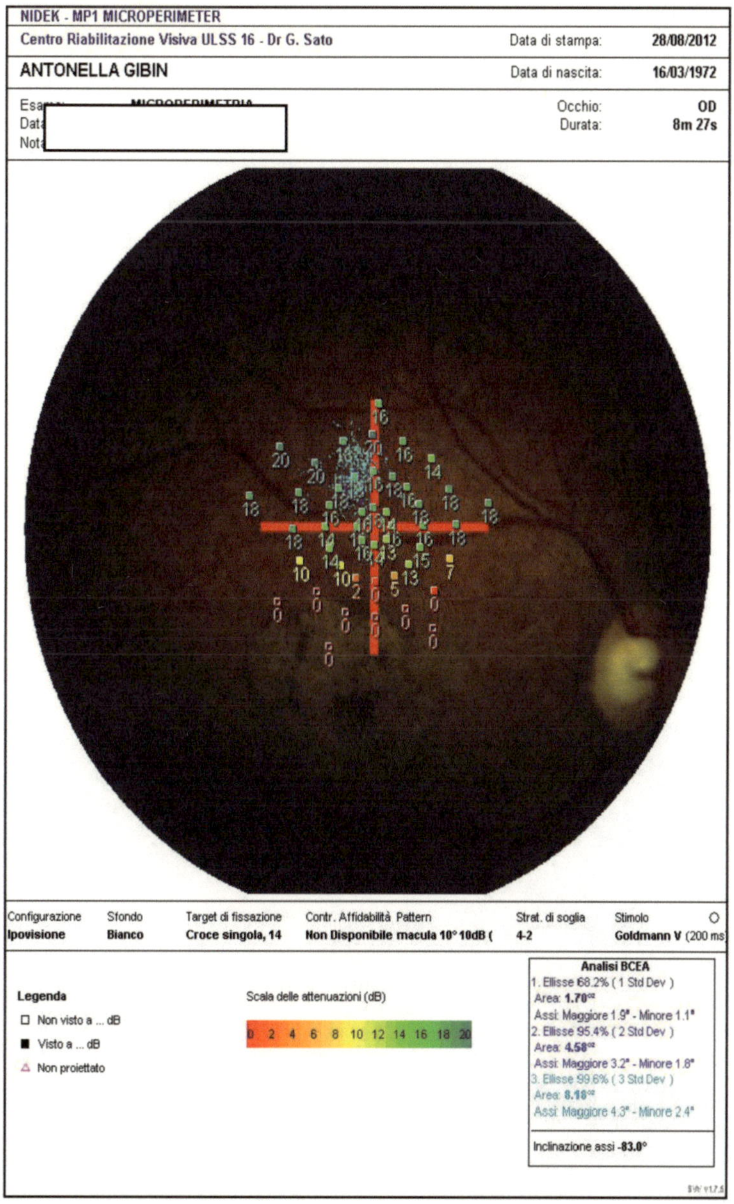

Figure 7.
Superior PRL in Stargardt disease.

MP enables precise assessment of the location and stability of fixation (PRL) in patients with maculopathy and also allows the shifting of PRL in the site of TRL (trained retinal locus) (**Figures 6** and 7).

The sight deficit area will be more or less extended in correlation to the retinal lesion extension and according to the PRL position (below, left, right and over the lesion) (**Figures 8** and **9**), and the reading difficulties may vary.

The most favorable situation for the reading activities is when the PRL is located over the atrophy.

Visual acuity depends on the site of PRL and from the stability of fixation.

The patient is trained, if he is not able and when the scotoma is more dense, and taught to fixate on the best available portion of the retina, where the PRL is better.

The patient will direct his sight a little above the target object (the words on the book).

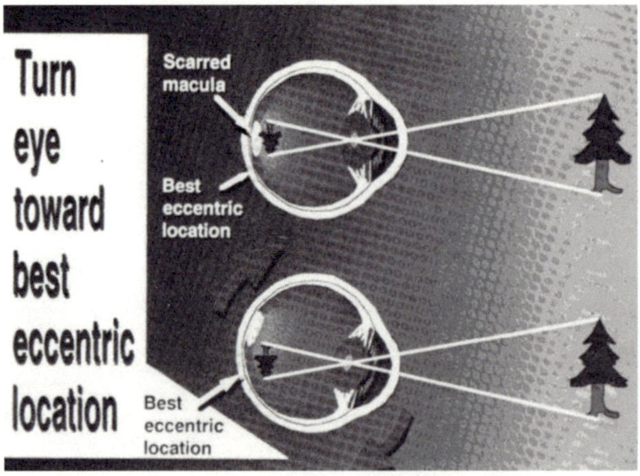

Figure 8.
Best eccentric fixation.

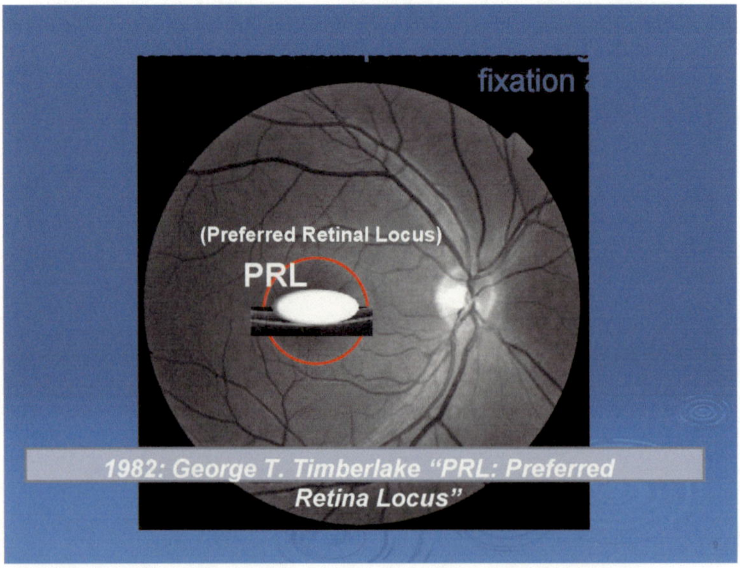

Figure 9.
Preferential retinal locus.

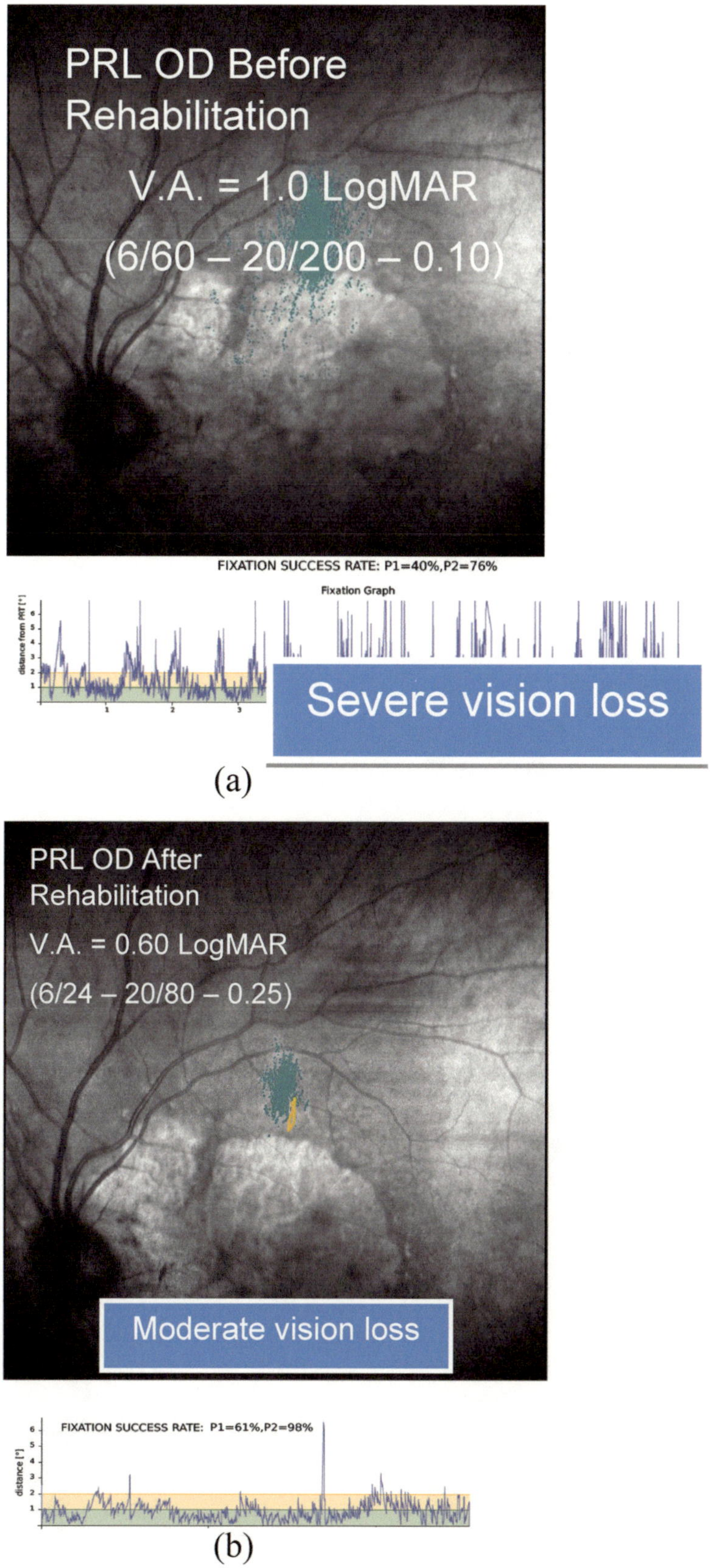

Figure 10.
(a) PRL above the retinal atrophy and (b) reduction of the area of ellipse of fixation in °q.

This type of low-vision rehabilitation is usually made with audiobiofeedback with microperimeter (**Figure 10a** and **b**).

The microperimeter employs an audiobiofeedback to help patients reach a new selected fixation position, with the purpose to increase fixation stability (**Figure 11**).

The examination of the fixation also allows us to assess whether the fixation chosen by the patient is to be strengthened or to be modified per site in order to improve a visual improvement (Retinal Locus Rehabilitated) (**Figure 11**).

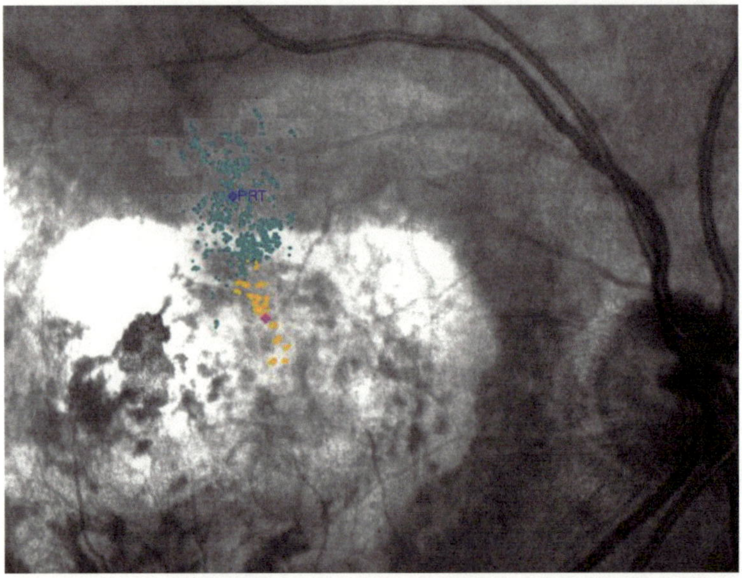

Figure 11.
Stabilization of fixation: a good use of peripheral vision retains a better quality of life.

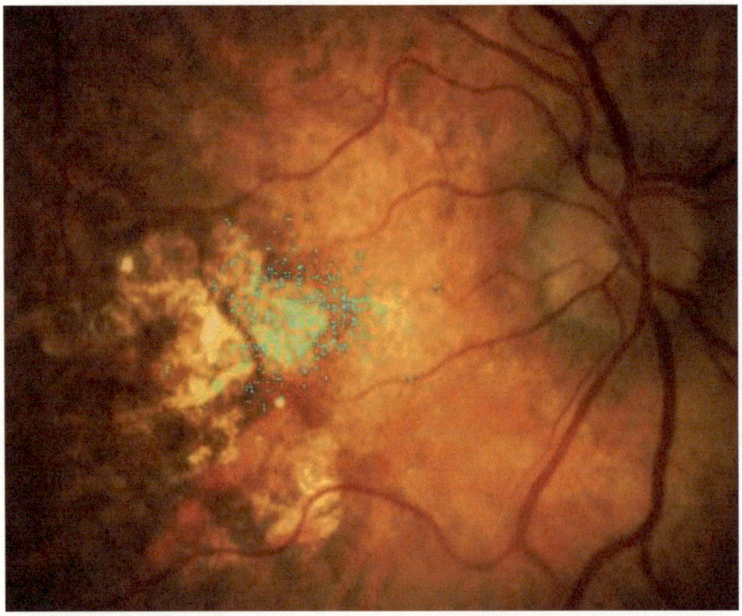

Figure 12.
Unstable eccentric fixation in ARMD.

After the localization of PRL and its level of stability or establishing the necessity to shift the PRL in another side of the nonatrophic retina (**Figure 12**), we must train PRL with reading exercise using the Backmann Formula [9].

Backman formula:

$$\text{TANG } D^{\circ} = X/RD.$$

$$X = \text{TANG } D^{\circ} \times RD.$$

where X is the distance on the reading paper between the text and point of fixation decentration; D° is the angle in degrees of the distance between the lesion fovea and the PRL; and RD is the reading distance in centimeters.

According to this formula, customized exercises are printed and the patient will practice with them at the Low Vision Center and then at home (**Figure 13**).

Only after a proper training session can the patient practice reading books or newspapers.

Reading coated paper is more difficult for it has many reflexes, newspapers for the low quality of the paper. The reading position must be ergonomically corrected, with reading stand vertical in front of the patient, with the possibility to put the elbows and with a correct illumination, to avoid dazzling, and to increase the contrast sensitivity, filter lenses may be used.

After the localization of PRL and the stabilization and/or the shifting with MP of the eccentric fixation, we must enhance the visual plasticity using neurovision training [13].

Perceptual learning (PL) paradigms have been successfully employed to treat a series of pathologies affecting central vision. Specifically, training observers for several weeks on basic visual tasks improved their visual abilities, such as visual acuity (VA) and the contrast sensitivity function (CSF) [14, 15]. One of the most efficient approaches consists in a contrast detection task of a low-contrast Gabor patch flanked above and below by high-contrast Gabor patches [15, 16].

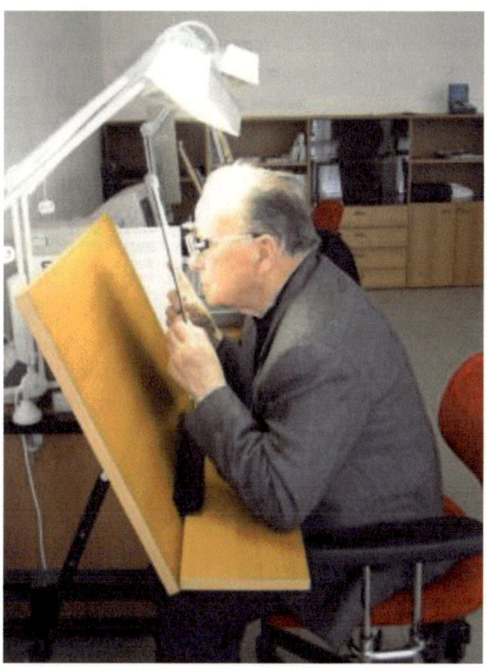

Figure 13.
Reading with aplanatic system.

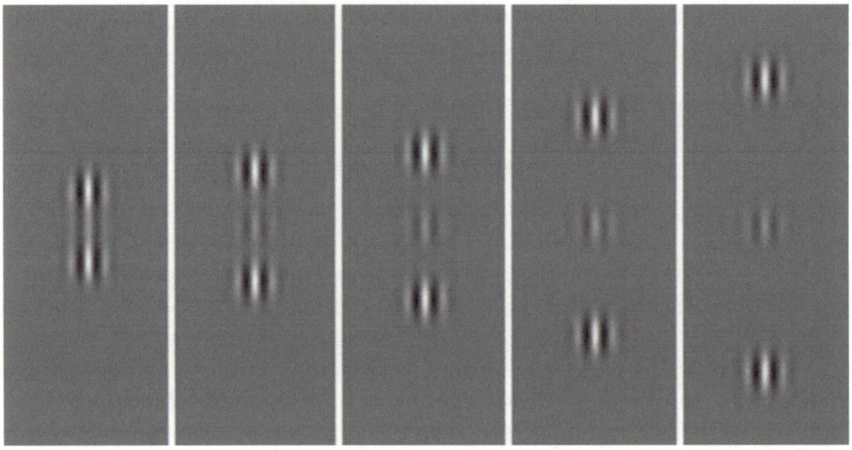

Figure 14.
Stimulus configuration used in the learning sessions. Only one spatial frequency is shown (i.e., 3 cpd). A central target Gabor is flanked by two high-contrast Gabor patches of the same orientation and spatial frequency. Panels from left to right show the five target-to-flankers distances trained: 2λ, 3λ, 4λ, 6λ and 8λ [13].

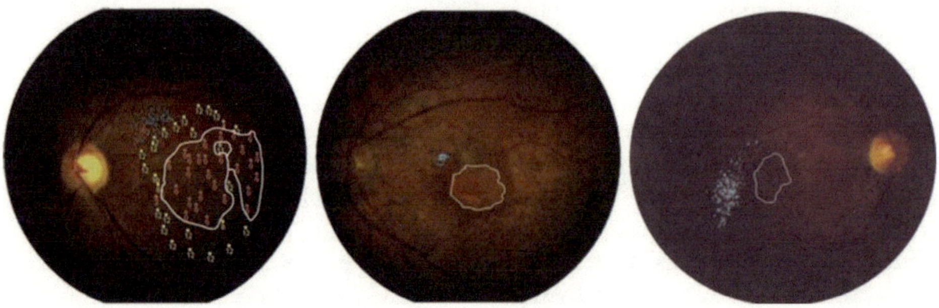

Figure 15.
MP of patients subjected to neurovision training: the blue points represent the dispersion of monocular fixation pattern that indicates the location of PRL, i.e., the part of the retina that is used by the patients during fixation tasks [13].

For foveal stimuli, it has been found that collinear flankers placed at a distance of 3–4 times the wavelength of the target Gabor (λ) enhance target detection, thus producing facilitation (i.e., lower contrast detection thresholds) (**Figure 14**).

Training on lateral interactions is effective in improving the residual visual functions in the periphery of the visual field of patients with maculopathy and eccentric fixation. Perceptual learning procedures produced significant improvements in the trained task and learning transferred to visual acuity and induced a significant improvement of the contrast sensitivity. Perceptual learning effects were retained between 4 and 6 months, suggesting long-term neural plasticity changes in the visual cortex (**Figure 15**).

The successive step in a low-vision rehabilitation patient is the choices of optic and/or visual aids.

3. Reading: physiopathology and rehabilitation of the reading process in low vision

Reading is the technical ability to perceive the words in a sequential way plus text understanding capability. Normal reading is composed of rapid eye movements

(SACCADES), 50 ms; and fixation pauses, 250 ms, saccade (50 ms). In the fixation pauses, there are 50 ms for text comprehension and 200 ms for programming the next saccade.

Normally, the perceptual area or sight field for reading is 3–4 letters to the left and 15 letters to the right of the fixation point. Decoding field or identification area or "VISUAL SPAN": number of letters of the smallest dimensions that can be recognized during one fixation. The normal sighted have a visual span of 8–12 letters.

The central 10° diameter of the visual field, which accounts for approximately 2% of the total visual field, is mapped onto nearly 50% of the primary visual cortex.

Visual acuity (yellow) decreases rapidly with increasing eccentricity (**Figure 16**) [5].

A person to have a good reading performance needs a window of visual field of at least:

≥2° to the right of the fixation point.

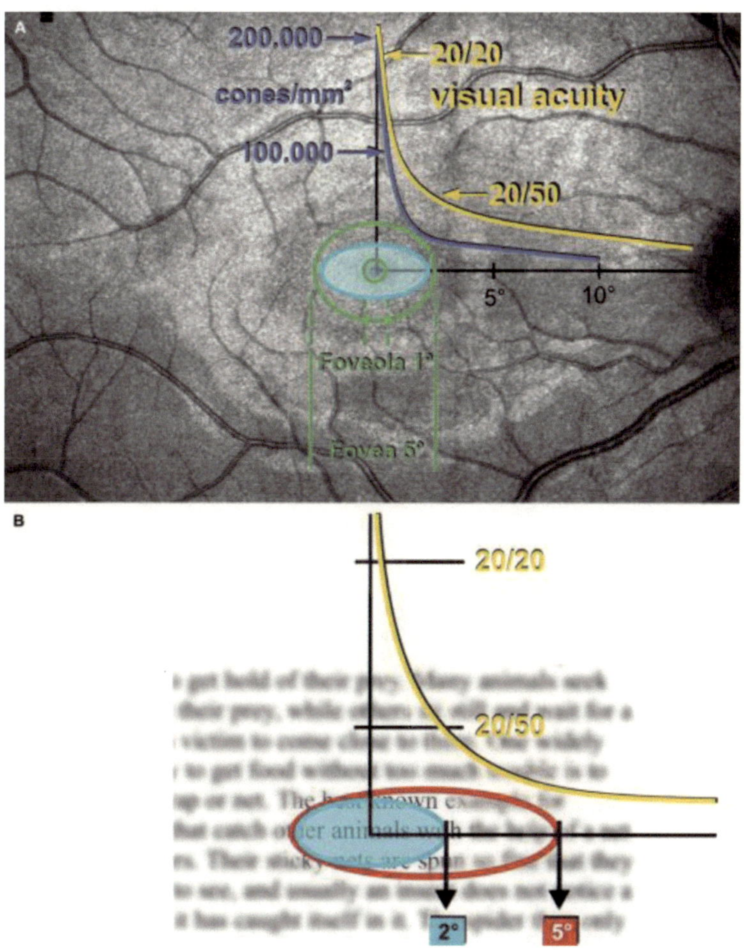

Figure 16.
(A) In normal subjects, the visual acuity (yellow) decreases rapidly with increasing eccentricity like the cone density (dark blue). The proportions of the foveola (1°, green circle) and the fovea (5° diameter, green oval) determine the minimum reading visual field (turquoise oval) of 2° to the right and left of fixation and 1° above and below fixation. (B) Because of the visual acuity curve (yellow), only in the minimum reading visual field (turquoise oval) can the text be perceived clearly. The total perceptual span (red oval) is extended up to 5° (or 15 letters) in the reading direction by parafoveal information processing [5].

In a low-vision patient with maculopathy, PRL may be located up, down, in the right or in the left of the macular atrophy.

The more favorable condition to reading is a PRL located above the macular atrophy that coincides with a PRL, seen at the way of visual field it is located below the scotoma. The patient must move the gaze or the eye up, down, right or left with respect to the object to be seen. Scotoma superior to the fixation point (PRL above the retinal lesion) represents the best location for the reading process.

Different conditions of scotoma/PRL location versus reading in low-vision patient are as follows:

1. Dense scotoma to the right of the fixation point: difficulties reading along a line (**Figure 17**).

2. Left of inferior scotomas to the fixation point scotomas: difficulties in finding the next line (**Figures 18** and **19**).

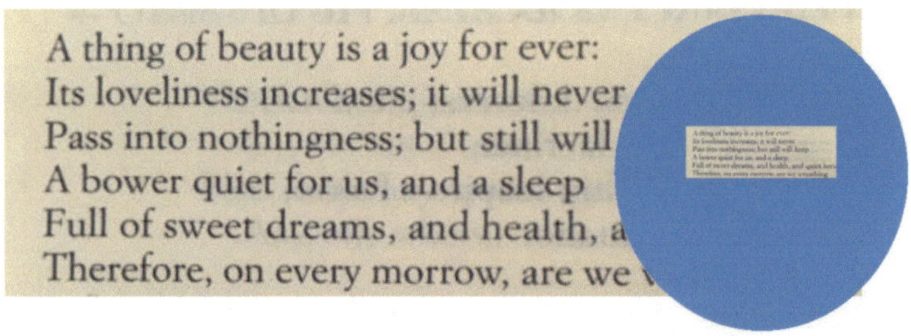

Figure 17.
Dense scotoma to the right of the fixation point: difficulties reading along a Line.

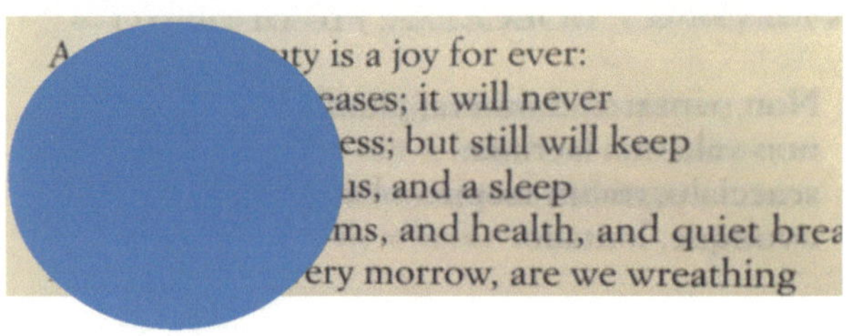

Figure 18.
Left scotomas to the fixation point scotomas: difficulties in finding the next line.

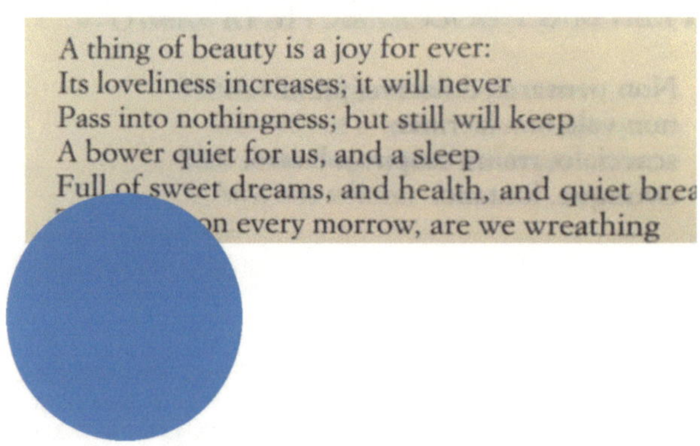

Figure 19.
Inferior scotomas to the fixation point scotomas: difficulties in finding 13 the next line.

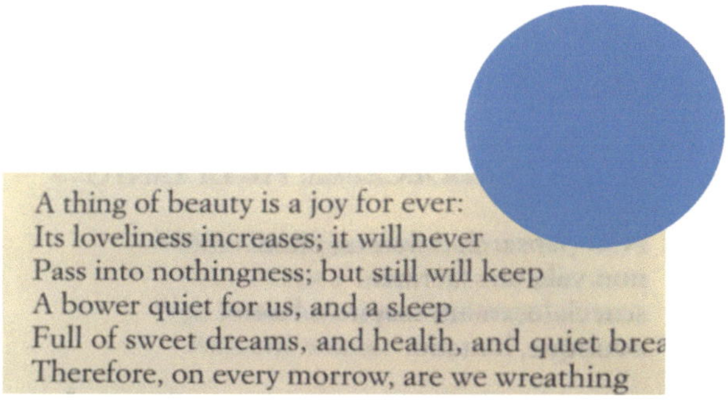

Figure 20.
Scotoma superior to the fixation point (PRL above the retinal lesion).

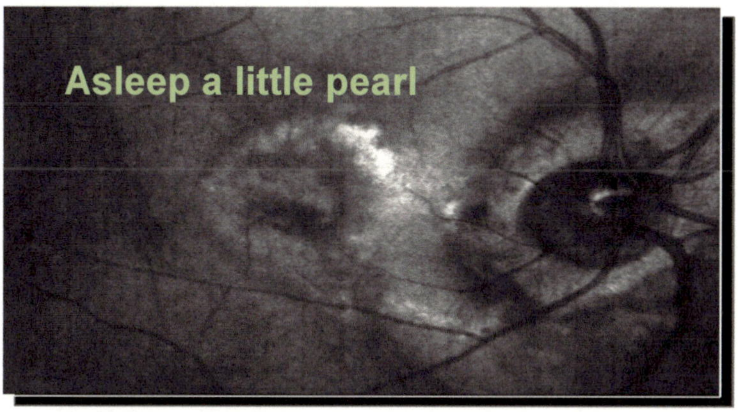

Figure 21.
PRL above the retinal lesion.

Scotoma superior to the fixation point (PRL above the retinal lesion) represents the best location for the reading process (**Figures 20** and **21**).

4. Optical aids

The purpose of low-vision rehabilitation is to recover the visual skills lost with visual impairment and first of all the possibility to read. After the first phase in which the patient is taught to fix in the PRL and the fixation is stabilized or moved to the best place for vision, we must begin the special training with optical devices [17].

4.1 Microscopic visual aids

Binocular hypercorrective prismatic lenses are used if the residual visual acuity is bilateral. The combination with the prism reduces the convergence effort for the short distance and can be associated with the correction of astigmatism. A filter lens of 450 nm can be used to increase the contrast and reduce the dazzling, and the power arrives to 16 diopters (**Figure 22**).

Monocular hypercorrective aplanatic lens is used if the residual visual acuity is monolateral. It is made of a polycarbonate ring holding two lenses facing each other

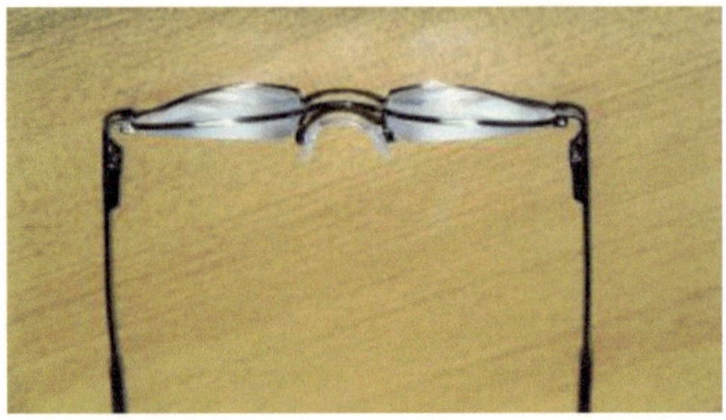

Figure 22.
Binocular hypercorrective prismatic lenses.

with the convex curve and the flat side external. In this way, the spherical aberrations are compensated.

The aplanatic monocular lens can have power from 2 up to 10×.

It combines an elevated magnifying power with an angle of 48°.

It is made of a polycarbonate ring holding two lenses facing each other with the convex curve and the flat side external.

In this way, the spherical aberrations are compensated (**Figures 23–25**).

When the patient needs to read and write or to use the PC keyboard and other electronic devices, he must use bifocal and trifocal AIDS (**Figure 26**).

An optic aid for intermediate distance is a pin-see (pince-nez) attachable to an eyeglass with a clip-on (**Figure 27**).

We can use also a telemicroscope. Adding a spherical positive lens in front of the Galilean telescope allows the patient to focus in intermediate and near distances, and this helps to work in near distance: reading, writing and other activities (**Figure 28**).

A simple aid may be also a magnifying glass neck-tight (**Figure 29**).

Electronic aids, electronic magnifying device [18–20].

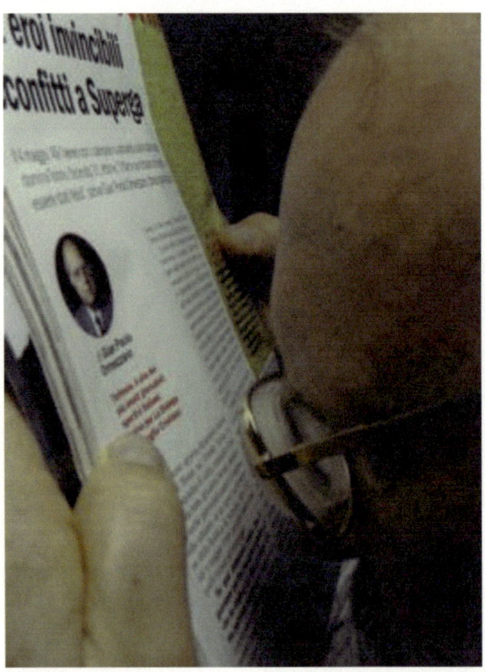

Figure 23.
Monocular hypercorrective aplanatic lens.

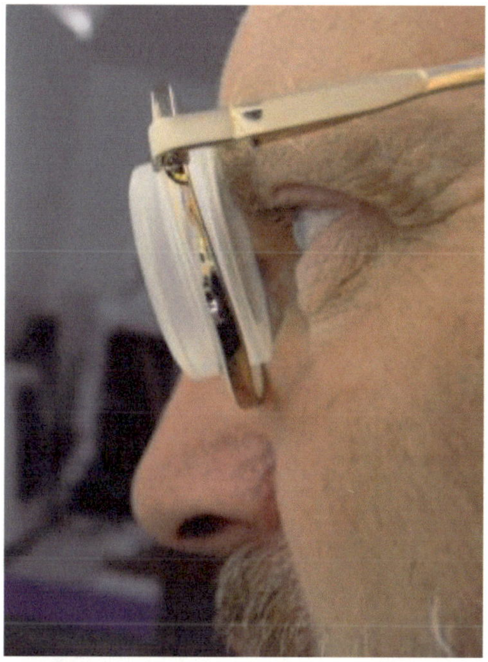

Figure 24.
Monocular hypercorrective aplanatic lens.

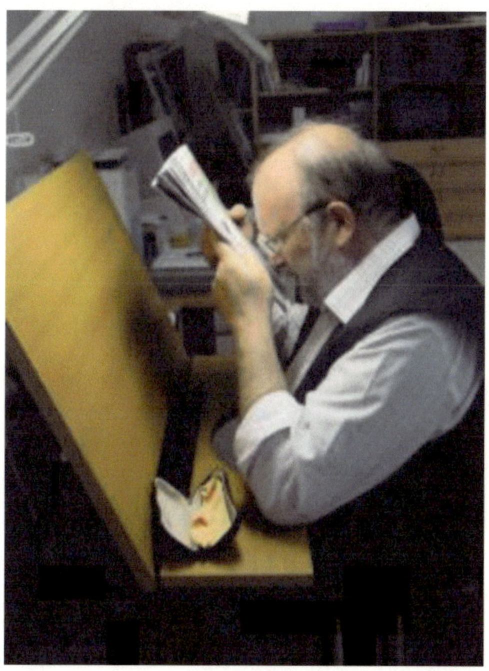

Figure 25.
Ergonomic table.

4.2 Close Circuit Tele Vision

Close Circuit Tele Vision (CCTV) is used when VA is less than 0.1 and when there is a dense absolute scotoma [21].

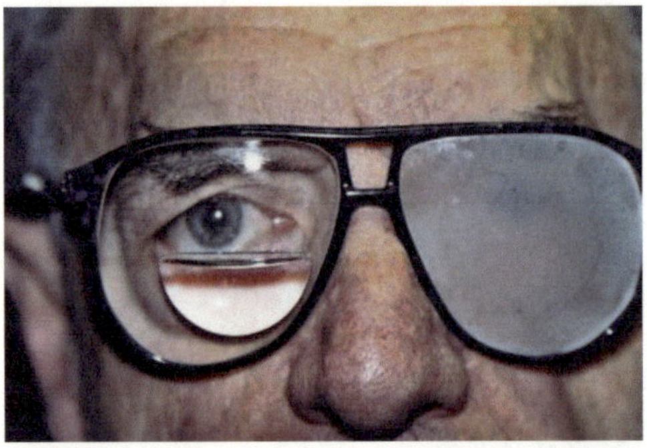

Figure 26.
Bifocal system (writing and reading).

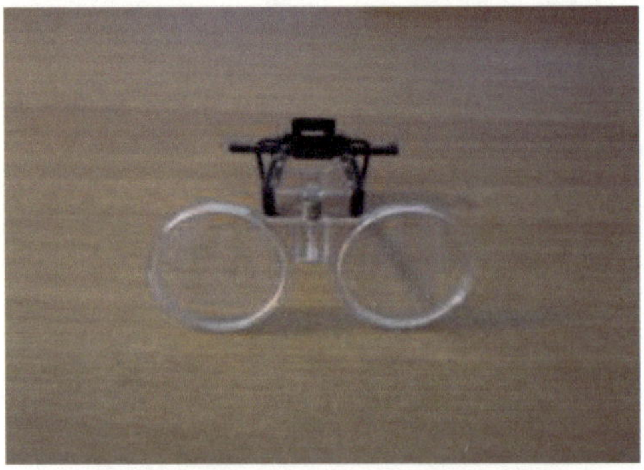

Figure 27.
Pin-see.

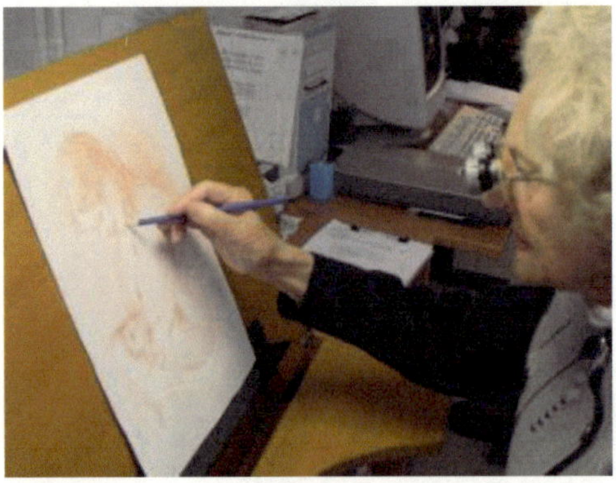

Figure 28.
Telemicroscope.

The use of CCTV restores reading ability and improves quality of life reducing depression in low-vision patients (**Figures 30–33**).

4.3 Aids for far vision: telescopes

4.3.1 Galilean telescope

It is made of a positive lens in the objective and with a negative lens in the eyepiece. It is an afocal optic system with visual field angle of 24° (**Figure 34**).

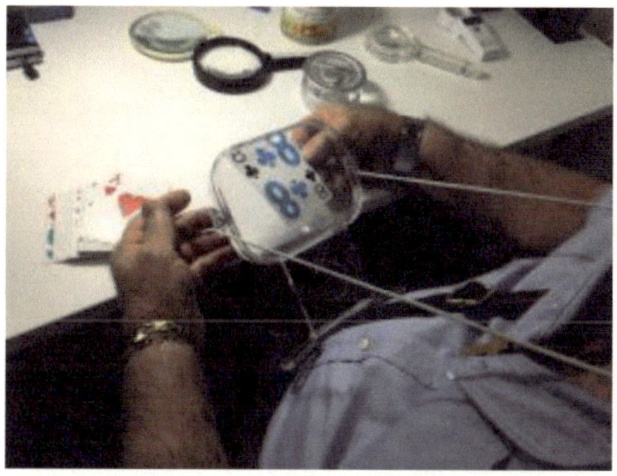

Figure 29.
Magnifying glass neck-tight.

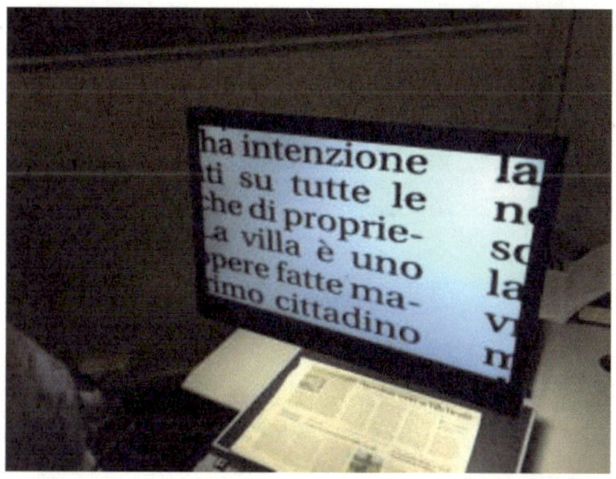

Figure 30.
CCTV.

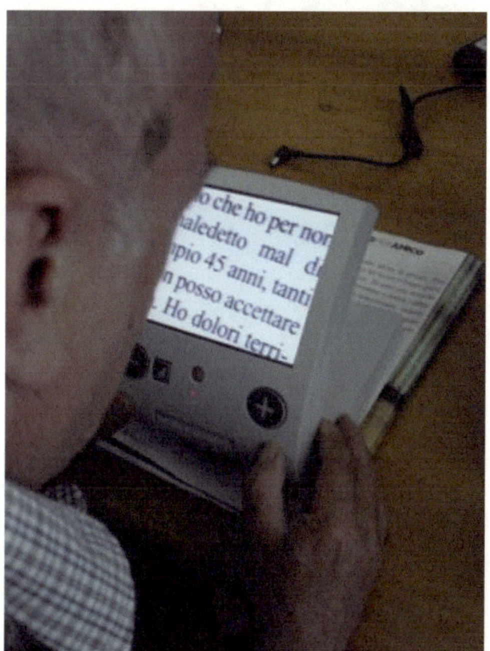
o che ho per nor
aledetto mal d
pio 45 anni, tanti
n posso accettare
. Ho dolori terri-

Figure 31.
Portable CCTV.

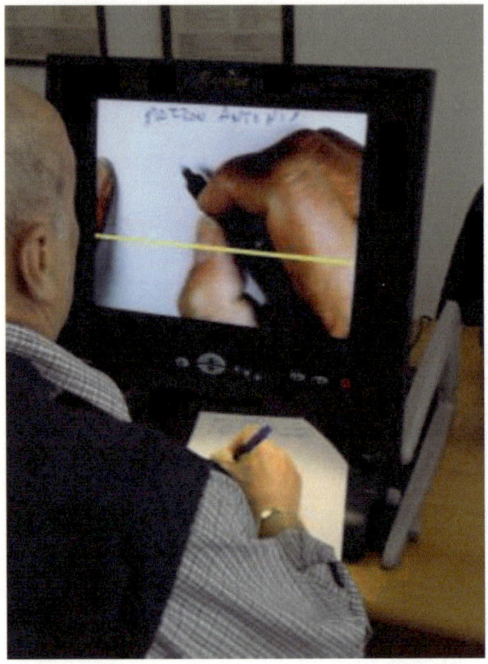

Figure 32.
Writing with CCTV.

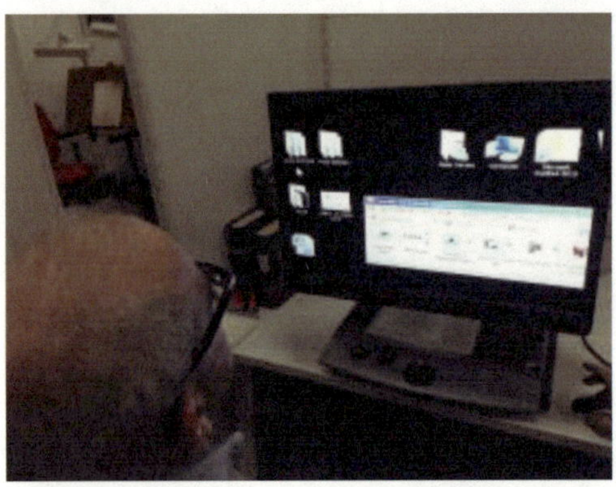

Figure 33.
Electronic magnifier with personal computer.

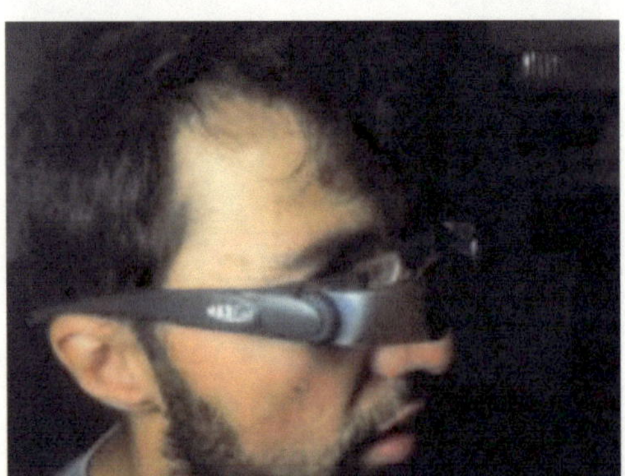

Figure 34.
Galilean telescope.

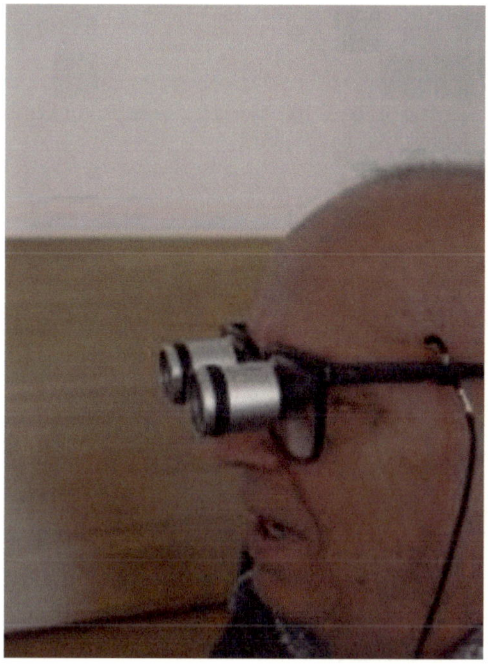

Figure 35.
Binocular Keplerian telescope.

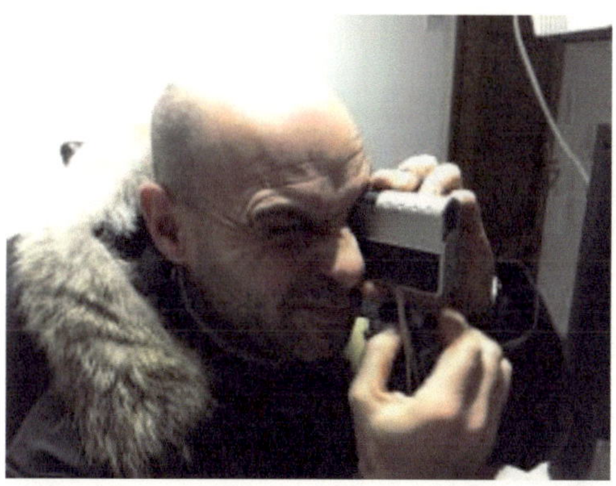

Figure 36.
Hand Keplerian telescope.

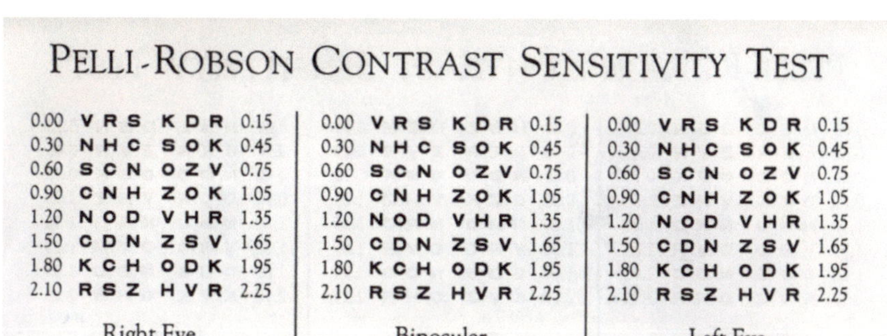

Figure 37.
Pelli-Robson contrast sensitivity test.

4.3.2 Keplerian telescope

It allows greater far magnification. It is composed of two positive lenses spaced from a distance equal to the sum of the two focal lengths (**Figures 35** and **36**).

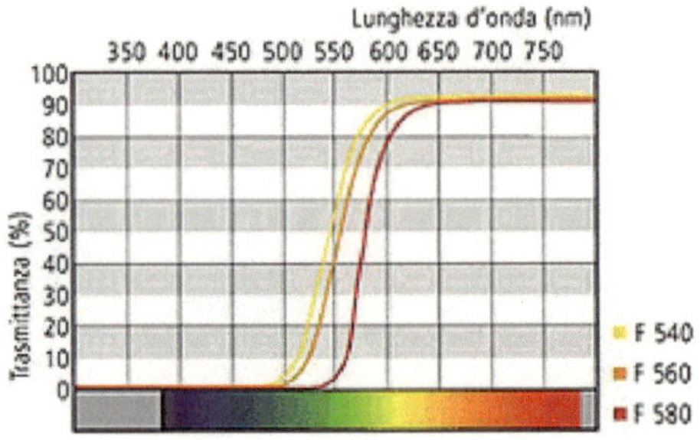

Figure 38.
Transmittance curves of 540–550-580 nm filter lens.

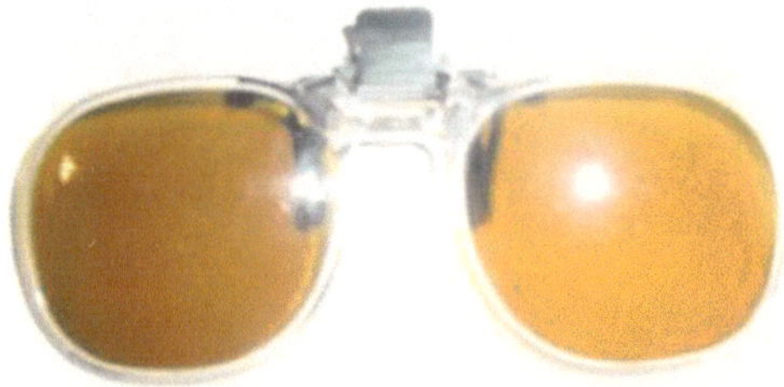

Figure 39.
511-nm filter lenses.

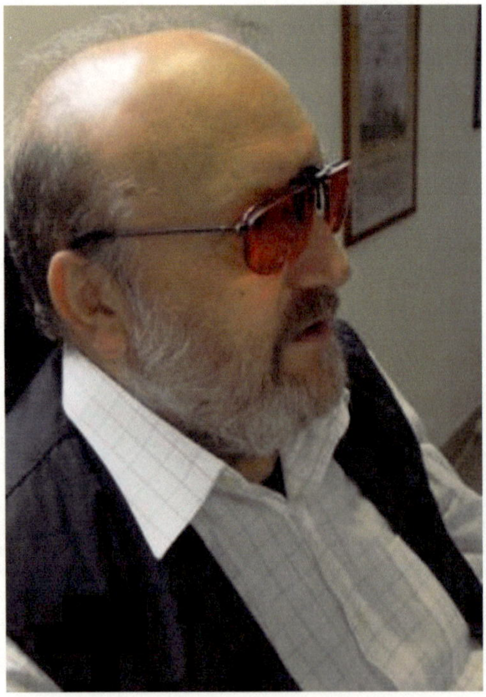

Figure 40.
550-nm filter lenses.

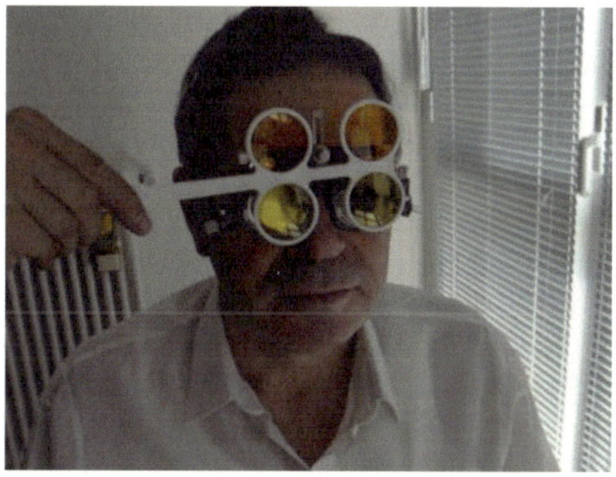

Figure 41.
Filter lenses test.

4.3.3 Filter lens

Low-vision patients in the most part of cases have dazzle, photophobia and a decrease in contrast sensitivity, so it is very important to evaluate the contrast sensitivity with Pelli-Robson test (**Figure 37**) and try out the filter lens starting from 400 nm with different grade of polarization [22–24].

Transmittance is a specific and fundamental feature of a filter lens and refers to the percentage of radiation that can pass through the lens related to the wavelength: a 100% of transmittance means that all the incident radiation on the lens passes through, while a 0% transmittance means that all the radiation is absorbed or reflected (**Figure 38**).

Filter lenses stop some wavelengths and some other get through.

A red-colored lens lets the red wavelength get through. Lenses have the color of the wavelength that passes through them.

For example, a 450-nm yellow lens blocks the wavelengths below 450 nm like the UV (phototoxic) and the Blu Light (diffusion and dazzling) (**Figures 39–41**).

5. Conclusions

Visual rehabilitation of low vision, with its various techniques, being able to recover visual disabilities, is likely to activate neuronal plasticity, which is the ability of neurons to undergo lasting changes in the efficiency of their synaptic transmission, a concept that is owed to Donald Hebb [25] who had the intuition that if two neurons are activated at the same time, the synapses between them are strengthened: "Neurons that fire together wire together."

In patients with central visual field scotoma, a large part of visual cortex is not adequately stimulated and the low-vision patients must use a new eccentric fixation area on intact peripheral retina: preferred retinal locus (PRL) that functions as a pseudofovea. Functional magnetic resonance imaging (fMRI) has been used to examine whether stimulating this pseudofovea leads to increased activation or altered activation patterns in visual cortex in comparison to stimulating a comparable peripheral area in the opposite hemifield (opposite PRL) [26]. The PRL and OppPRL were stimulated with flickering checkerboard stimuli and object pictures during fMRI measurement and the result shows that stimulation with pictures of everyday objects led to overall larger BOLD (blood oxygen level dependent) responses in V1 visual cortex compared to that evoked by stimulation with flickering checkerboards. BOLD responses to stimulation of the PRL with object pictures were significantly enhanced in comparison to stimulation of the OppPRL area, and a stable eccentric fixation with the PRL was associated with a higher BOLD signal in visual cortex.

The first step in low-vision rehabilitation in maculopathy is to find the preferential retinal locus (PRL) with microperimetry, stabilize the PRL and, if necessary, shift PRL to a better area useful in reading, using audiobiofeedback. Then, with neurovision training (NVT) and perceptual learning, we can increase the neuronal wire and further improve the visual quality, the contrast sensitivity and the VA.

After these neurovisual rehabilitations, we must consider visual aids for all the visual activity requests from the patient: reading, writing, watching TV, walking, the possibility of orientation and movement, manual work, daily activity like cooking and moving in the house.

The low-vision patient is a person and we must consider all his appearances: visual, physical, psychological and social life [27–30].

Author details

Giovanni Sato* and Roberta Rizzo
Low Vision Rehabilitation Center, Padova, Italy

*Address all correspondence to: giovanni.sato@aopd.veneto.it

References

[1] Timberlake GT, Mainster MA, Webb RH, Hughes GW, Trempe CL. Retinal localization of scotomata by scanning laser ophthalmoscopy. Investigative Ophthalmology & Visual Science. 1982; **22**(1):91-97

[2] Sunness JS, Applegate CA, Haselwood D, Rubin GS. Fixation patterns and reading rates in eyes with central scotomas from advanced atrophic age-related macular degeneration and Stargardt disease. Ophthalmology. 1996;**103**(9):1458-1466

[3] Cummings RW, Rubin GS. Reading speed and saccadic eye movements with an artificial paracentral scotoma. Investigative Ophthalmology and Visual Science. 1992;**33**(Suppl):1418

[4] Fletcher DC, Schuchard RA. Preferred retinal loci relationship to macular scotomas in a low-vision population. Ophthalmology. 1997; **104**(1997):632-638

[5] Trauzettel-Klosinski S. Rehabilitation for visual disorders. Journal of Neuro-Ophthalmology. 2010;**30**(1):73-84

[6] Nilsson UL, Frennesson C, Nilsson SE. Patients with AMD and a large absolute central scotoma can be trained successfully to use eccentric viewing, as demonstrated in a scanning laser ophthalmoscope. Vision Research. 2003 Jul;**43**(16):1777-1787

[7] Nilsson UL, Nilsson SEG. Rehabilitation of the visually handicapped with advanced macular degeneration. Documenta Ophthalmologica. 1986;**62**(1986):345-367

[8] Bäckman Ö, Inde K. Low Vision Training. Malmö, Sweden: Hermods; 1979

[9] Backman O, Inde K. In: Broggini M, editor. Riabilitazione visiva del paziente ipovedente a cura del dott. Fabiano Editore; 1979

[10] Cassels NK et al. The use of microperimetry in assessing visual function in age-related macular degeneration. Survey of Ophthalmology. 2018

[11] Molina-Martín A, Pérez-Cambrodí RJ, Piñero DP. Current clinical application of microperimetry: A review. Seminars in Ophthalmology. 2018;**33**(5):620-628

[12] Giacomelli G, Virgili G, Giansanti F, Sato G, Cappello E, Cruciani F, et al. Clinical and microperimetric predictors of reading speed in low vision patients: A structural equation modeling approach. Investigative Ophthalmology & Visual Science. 2013;**54**(6): 4403-4408. DOI: 10.1167/iovs.12-10734

[13] Maniglia M, Pavan A, Sato G, Contemori G, Montemurro S, Battaglini L, et al. Perceptual learning leads to long lasting visual improvement in patients with central vision loss. Restorative Neurology and Neuroscience. 2016; **34**(5):697-720

[14] Polat U, Ma-Naim T, Belkin M, Sagi D. Improving vision in adult amblyopia by perceptual learning. Proceedings of the National Academy of Sciences of the United States of America. 2004;**101**(17): 6692-6697

[15] Polat U, Sagi D. Spatial interactions in human vision: From near to far via experience-dependent cascades of connections. Proceedings of the National Academy of Sciences of the United States of America. 1994;**91**(4): 1206-1209

[16] Casco C, Guzzon D, Moise M, Vecchies A, Testa T, Pavan A. Specificity and generalization of perceptual learning in low myopia.

Restorative Neurology and Neuroscience. 2014;**32**(5):639-653

[17] Virgili G, Acosta R, Bentley SA, Giacomelli G, Allcock C, Evans J. Reading aids for adults with low vision. Cochrane Database of Systematic Reviews. 2018;**4**:CD003303

[18] Morrice E, Johnson AP, Marinier JA, Wittich W. Assessment of the Apple iPad as a low vision reading aid. Eye (London, England). 2017;**31**(6):865-871

[19] Burggraaff MC, van Nispen RM, Knol DL, Ringens PJ, van Rens GH. Randomized controlled trial on the effects of CCTV training on quality of life, depression, and adaptation to vision loss. Investigative Ophthalmology & Visual Science. 2012;**53**(7):3645-3652

[20] Harland S, Legge GE, Luebker A. Psychophysics of reading. XVII. Low-vision performance with four types of electronically magnified text. Optometry and Vision Science. 1998; **75**(3):183-190

[21] Beckmann PJ, Legge GE. Psychophysics of reading—XIV. The page navigation problem in using magnifiers. Vision Research. 1996; **36**(22):3723-3733

[22] Eperjesi F, Fowler CW, Evans BJ. Do tinted lenses or filters improve visual performance in low vision? A review of the literature. Ophthalmic and Physiological Optics. 2002;**22**(1):68-77. Review

[23] Chung ST, Legge GE. Comparing the shape of contrast sensitivity functions for normal and low vision. Investigative Ophthalmology & Visual Science. 2016;**57**(1):198-207

[24] Giacomelli G, Volpe R, Virgili G, Farini A, Arrighi R, Tarli-Barbieri C, et al. Contrast reduction and reading: Assessment and reliability with the reading explorer test. European Journal of Ophthalmology. 2010;**20**(2):389-396

[25] Hebb D. The Organization of Behavior. New York: Wiley & Sons; 1949

[26] Plank T, Frolo J, Brandl-Rühle S, Renner AB, Jägle H, Greenlee MW. fMRI with central vision loss: Effects of fixation locus and stimulus type. Optometry and Vision Science. 2017; **94**(3):297-310

[27] Legge GE, Chung STL. Low vision and plasticity: Implications for rehabilitation. Annual Review of Vision Science. 2016;**2**:321-343

[28] Sagi D. Perceptual learning in vision research. Vision Research. 2011;**51**(13): 1552-1566

[29] Sabel BA, Flammer J, Merabet LB. Residual vision activation and the brain-eye-vascular triad: Dysregulation, plasticity and restoration in low vision and blindness—A review. Restorative Neurology and Neuroscience. 2018; **36**(6):767-791

[30] Colenbrander A, Fletcher DC. Vision rehabilitation. Journal of Neuro-Ophthalmology. 2018;**38**(2):135-137

Chapter 20

Biometric Systems and Their Applications

Souhail Guennouni, Anass Mansouri and Ali Ahaitouf

Abstract

Nowadays, we are talking more and more about insecurity in various sectors as well as the computer techniques to be implemented to counter this trend: access control to computers, e-commerce, banking, etc. There are two traditional ways of identifying an individual. The first method is a knowledge-based method. It is based on the knowledge of an individual's information such as the PIN code to allow him/her to activate a mobile phone. The second method is based on the possession of token. It can be a piece of identification, a key, a badge, etc. These two methods of identification can be used in a complementary way to obtain increased security like in bank cards. However, they each have their weaknesses. In the first case, the password can be forgotten or guessed by a third party. In the second case, the badge (or ID or key) may be lost or stolen. Biometric features are an alternative solution to the two previous identification modes. The advantage of using the biometric features is that they are all universal, measurable, unique, and permanent. The interest of applications using biometrics can be summed up in two classes: to facilitate the way of life and to avoid fraud.

Keywords: biometry, object detection, recognition, security

1. Introduction

The increasing performance of computers over the last decade has stimulated the development of general-purpose computer vision algorithms. One of the major problems of computer vision is object recognition tasks, to which special attention is paid. This is due to the desire to create artificial intelligent systems. The first step toward any kind of intelligence is perception, followed by reasoning and action.

Human perception is based on visual perception. Since intelligent artificial systems are primarily inspired by human perception and reasoning, we can conclude that visual perception is an important source of information for many potential systems.

Recently, there was a raising interest on eye tracking technology. This is mainly due to the industrial growth of many domains such as augmented reality, smart cars, and web applications' testing for which a solid eye tracking technology is essential. Eye movement recognition, combined with other biometrics such as sound recognition, can enable a smooth interaction with virtual environments.

A good example of a smart system is the autonomous car. It perceives the surrounding world and the signs while adapting her behavior to changing situations. Such a car contains a lot of different sensors, which help to perceive the necessary information.

IntechOpen

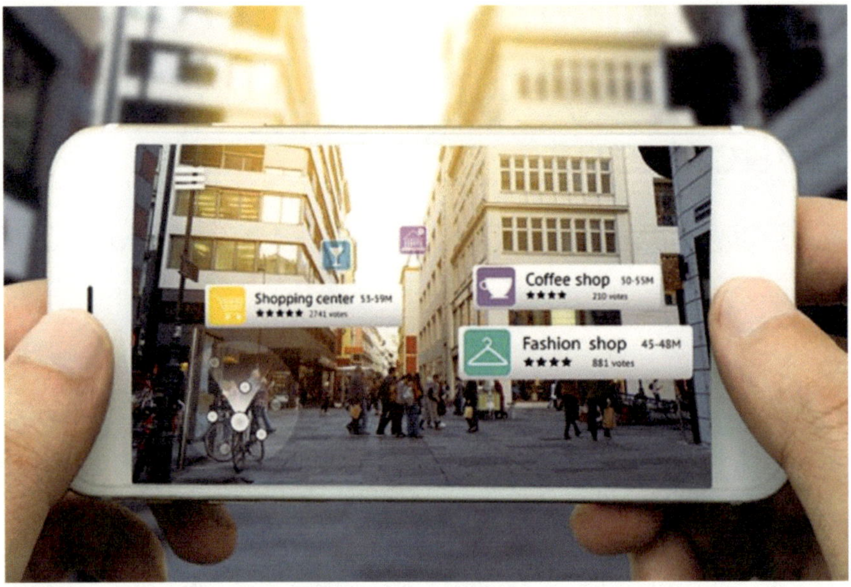

Figure 1.
Augmented reality.

The visual perception of the surrounding world is among the most important. It could be used to recognize pedestrians on the street, cars, animals, or even unspecified objects on the road, which could pose a potential threat to human life.

Improving and developing object recognition algorithms will help improve not only artificial intelligent systems but many other useful applications in today's world. Other examples of application of this system can be extended to the tourist industry where applications of augmented reality (**Figure 1**) are becoming more and more popular especially after the widespread use of smartphones. In addition, the field of video surveillance is also a possible extension of object detection algorithms because of the need for quick and timely detection of different video scenes captured by cameras.

Indeed, scene comprehension includes many separable tasks ranging from object recognition to the categorization of scenes and events. Object detection is a complex discipline that can be divided into three main directions:

- Image classification: The search for images in the majority of search engines is a typical case of image classification algorithms.

- Object detection: The location of the object on the request is one of the desired information in many of the systems mentioned.

- Segmentation of objects: Which pixels belong to which objects? It is more precisely compared to object detection for obvious reasons.

2. Issues and challenges

Object detection is a difficult task mainly because of possible changes in the appearance of the object due to different consequences. The design of the potential method must consider the possible difficulties:

- Intra-class variations: An object type can have a large number of variations (**Figure 2** illustrates different types of chairs). This can pose a problem by using specific features, which do not cover all possible object variations.
- Luminance conditions: Variations in luminance conditions change the appearance of the object, mainly in color and reflection.
- Point of view: The majority of objects in the images are in three dimensions. The images are only two dimensions, which means that we can only see a particular view of the given object. The same object may differ from other points of view, which we must also be aware of. Different views of the same object cause the invisibility of different features. Not all features are visible from a single point of view.
- Scale: The size of the object may differ, and there is a desire to be able to detect what the object gives to any size or scale.
- Location: It is much easier if you know where the desired object is. The situation differs if you have a prior knowledge of the location of the object and no information about it or if you know that the image contains only one object, located in the center of the image.
- Orientation: Humans do not have obvious problems recognizing the same object with a different orientation, but many algorithms do. Invariance to this possibility is often crucial.
- Occlusion and truncation: Occlusion from one object to another often causes a lot of inconvenience. Sometimes even humans do not see enough features of the object to recognize correctly. Truncation is the same problem when you do not see certain parts of the object, because they are out of the picture.
- Footprint: The background is almost nonexistent; an image contains only one chair. This situation is not typical in a real world. When you take the image of an object, there are almost always many other objects in the background, in which the recognition algorithm is usually not interested. The scene is often very complex, and it is difficult to recognize the object/objects desired among other objects.
- Out of context: Context is often used to increase the likelihood of certain categories of common occurrences. For example, cars and roads are often associated, but we cannot rely too much on context because sometimes it can be misleading.
- Multiple instances: The image often contains several objects of the same category. Some algorithms can identify regions of different categories in the image, but they cannot identify individual instances of the same object category.
- Pose: One of the biggest challenges is the invariant detection of the pose. Many objects change their appearance by changing their shape. For example, it is desirable to detect a person in any posture of their body [1].
- Instance level recognition vs. object class recognition. It is necessary to realize the difference between these problems. It is obvious that different methods are needed to recognize the human face in general and the person who uses the face.

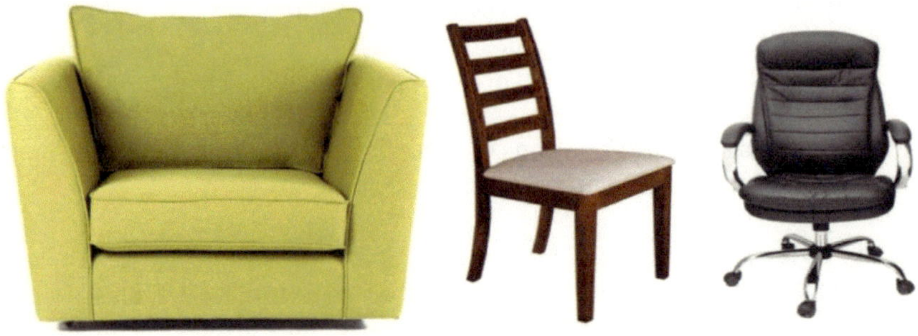

Figure 2.
Image search results.

After analyzing the potential problems associated with recognition tasks, we believe that the direction to follow in imitating the human visual perception system is natural. The first moment of human comprehension of the image is a very general activity that analyzes the basic categories (buildings, men, cars, etc.). After getting the big picture, his attention focuses on the things that interest him. While focusing, humans observe objects of interest to enrich more details and see and recognize more features. A feature is a general term for describing a particular part of the object in order to enrich its appearance. A human has special predispositions on several objects (e.g., faces) and on situations (mainly of the danger and movement type) on which he is more sensitive to recognize. The typical situation is when you see someone away from you and you can recognize that it is a person. As you get closer, by focusing on this person, you are enriching and recognizing more and more elements that make it possible to distinguish whether he is a known person and to detect his name. Humans can do instance-level recognition as in the case presented, but they must first distinguish the object category to optimize the subsequent search.

3. Biometric systems overview

3.1 History of biometrics

Biometrics has been a concern for centuries. Proving one's identity reliably was done using several techniques. From prehistory man knew the uniqueness of fingerprints, which meant that signatures by fingerprints were sufficient to prove the identity of an individual. Indeed, two centuries before Christ, the Emperor Ts-In-She authenticated certain sealed with the fingerprint.

At the beginning of the nineteenth century, in France, Alphonse Bertillon launched the first steps of the scientific police. He proposed the first method of biometrics that can be described as a scientific approach: bertillonage allowed the identification of criminals through several physiological measures.

At the beginning of the twentieth century, biometry was rediscovered by William James Herschel, an English officer who had the idea of having his subcontractors sign their fingerprints to find them easily in case of unhonored contracts. As a result, police departments have begun using fingerprints as a unique and reliable feature to identify an individual.

Biometrics is constantly growing especially in the field of secure identity documents such as the national identity card, passport, or driving license. This technology is running on new platforms, including chip cards based on the microprocessor.

3.2 Biometric market development

The biometric market has undergone a great development thanks to the great number of advancement and innovation that this field has experienced in recent decades. This development is increasing as a result of the security concerns of several countries, which has pushed investment in this area and the widespread use of biometric solutions in several social and legal fields.

As shown by the statistics in **Figure 3** between 2007 and 2015, there has been a considerable increase in the share of the private sector market due to the growing need for biometric solutions in this sector especially for smartphone and camera manufacturers.

According to ABI Research [2], the global biometric market will break the $30 billion mark by 2021, 118% higher than the 2015 market. In this context, consumer electronics, and smartphones in particular, are boosting the biometric sector: it is expected to sell two billion onboard fingerprint sensors in 2021, for an average annual increase of 40% in 5 years.

3.3 Biometric systems

A biometric system is a system that allows the recognition of a certain characteristic of an individual using mathematical algorithms and biometric data. There are several uses of biometric systems. There are systems that require enrollment upstream of users. Other identification systems do not require this phase.

- Enrollment mode is a learning phase that aims to collect biometric information about who to identify. Several data acquisition campaigns can be carried out to ensure a certain robustness of the recognition system to temporal variations of the data. During this phase, the biometric characteristics of individuals are captured by a biometric sensor, and then represented in digital form (signatures), and finally stored in the database. The processing related to the enrollment has no time constraint, since it is performed "off-line."

- The verification or authentication mode is a "one-to-one" comparison, in which the system validates the identity of a person by comparing the biometric data entered with the biometric template of that person stored in the system's database. In such a mode, the system must then answer the question related to the identity of the user. Currently the verification is carried out via a personal identification number, a user name, or a smart card.

- The identification mode is a "one-to-N" comparison, in which the system recognizes an individual by matching it with one of the models in the database. The person may not be in the database. This mode consists of associating an identity with a person.

Figure 4 presents the architecture of a biometric system, which consists of the following elements:

- The capture module that represents the entry point of the biometric system and consists in acquiring the biometric data in order to extract a digital representation. This representation is used later in the following phases.

- The module of signal processing makes it possible to optimize the processing time and the digital representation acquired in the enrollment phase in order to optimize the processing time of the verification phase and the identification.

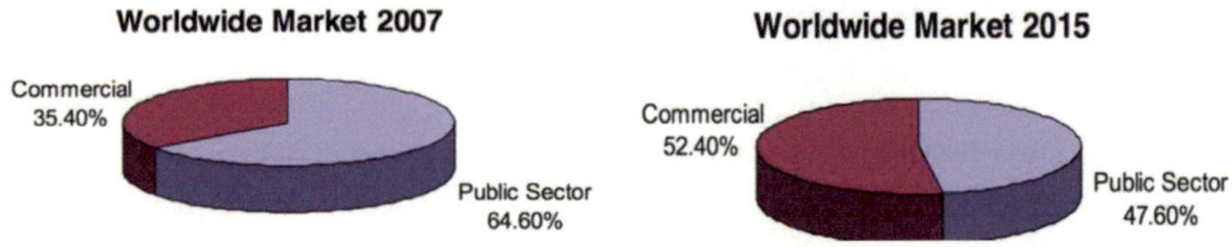

Figure 3.
Distribution of the global biometric market.

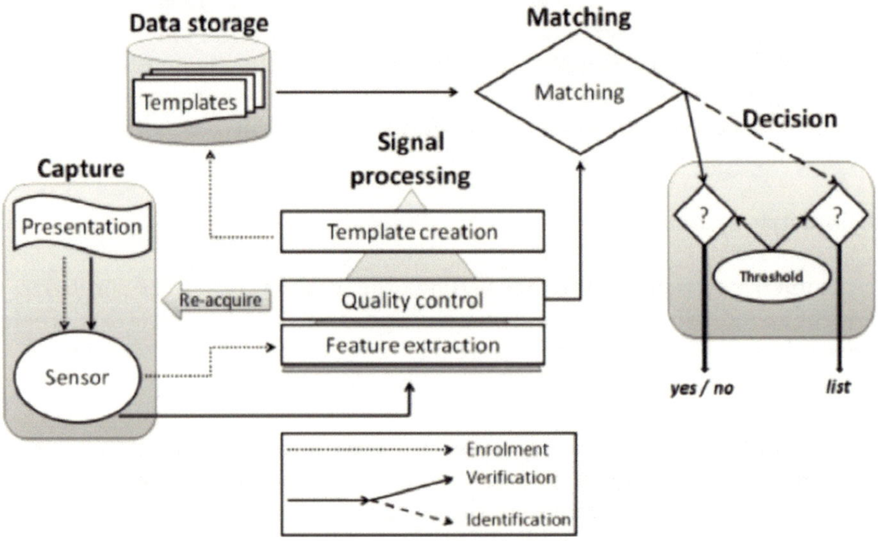

Figure 4.
Biometric system architecture.

- The storage module that contains the biometric templates of the system enrollees.
- The matching module that compares the data extracted by the extraction module with the data of the registered models and determines the degree of similarity between the two biometric data.
- The decision module that determines whether the similarity index returns through the matching module is sufficient to make a decision about the identity of an individual.

4. Performance of biometric systems

4.1 Performance evaluation

For the evaluation of the precision of a biometric system, which makes it possible to measure these performances, numerous attempts have been made on the system, and all the similarity scores are saved.

By applying the variable score threshold to similarity scores, the pairs of false recognition rate (FRR) and false acceptance rate (FAR) can be calculated. The false recognition rate, or FRR, is the measure of the likelihood that the biometric system will incorrectly reject an access attempt by an authorized user. It is stated as the ratio of the number of false recognitions divided by the number of identification attempts. On the other hand, the false acceptance rate, or FAR, is the measure of the likelihood that the biometric system will incorrectly accept an access attempt by an unauthorized user. It is stated as the ratio of the number of false acceptances divided by the number of identification attempts.

The results are presented either as such pairs, i.e., FRR at a certain level of FAR or as the graph in **Figure 5**. The rates can be expressed in several ways, for example, in percentages (1%), in fractions (1/100), in decimal format (0.01), or using powers of ten ($10p^2$). When comparing two systems, the most accurate shows a lower FRR equal to FAR level. Some systems do not report the similarity score, only the decision. In this case, it is only possible to win a single FRR/FAR pair (and not a continuous series) as a result of a performance evaluation. If the mode of operation (the security level) is adjustable (i.e., we have a means of controlling the scoring threshold used internally), the performance evaluation can be performed repeatedly in different modes to get other FRR/FAR pairs.

4.2 Evaluation mode

There are three modes of performance evaluations, which are technology, scenario, and operational evaluation. When evaluating biometric algorithms, technological evaluations are the most common and often the most feasible. Since this type of evaluation is done using saved samples, the results are reproducible, and the evaluation is not a tedious or complicated process.

- Technological evaluation: Evaluation using recorded data, e.g., previously acquired fingerprints

- Scenario evaluation: End-to-end evaluation of the system using a prototype or simulated environment

- Operational evaluation: Evaluation in which the performance of a complete biometric system is determined in an application environment with a specific population

The biggest disadvantage of technological evaluations is that they do not necessarily reflect the final conditions of use of the system. For this reason, it is important to collect a set of samples of the conditions of use of the target system when preparing an assessment.

4.3 Database

Registered samples used in technology assessments are collected in databases. Data collection is performed using a group of volunteers, at least some of whom provide multiple acquisitions of the same biometric modality (e.g., the same finger) to have relevant attempts. To make collection efficient, samples of several objects can be collected from each volunteer, for example, every ten fingers. The characteristics of the database have a great impact on the results of an evaluation. As previously stated, with the exception of the capabilities of the biometric algorithm, the amount of available information can be used to characterize the objects.

4.4 Degree of confidence

To be able to make an assertion about the FRR 1% @ FAR 1 / 1 000 000 (i.e., when the system operates in a mode where one out of one million impostor attempts

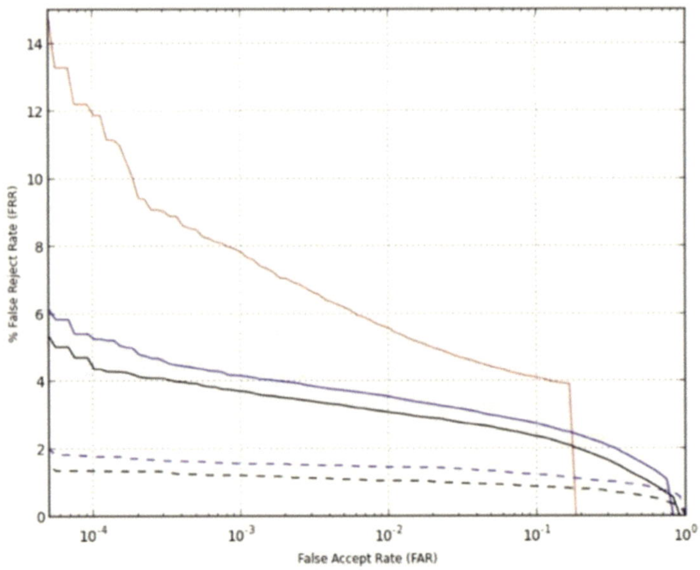

Figure 5.
DET graph sample.

is-falsely-considered a match, one percent of the genuine attempts would fail) it at least one million impostor attempts (user sticking perfectly to another person's template). It is not difficult to understand that the uncertainty of such an assertion would be rather high. The result depends heavily on how the two most similar samples in the database are scored. When comparing and viewing a DET (detection error trade-off) graph, it is important to understand that the uncertainty is higher on the side of the edges of the image. The number of comparisons made is only an important factor affecting confidence. The key to getting better statistical significance is to make as many uncorrelated attempts as possible.

5. Applications of biometric systems

Biometric systems can be used in a large number of applications. For security reasons, biometrics can help make transactions, and everyday life is both safer and more practical. The following domains use biometric solutions to meet their respective needs:

- Legal applications:
    - Justice and law enforcement: Biometric technology and law enforcement have a very long history, and many very important innovations in identity management have emerged from this beneficial relationship. Today, the biometrics applied by the police force is truly multimodal. Fingerprint, face, and voice recognitions play a unique role in improving public safety and keeping track of the people we are looking for.
- Government applications:
    - Border control and airport: A key area of application for biometric technology is at the border. Biometric technology helps to automate the process of border crossing. Reliable and automated passenger screening initiatives and automated SAS help to facilitate international passenger travel experience

while improving the efficiency of government agencies and keeping borders safer than ever before.

- Healthcare: In the field of healthcare, biometrics introduces an enhanced model. Medical records are among the most valuable personal documents; doctors need to be able to access them quickly, and they need to be accurate. A lack of security and good accounting can make the difference between timely and accurate diagnosis and health fraud.

• Commercial applications:

- Security: As connectivity continues to spread around the world, it is clear that old security methods are simply not strong enough to protect what is most important. Fortunately, biometric technology is more accessible than ever, ready to provide added security and convenience for everything that needs to be protected, from a car door to the phone's PIN.

- Finance: Among the most popular applications of biometric technology, financial identification, verification, and authentication in commerce help make banking, purchasing, and account management safer and more convenient and responsible. In the financial area, biometric solutions help to ensure that a customer is the person he/she claims to be when accessing sensitive financial data by entering his/her unique biometric characteristics and comparing them to a model stored in a device or on a secure server. Banking solutions and the payment technologies available today use a wide range of biometric modalities: fingerprints, iris, voice, face, fingerprint, palm veins, behavior, and other types of biometric recognition are all used alone or combined in a multifactorial manner as a system, to lock accounts and serve against fraud.

- Mobile: Mobile biometric solutions live at the intersection connectivity and identity. They integrate one or more biometric terms for authentication or identification purposes and take advantage of smartphones, tablets, other types of handhelds, wearable technology, and the Internet of things for versatile deployment capabilities. Thanks to the versatility brought by modern mobile technology, as well as the proliferation of mobile paradigms in the consumer, public, and private world, mobile biometrics is becoming more and more important.

- Eye movements tracking applications:

  1. Automotive industry: there is an established relationship between eye movement and attention. Thus, tracking the car driver's eye movements can be very helpful in measuring the degree of sleepiness, tiredness, or drowsiness. The sleepiness of the driver can be detected by analyzing either blink duration and amplitude or the level of gaze activity [3].

  2. Screen navigation: one of the most important applications for people with disabilities is screen navigation. Using cameras, the application can track a person's eye movements in order to scroll a web page, write text, or perform actions by clicking on buttons on a computer or mobile devices. Therefore, this kind of application is gaining more attention recently due the rapid development and the growing need of new means of screen navigation especially on mobile devices platforms.

3. Aviation: the flight simulators track the pilot eye and head movement in order to analyze the pilot's behavior under realistic circumstances. This simulator is capable of evaluating a pilot's performance based on his eye movements combined with other information. It can be also used as an important training tool for new pilots in order to help them to look at the primary flight display (PFD) more regularly in order to monitor different airplane indicators.

5.1 Detection and recognition of dynamic shapes

Detection of dynamic forms is a very important research area that is rapidly evolving in the field of image processing. The goal is to recognize the shapes of objects in an image or in a sequence of images from the information relating to their shapes. In fact, shape is one of the most differentiating features in an image. However, the description and representation of an image remain a major challenge to perform the recognition task.

The quality of a descriptor is represented by its intelligence and ability to distinguish the different forms in a reliable manner despite the geometric variations related to translation and rotation.

On the other hand, a reliable descriptor must withstand the various changes that affect the shape of an object such as noise and distortion that can actually alter the shape and make the recognition task more complicated.

5.2 Representation and description of planar shapes

The form representation and description techniques can be generally split into two main classes of methods: contour-based methods and region-based methods. This ranking depends on how the shape features are extracted: from only the outline or the entire region of the shape. For each category, the different approaches are divided into global approaches and local (structural) approaches. This subclassification is based on the representation of the form that depends on the whole form or parts of the form (primitives). These approaches can also be distinguished according to the spatial or transform processing space, in which the shape characteristics are calculated. Global methods are not always robust against occlusions and image noise. In addition, they require an entire and correct segmentation of objects in the images. In general, the segmentation process results in partitioning objects into regions or contour parts that do not necessarily correspond to whole objects.

The contour-based approaches only exploit the boundary of the object for the characterization of the form by ignoring its inner content. The most commonly used representation in contour-based recognition methods is the signature of the form [4]. For a given form, the signature is essentially a representation based on the parameters 1D of the contour of shape. This can be done using a scalar value of the radial distance, angle, curvature, or velocity function. Let us note here that the signature of an entire form (closed curve) is often a periodic function; this will not be the case of a part of form (open curve) for which the two ends are not contiguous. Outline-based descriptors include Fourier descriptors [5, 6], the wavelet descriptors [7, 8], the multi-scale curvature [9], the shape context [10], the contour moments [11], and the symbol chain [12, 13]. Since these descriptors are calculated using only the pixels of the contour, the computational complexity is low, and their characteristic vectors are generally compact.

In region-based approaches, all pixels of the object are considered for characterization of the shape. This type of methods aims to exploit not only the information of the shape boundary but also that of the inner region of the form. The majority of region-based methods use moment descriptors to describe shapes such as Zernike moments [14], Legendre moments [15], or invariant geometric moments [16]. Other methods include grid descriptors [17] or shape matrix [18]. Since the region-based descriptor makes use of all the pixels constituting the shape, it can effectively describe various forms in a single descriptor. However, the size of the region-based features is usually large. This descriptor leads to a computing time that remains considerable.

It remains to emphasize that the description of the forms based on the contour is considered more relevant than that based on the region because the shape of an object is essentially distinguished by the border. In most cases, the central part of the object does not contribute much to pattern recognition [13].

6. Conclusion

In this chapter, we presented different biometric techniques used in the industrial world as well as their performances.

We started with an overview of biometric systems as well as an overview of biometrics. Then we presented the different issues and challenges related to implementation of such systems.

After that, we presented a performance evaluation of different biometric systems given the issues and challenges previously stated. Then we presented an overview of some important biometric elements such as the databases and the degree of confidence. Furthermore, a detailed analysis of different domains of application of several biometric techniques was presented with a focus on eye movement tracking techniques.

Finally, the different approaches of recognition of dynamic and planar shapes were discussed in the last paragraph.

Conflict of interest

We have no conflicts of interest to disclose.

Author details

Souhail Guennouni[1]*, Anass Mansouri[2] and Ali Ahaitouf[1]

1 Renewable Energy and Smart Systems Laboratory, Faculty of Science and Technology, Sidi Mohammed Ben Abdellah University, Fez, Morocco

2 Renewable Energy and Smart Systems Laboratory, National School of Applied Sciences, Sidi Mohammed Ben Abdellah University, Fez, Morocco

*Address all correspondence to: mrsouhail@gmail.com

References

[1] Shotton J et al. Real-time human pose recognition in parts from single depth images. In: Computer Vision and Pattern Recognition (CVPR), 2011 IEEE Conference. IEEE; 2011. pp. 1297-1304

[2] David P. Fueling innovation beyond security—bio-metrics in payments. Available from: https://www.abiresearch.com/market-research/product/1031105-fueling-innovation-beyond-security-biometr [Accessed: 01 February 2018]

[3] Barbuceanu F, Antonya C. Eye Tracking Applications. In: Bulletin of the Transilvania University of Brasov. Engineering Sciences. Series I 2. 2009. p. 17

[4] Quinlan JR. C4.5: Programs for Machine Learning. Elsevier; 2014

[5] Boykov Y, Veksler O, Zabih R. Fast approximate energy minimization via graph cuts. IEEE Transactions on Pattern Analysis and Machine Intelligence. 2001;**23**(11):1222-1239

[6] Ballerini L et al. A query-by-example content-based image retrieval system of non-melanoma skin lesions. In: MICCAI International Workshop on Medical Content-Based Retrieval for Clinical Decision Support. Springer; 2009. pp. 31-38

[7] LeCun Y et al. Back propagation applied to handwritten zip code recognition. Neural Computation. 1989;**1**(4):541-551

[8] Platt J et al. Probabilistic outputs for support vector machines and comparisons to regularized likelihood methods. Advances in Large Margin Classifiers. 1999;**10**(3):61-74

[9] Hao F, Qiu G, He H. Feature combination beyond basic arithmetics. In: BMVC; Citeseer. 2011. pp. 1-11

[10] Sivic J, Zisserman A. Video Google: A Text Retrieval Approach to Object Matching in Videos. IEEE; 2003. p. 1470

[11] Tomasz A. Using contour information and segmentation for object registration, modeling and retrieval [PhD thesis]. Dublin City University; 2006

[12] Shotton J, Johnson M, Cipolla R. Semantic text on forests for image categorization and segmentation. In: Computer Vision and Pattern Recognition, 2008 (CVPR 2008). IEEE; 2008. pp. 1-8

[13] Leibe B, Leonardis A, Schiele B. Combined object categorization and segmentation with an implicit shape model. In: Workshop on Statistical Learning in Computer Vision, ECCV. Vol. 2.5. 2004. p. 7

[14] Bengio S, Weston J, Grangier D. Label em-bedding trees for large multi-class tasks. In: Advances in Neural Information Processing Systems. 2010. pp. 163-171

[15] Zhang P, Peng J, Domeniconi C. Kernel pooled local subspaces for classification. In: IEEE Transactions on Systems, Man, and Cybernetics, Part B (Cybernetics) 35.3. 2005. pp. 489-502

[16] Fergus R, Perona P, Zisserman A. A Sparse Object Category Model for Efficient Learning and Exhaustive Recognition. IEEE; 2005. pp. 380-387

[17] Theocharides T, Vijaykrishnan N, Irwin MJ. A parallel architecture for hardware face detection. In: ISVLSI. Vol. 6. Citeseer; 2006. p. 452

[18] Kullback S, Leibler RA. On information and sufficiency. The Annals of Mathematical Statistics. 1951;**22**(1):79-86

Chapter 21

Eye Movements during Barking at Print

Tanya Beelders and Angela Stott

Abstract

In order for educational software coupled with eye-tracking capability to respond with pedagogical appropriateness to a reader's eye movements, reading metrics must be validly interpreted. These metrics and the types of reading they diagnose, for example, scanning, skimming and reading for meaning, come largely from reading fiction texts in a home language. The use of existing classification systems for disadvantaged South African learners did not yield consistent and credible classification of these learners' reading. This could be attributed to learners barking at print, that is, decoding the text without comprehending what they were reading beyond the word level. Eye movements of barkers and non-barkers were analysed and no statistically significant differences were found. Barking at print was found to be distinct from mindless reading and mind-wandering, as well as other reading types for both first and second languages. Barking is characterised by slow reading with few regressions, average fixation durations typical of second language reading, and variability in eye-movements between lines of text. This work is significant in that it establishes that eye-movement during barking at print is distinct from other categories of reading. However, further research is needed before valid applications can be made from this work.

Keywords: reading, eye-tracking, eye movements, barking

1. Introduction

Eye-tracking has the potential to enhance learning, for example through incorporation in intelligent learning technologies which make use of artificial intelligence which acts on data gathered from a user to alter the user experience in a personalised manner to optimise learning [1]. Although incorporation of eye tracking technology into such systems is still in its infancy, such technology has already been shown to, for example: improve attention during engagement with intelligent tutoring systems for learning Biology [2], Geography [3] and Computer Programming [4]; Respond to mind-wandering during reading [5]; Detect engagement in metacognitive processing [6]; Predict affect [7]. Particularly if future uses of such technology are aimed at reading-improvement, the software creators must be able to interpret the correspondence between eye-movement metrics and the type of reading the user is undergoing, validly. A well-developed categorisation system does exist for this purpose for a variety of reading types, such as skimming, scanning and reading for meaning at various grade levels, for English home language readers reading fiction, which will be discussed in detail in a subsequent section. Data we collected from a group of poor South African learners reading a science text in English, which is not their home language, however, could not credibly be categorised using these existing systems, exposing a gap in the literature addressed in this article. This chapter will proceed by giving background on the problem under investigation as well as related studies. This will be followed by a brief discussion on the methodology and an in-depth discussion of the data analysis. The paper will conclude by summarising the significance and limitations of the study.

2. Problem statement

The poorest 80% of South African learners possess, on average, reading skills which rank among the worst in the world [8]. For example, 60% of South African grade 6 learners are unable to read with comprehension in any language [9]. Pretorius and Spaull [10] identify inability to decode text accurately as the primary problem, with barking at print being an additional problem among many of those relatively stronger learners who are at least able to undergo text-decoding. Barking at print refers to engaging in decoding with little to no comprehension of what the text means on a global level, although the meaning of individual words or even groups of words may be comprehended [11]. Such a reading style is consistent with the engagement in superficial textual strategies that strongly characterises poor South African learners' multiple-choice answering patterns [12], for example choosing options containing terms common to or with superficial similarity to the question or to terms in an associated comprehension passage. Barking at print is not unique to South African learners, with the term having been coined by Samuels [13] in the United States, and reports on barking at print even including presence among relatively high achieving learners in what could be considered good schools in affluent areas (see, e.g. [14]). However, given the high prevalence of barking at print among poor South African learners, whom we have easy access to due to our engagement in various intervention programmes for such learners, we are well situated to investigate this reading phenomenon.

Despite the firm establishment of barking at print in education literature, the nearest correspondence in eye-tracking literature is mindless reading, researched by observing participants reading nonsense-text, i.e. text having no meaning in any language [15], as well as reading during mind-wandering (e.g. [5]). Both mindless reading of nonsense text and reading during mind-wandering differ in a number of ways from non-mind-wandering barking at print written in a language which the reader does understand, at least to some extent. These differences include motivation, perceived purpose and prior exposure and expectations to perform each of these activities. Therefore, the findings of mindless reading and mind-wandering research may not correspond to barking at print, and if this is found to be the case, then obviously the usefulness of the existing literature, at least for mindless reading, to applications such as intelligent learning technologies, is limited and a new and more useful set of metrics associated with decoding without comprehension is needed. Further, the eye-tracking metric guidelines resulting from research related to mindless reading and mind-wandering are restricted to gaze length, so that even should barking at print prove to be similar to mindless reading or mind-wandering, there is a gap in the literature about other eye-movement metrics during such reading.

In this study the eye-movement characteristics of 67 grade 8 and 9 South African learners from financially and educationally impoverished backgrounds were examined during silent reading of science text in English, their second language. Based on their comprehension scores, these participants are divided into three groups: barkers (n = 23), poor readers (n = 25) and moderate readers (n = 19). Statistical analyses were then performed on the eye-movement characteristics of the barkers relative to that of the other groups of participants, as well as descriptive analyses of the differences between barking and existing literature about other types of reading. For this purpose the following research questions are applicable:

1. How do the reading eye-movements of those participants who were barking at print compare to those of their peers of two levels of reading proficiency?

2. What are the eye movement characteristics of those participants who were barking at print?

3. How do the eye-movement characteristics of barking at print compare to those published for skimming, scanning and reading for meaning at various levels of proficiency?

3. Background

3.1 Reading

If one is able to read, it means one can look at a word and process its meaning [16]. Rauding, derived from reading and auding, means the ability of a person to understand most of the thoughts contained within the material they are reading [16]. During rauding the eyes move across the lines of words allowing consecutive words to be perceived without needing to concentrate on where the eyes will move next. There are 5 basic reading processes, referred to as gears 1–5, where rauding or gear 3 is the process used most often. Readers can control the rate of input [17] thus the different gears are characterised by different reading speeds, averaging from 138 wpm to 600+ wpm for college students [16]. The goal of the reader determines the gear they use to process the material [16] which changes the reading behaviour [17]. A person's rauding rate is the fastest speed at which they able to successfully process relatively easily text [16]. The average rauding rate for grade 8 and 9 learners is 205 and 219 wpm respectively [16].

While fluency does not guarantee comprehension, it is essential to be able to comprehend [18]. The four levels of reading which are still applicable today were introduced in 1946 and are as follows: (1) the independent level, (2) the instructional level, (3) the frustration level and (4) the probable capacity level [19]. The fourth level is based on material which is read to a student but the first three are based on the decoding and comprehending ability of the student when reading a text [19], and are therefore focussed on in this article. The word-reading accuracy and comprehension of the first 3 levels are given in **Table 1**. Readers who are able to read at the independent and instructional levels are likely to be able to self-direct their learning through reading, although those at the instructional level would do so sub-optimally unless provided with explicit help. Readers operating at the frustration level are unlikely to engage in voluntary reading activity, given the large amount of effort required.

3.2 Eye movements during reading

The basic eye movements relevant to reading and visual search are fixations and saccades. Fixations are periods during which the eye is held relatively still in order to focus on an object [20]. Fixations typically last between 200 and 300 ms but the duration is dependent on the task [20]. For example, when reading in English, the

	Decoding accuracy (%)	Comprehension (%)
Independent level (level 1)	99	90
Instructional level (level 2)	95–99	75–89
Frustration level (level 3)	≤90	≤50

Table 1.
Reading classification according to Halladay [19].

mean fixation duration is 225–250 ms [21]. Fixation duration refers to the time, in milliseconds, that the eyes dwell on an object. Between fixations, saccades are used to move the eyes to an object of interest. Saccades are high velocity ballistic movements during which visual acuity is suppressed [20]. Saccadic amplitude is a measurement of the length of the saccades and can be measured in terms of visual angle, and refers to the eye span which can be deduced from the jumps (saccades) made by the eyes across the text. When reading text, the saccade length is generally measured in terms of character spaces ([22] as cited in [21]). Average saccade length when reading English is 7–9 characters [20] or 8–9 characters as reported in a later study [21].

Regressions refer to eye movements in the opposite direction of the reading movement. A regression can be a correction when a saccade overshoots the desired text or it can be used to re-read text. Good readers are skilled at using regressions to reposition their eyes where they would like to in order to reinforce something or to gain clarity if they lack understanding, but poor readers are inclined to struggle to use regressions accurately and efficiently and will trace indiscriminately backwards through the text [23]. While the difficulty of the text does influence the number of regressions, it is typical for L1 readers to perform regressions for 10–15% of the time while reading fiction [21].

3.3 Reading behaviour

Reading can be measured in fixation progress by determining how many characters the reader advances with each saccade [24, 25]. On average, the fixation will fall just left of the word centre [26, 27]—this is referred to as the preferred viewing location [26]. Some studies have found that readers do not fixate on every word while others have found that readers do indeed fixate on almost every word, with readers tending to skip short words [17]. When speed reading or skimming more words are skipped as a natural process [17]. When reading linearly, readers may skip to the next piece of text if they find that the current piece they are reading is no longer giving enough information [28].

Literature suggests that eye movements are useful in detecting reading difficulty and analysing reading behaviour. As readers progress from beginner to skilled (adult) levels, their reading speed [29] and mean saccadic amplitude [30] increase while the number of fixations their eyes make per 100 words, their mean fixation duration and the frequency of their regressions [20] decrease. Reading difficulty is characterised by longer fixation durations, more regressions and shorter saccades [31]. The length of the regression can also highlight whether the reader is experiencing difficulty or not, namely short regressions within a word show lack of understanding of that particular word. Longer regressions show a lack of understanding of the text. Regression percentage is the number of regressions divided by the number of fixations made, expressed as a percentage. It also appears that the number of words per fixation differs according to the difficulty of the text presented. When reading a passage with a difficulty appropriate to the age of the reader, there is an average of 1.2 words per fixation. If the text is easier than the age level of the reader, then the number of words per fixation has a higher average [17].

During reading studies, measurements such as first fixation duration, single fixation duration, and gaze duration are often used instead of average fixation duration since readers do not generally only fixate on a word once and words are often skipped during the course of reading the text [21]. It is possible that skipped words may be perceived in the prior fixation and words that are fixated on more than once are likely done so in order to process their meaning [21]. Perceptual span can also be considered a key feature to take into account since this indicates how much the reader can "see" when pausing over a word [21]. English first language (L1) readers appear to be able to perceive a range starting 3–4 characters to the left of the fixation and ending 14–15 characters to the right of the fixation [21]. Vocabulary size has a significant effect on the total time spent on words but not on the initial processing of the word [32].

The amount of time spent on a word is affected by the ease or difficulty with which the word is processed and other variables [21]. Fixation durations are strongly influenced by the frequency of the word (high frequency words have shorter durations), the predictability of the word being read, the number of meanings the word has, when the meaning of the word was acquired, semantic relations between the word and preceding words and how familiar the word is to the reader (multiple sources as cited in [21]). The length of a word correlates with the likelihood that the reader will fixate on the word again and the likelihood that the reader will skip the word [33]. Words with high frequency are more likely to be skipped than words with low frequency [34] and low frequency words receive more initial processing time than high frequency words [35]. Predictable words are also more likely to be skipped than unpredictable words [36, 37] and they also have a shorter fixation duration [37]. More attention and cognitive effort are required for unfamiliar words than familiar words [32] and while familiar words in L1 and L2 (second language) require similar processing times, unfamiliar words in L1 increase the cognitive load [32]. Unfamiliar words are read slower than familiar words in terms of fixation durations and they are read "more times"—in other words regressions to unfamiliar words are more common than to familiar words [35]. Similarly, when reading in L2, unfamiliar words have a higher fixation duration than familiar words and are visited more than familiar words [38]. However, in this instance the initial processing time between familiar and unfamiliar words is not significantly different [38].

Eye movement measurements can also be evaluated on the first and second pass—the first pass being the first time the word is read and the second pass being the subsequent time the word/piece is read if the reader regresses to that word/piece [39]. First fixation duration, single fixation duration and the likelihood that the word will be refixated are indicators of the difficulty of the word experienced during the initial reading while gaze duration is an indicator of the difficulty experienced in identifying the word [40]. Second pass duration indicates late measures of word difficulty and total fixation time can be used to measure comprehension difficulty [40].

3.4 Behaviour in different types of reading

The measurements discussed in the previous section were presumably measured for readers reading in English, which in all likelihood was their first language. Reading in a second or third language may be characterised by different behaviour and there are different types of reading which can be conducted.

For instance, since reading behaviour is coupled with cognitive processing, it stands to reason that eye movements can indicate when attention is low. Fixation durations are indicative of the amount of processing which is occurring, with longer fixations on words that require more processing [17]. Words which require more processing are infrequent words, while longer fixations are seen when making inferences at the end of a sentence and when integrating information from important clauses [17]. As a means to detect mindless wandering, or low attention while reading, eye movement behaviour at the end of phrases or sentences can be used—the natural slowing down in reading which occurs in order to integrate the words does not occur when attention is low [41]. Additionally, the variability in fixation durations caused by word length and frequency is lower when the reader is not paying attention [41]. Hence, when the mind of the reader wanders, there are short fixations on low frequency words and long fixations on high frequency words [41]. Fixations are also fewer and longer and eye behaviour is more erratic when the mind wanders [42]. First fixation durations, total gaze duration and total viewing time are shorter for normal reading than for wandering [42]. Additionally, when the mind wanders, readers are less likely to make fixations and regressions on text and more likely to fixate on areas other than the text [42]. The number of saccades and fixations drops when the mind wanders and there are less and shorter within-word regressions [43].

When scanning transformed text as opposed to reading, fixations are longer and saccades are shorter [15]. In this instance, transformed text refers to the practice of replacing all alphabetic characters with the letter z but preserving casing and punctuation among other characteristics [15]. Participants were requested to pretend to read the transformed text [15] in order to simulate scanning. In contrast, skimming normal text for proofreading is characterised by shorter fixations, and longer saccades than when reading text for understanding [21]. Readers also tend to read the start of the text more thoroughly than the second half and readers first skim the entire text before reading it [28]. When reading in a second language (L2), reading times are longer and readers exhibit more fixations, shorter saccades and less word skipping than when they read in their first language (L1) [44]. Furthermore, L2 readers of Afrikaans text required an average of one fixation per syllable [45]. Fixation durations for L2 readers were longer, averaging 313 and 331 ms for an easy and difficult text respectively [45]. The increased fixation times in L2 could be attributed to the fact that L2 processing requires more cognitive load than L1 [32]. One of the purposes of this research is to understand whether the reading ability of South African township learners can meaningfully be classified using the guidelines developed in publications such as those referred to above.

In a comprehensive study eye movement behaviour was investigated for the different types of reading. This study will be discussed in greater depth for the purposes of this chapter. Regular reading, or reading for comprehension, is defined as reading a piece of text as one would normally read [46] as cited [47]. Thorough reading is reading to learn and is used to read text in a manner which will allow them to learn the content, perhaps in order to write a test about the content [48] as cited in [47]. Skimming, also known as reading for gist, means the reader must read the text as quickly as possible while still trying to understand the content [46] as cited in [47] and spell checking is the type of reading which is conducted in order to detect spelling errors in a text [49].

Thorough reading exhibits longer reading times and more rereading which results in higher comprehension scores [47]. When skimming, participants exhibit longer saccades, short fixations and skip more words [47]. Additionally, the total reading time is shorter and comprehension is lower [47]. When reading in order to achieve spell checking, saccades are short, fixation durations are long and fewer words are skipped [47]. Comprehension scores are lower and total reading times are longer [47]. Overall thorough reading was less uniform than regular reading, skimming was faster and more uniform and spell checking was slower and more uniform [47].

3.5 Summary of reading behaviour indicators

In summary, reading difficulty is characterised by long fixations, higher incidence of regressions and shorter saccades. Similarly, scanning transformed text results in longer fixations and shorter saccades but skimming results in shorter fixations and longer saccades. When reading in a second language, readers exhibit more fixations, shorter saccades and less word skipping and unfamiliar words cause higher fixation durations and are visited more. Unfamiliar words in L1 require more cognitive processing and hence they are read slower and cause more regressions.

Thorough reading has more visits on words and more vertical saccades and has a pattern similar to regular reading. When skimming, fixation durations are much shorter, while saccades are much larger and there are fewer regressions. In contrast, spell checking shows an increase in fixation duration and smaller saccades and an increase in first pass metrics.

4. Methodology

4.1 Sample and data collection

The 67 grade 8 and 9 learners who form the sample for this study attended two schools in densely populated areas of extreme poverty and high unemployment, 50 km from the nearest town, Bloemfontein, in South Africa. The sample was relatively academically strong for the context, since 50 of the learners had been identified, by their teachers, as being among the strongest in mathematics and natural sciences in their class, with the others being randomly chosen to increase the ability range. Each participant read a comprehension text about lighting, with a Flesch-Kincaid reading difficulty level [50] of grade 9, and answered four multiple choice questions about this text, individually, on a computer fitted with a Tobii TX300 eye-tracker. Tobii Studio 3.4.5, installed on the computer, was used for data extraction, including the generation of a screen-capture video showing eye-movements and mouse clicks, for each learner. The data collected for this article were obtained as the learners engaged with two screens. Screen 1 consisted of 5 lines of text about lighting, with an illustrative diagram below the text. Screen 2 was divided into two with the left-hand half being a repeat of the first screen and the right-hand half displaying the multiple choice questions one at a time. The learner progressed through the four questions once he/she had answered a question correctly.

Consistent with Pretorius and Spaull's [10] statistics about poor South African learners' reading abilities, 2 of the original 69 learners in this relatively strong sample did not even show evidence of being able to decode the text they were given to read since they moved their eyes randomly around the screen for a while before claiming they had finished reading. These 2 learners were therefore excluded from this study. The remaining 67 learners' eyes did track the text systematically, at least for parts of the text, suggesting, to the extent to which this is possible from eye tracking data, that they were engaging in text decoding, and so were admitted into the sample for this study.

These learners were divided into the categories shown in **Table 2**, which is based on the learners' reading behaviour and comprehension scores, informed both by a qualitative analysis of the learners' eye movements during the question answering process and by the scores the software displayed in response to their choices. Guessing was inferred if the learner did not read sufficient text in the question or

Category		n		Criteria	
Barkers	Jumping	10	23	Learner either guessed or used superficial text-matching for all 4 questions on screen 2	Eyes tracked some text and jumped over other text on screen 1
	Regular	13			Eyes faithfully tracked the entire text on screen 1
Poor readers		25		Comprehension score was below 75%. Learner may have guessed or used superficial text-matching for some, but not for all, of the 4 questions on screen 2	
Moderate readers		19		Comprehension score was 75% or higher for screen 2	

Table 2.
Division of the sample into reading categories.

chosen distractor to be able to answer the question with comprehension. Use of superficial text matching was inferred if the learner chose the distractor designed to have superficial ties to the question and comprehension text. For example, for the question "Why do you know that conditions are right for lightning if you feel your hair standing up in a storm?", the distractor "This means that you have a tingling feeling." has superficial correspondence to the text: "If you ever feel your hair standing up or get a tingling feeling during a storm it could mean charges are moving onto you and you may be in danger of being hit by lightning!". The comprehension score was derived as the average of the four scores obtained for the four-question multiple choice test, where each of these four scores was obtained as follows: If the learner engaged in guessing, inferred as described above, he/she was assigned 0% for that question. Otherwise, the learner was assigned 100% if he/she answered the question correctly on his/her first attempt, with 25% being subtracted for each successive incorrect attempt at the answer.

This classification system groups those who could be described as reading at the instructional or independent levels, according to Halladay's [19] comprehension criterion, together in the group 'Moderate readers'. The 23 barkers did not answer any of the 4 multiple choice questions correctly on the first attempt, except for a few cases of lucky guessing, i.e. happening to choose the correct option despite not having read the text of the option chosen or, frequently, even the question itself. From this we can deduce their comprehension of the text was minimal, well below the 50% minimum for inclusion in Halladay's [19] frustration level. The poor readers showed at least some evidence of trying to answer the questions from comprehension, rather than guessing or superficial text-matching, but were clearly poor comprehenders. They fall into the upper end of Halladay's [19] frustration level as well as in the unnamed category between the frustration and instructional levels. It should be noted that it is impossible, from the data at our disposal, to apply the decoding accuracy section of Halladay's [19] classification system. We assume that evidence of the eyes systematically tracking the text is indicative of engagement in a high degree of decoding accuracy. Particularly for the jumping barkers, whose eyes only tracked some of the text systematically, this assumption may not be valid.

4.2 Metrics

The following metrics were extracted from the eye-tracking data gathered as the learners read the 5-line text about lighting on screen 1:

- Reading speed: similar to the method in [47] reading speed was calculated as milliseconds per character calculated using the total time the participant read the passage.

- Fixation duration: this indicates the length of fixations during the reading and is measured in milliseconds. The fixation duration was calculated as the mean fixation duration for each participant. For this measure, both those who were jumping and using regular barking were included.

- Fixation count: the total number of fixations captured during the reading process. Additionally the number of fixations per word was also calculated. This gives an indication of the distribution of the fixations over the piece and, on average, how many fixations were required per word in the piece. For this measure, those who were jumping were removed as they would naturally have less fixations as a result of their behaviour. Consequently, they would have much fewer fixations and this would not be due to them experienced no difficulty in reading, but rather in skipping large areas of the text without attempting to read it.

- Saccadic amplitude: as previously mentioned, the saccadic amplitude measures the distance between successive fixations. The mean saccadic amplitude per participant was calculated over the whole reading piece. Saccades which were longer than 8 degrees were considered to be a line sweep and were discarded. However regressive saccades were not discarded from this measurement. In this instance, participants who were jumping were also removed from the analysis, as they have very large saccades in order to facilitate their skipping behaviour. Even though the saccades were shorter than the length estimated for a line sweep, they would be fairly large and may unnecessarily skew the data.

- Number of regressions: the total number of regressions was counted manually for each participant and defined as any fixation that has an upward and left movement in order to fixate on a piece of text that was previously read.

- First fixation duration: the mean first fixation duration was calculated for each participant and each word as an indication of the length that was required per word on the first pass read.

- Visit count: the mean number of visits to each word was calculated for each participant as an indication of how many times, on average, each word is looked at. A visit is defined as distinct viewings of the word, in other words, separate fixations on each word within a single reading of the word constitutes a single visit. In order for another visit to be registered, the participant must read another word and return to a previously read word. As with fixations, the jumping barkers were removed for this analysis.

4.3 Data analysis

As briefly mentioned above, for the analysis of all duration metrics, reading speed and regressions, the regular barkers and the jumping barkers were classed as a single category collectively referred to as "Barkers". Since the jumping barkers exhibited large saccades and few fixations as a result of their inherent reading behaviour which differs from regular barking they were excluded from the remaining metric analyses and only the barkers and non-barkers were analysed. Thus for fixation and visit count and saccadic amplitude, the jumping barkers were excluded. The non-barkers were then further subdivided based on their comprehension scores as per the reading levels of Halladay [19] as frustration readers—comprehension scores lower than 75%—and instructional and independent readers were grouped together as moderate readers. To answer the first research question, regarding the comparison of the barkers' eye movements during reading with that of their peers, Kruskal-Wallis statistical tests were performed between the three groups for each reading metric. A Friedman ANOVA was also applied to the per-line reading metrics of each group to determine whether reading behaviour varied significantly between the lines. For both these analyses, $p < 0.05$ is taken as showing statistical significance. Descriptive analyses were performed to answer the remaining research questions, with gaze plots and comparisons between average measurements and those found in the literature drawn on to guide such descriptions.

5. Results

5.1 Qualitative discussion

The images below are gaze plots and serve to qualitatively illustrate the different reading behaviours which were evident in the sample.

Figure 1 is a gaze plot of the strongest reader in the group. From this it can clearly be seen that the reader fixated on most words. Durations, as reflected by the size of the fixation points, fluctuate within acceptable ranges. Some fixations are slightly offset but it can clearly be seen that reading is occurring at a steady pace with regular reading behaviour.

Figure 2 is an example of one of the jumping barkers who is clearly not reading but rather exhibiting clusters of fixations interspersed with large saccades—or

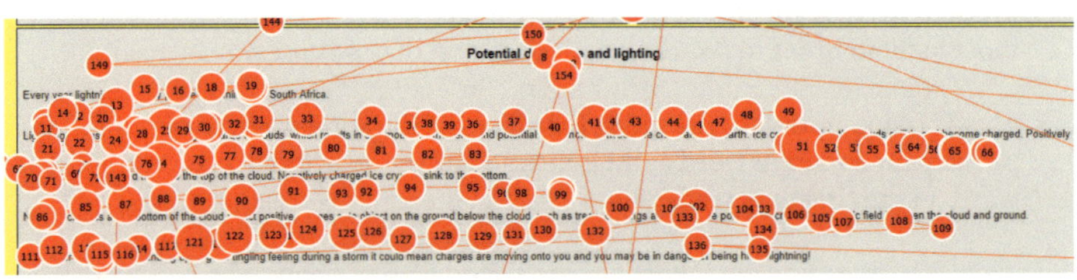

Figure 1.
The gaze plot of the strongest of the learners in the 'moderate reader' category.

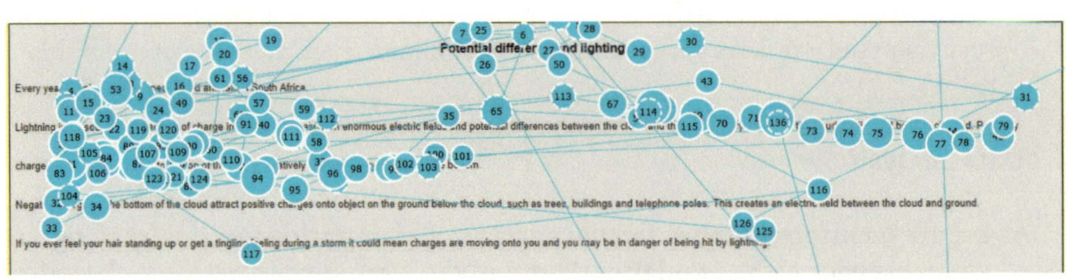

Figure 2.
The gaze plot of one of the 'jumping barkers'.

jumps. Fixations are more erratic and spread wildly over the body of the text and no regular pattern is discernible except in short spurts hence they are not habitual barkers but instead tend to skip large parts of the text. Durations also remain fairly constant for this jumper.

Figure 3 is one of the regular barkers, but here it can be seen that the fixations closely relate to regular reading. There is a regular pattern, fixations are spread over the whole text and on each word the durations fluctuate. This type of pattern is representative of the majority of the barkers and it can be deduced that the behaviour very closely mimics proper reading.

5.2 Reading metrics for whole text

This section discusses the metrics which were analysed for the whole text while the participants read screen 1, thus no distinction was made on the word level and the entire text piece was treated as a single AOI. **Table 3** shows these metrics,

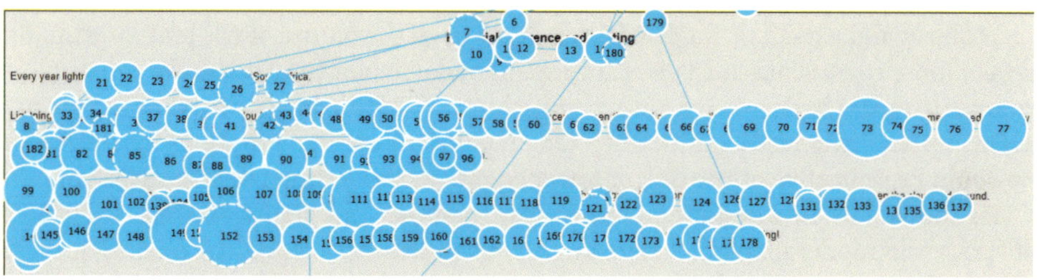

Figure 3.
The gaze plot of one of the 'regular barkers'.

	N	Reading speed (ms per character)	Mean fixation duration (ms)	Regressions (n)	Regression %
Barkers*	23	$\bar{x}$ = 88.9 sd = 29.1	$\bar{x}$ = 296.8 sd = 63.2	$\bar{x}$ = 14.9 sd = 7.8	$\bar{x}$ = 9.0 sd = 3.5
Poor readers	25	$\bar{x}$ = 85.7 sd = 19.6	$\bar{x}$ = 310.9 sd = 42.8	$\bar{x}$ = 17.9 sd = 11.0	$\bar{x}$ = 10.5 sd = 5.3
Moderate readers	19	$\bar{x}$ = 88.1 sd = 33.1	$\bar{x}$ = 309.0 sd = 66.0	$\bar{x}$ = 21.2 sd = 10.8	$\bar{x}$ = 12.3 sd = 5.8
Kruskal-Wallis		$H(2) = 0.3, p > 0.05$	$H(3) = 0, p > 0.05$	$H(3) = 0,$ $p > 0.05$	$H(3) = 0,$ $p > 0.05$
Expected values		Thorough reading 56 ms/c Skimming 26 ms/c Spell checking 62 ms/c Regular reading 45 ms/c	Thorough reading 196 ms Skimming 192 ms Spell checking 221 ms Regular reading 197 ms English L1 200–250 ms Afrikaans L2 300+ ms		English L1 10–15%

Barkers includes jumping and regular barkers due to the nature of these metrics.

Table 3.
A summary of the analysis for the metrics calculated over the whole piece of text for all participants.

together with the range of expected values that could be obtained from previous literature. The ranges were read from graphs that were reported and as such are approximate values which will be used for reference to aid the comparison.

Since the reading speed is measured as milliseconds per characters, higher values actually indicate a slower reading speed in this instance. From the mean values in the table above, it can be seen that the reading speed is slightly lower for the barkers than the readers, but not significantly so. Surprisingly, the poor readers had the fastest speed. Fixation durations are lower for the barkers than the other groups and they have fewer regressions and a lower regression percentage. For English first language silent reading it is accepted that the average fixation is between 200 and 250 ms. When experiencing reading difficulty, fixations will be longer, hence this could be indicative of the nature of the text and the attempt to process and understand the text. However, for these participants, English is not their first language but it is their language of instruction. As such, the fixation durations are closer to what would be expected from a second language reader as evidenced in [45]. Interestingly the barkers had the lowest fixation duration perhaps indicating the lower cognitive processing that was occurring. Regression percentage of the moderate readers is in line with what one would expect of English L1 reading. Given the nature of the text, one might expect more regressions as readers attempt to make sense of the scientific content. Poor readers and barkers have fewer regressions, which is contrary to what is expected when experiencing reading difficulty. Once again, the contrary findings for the barkers could be indicative of the lack or lower cognitive processing which is occurring.

As shown in **Table 4**, barkers have fewer fixations and longer saccades than the poor and moderate readers, although not significantly so. For L2 reading it is expected that saccades will be shorter and there will be more fixations. Skimming exhibits larger saccades while spell checking has shorter saccades. Therefore, the saccadic amplitude is contradictory to previous findings and veers towards skimming behaviour. The fact that regressive saccades were included in the data could account for the larger saccadic amplitude if the regressions were large. However, barkers had fewer saccades and therefore the longer saccades perhaps indicates the tendency not to concentrate on words in order to assimilate them but instead to mimic the behaviour of reading and thus not always to exhibit the saccade amplitude required to process and understand words. The actual nature of the saccades should be investigated in more depth in order to determine whether the cause is large backwards or forwards regressions. What should be kept in consideration is that, on average, the difference is very small and could thus not be on a scale that makes a difference to the number of fixations per word which will be analysed next.

	N	Fixation count (n)	Saccadic amplitude (visual angle)
Regular barkers*	13	$\bar{x}$ = 163.2, sd = 25.0	$\bar{x}$ = 1.9, sd = 0.1
Poor readers	25	$\bar{x}$ = 165.9, sd = 37.1	$\bar{x}$ = 1.8, sd = 0.1
Moderate readers	19	$\bar{x}$ = 175.9, sd = 44.1	$\bar{x}$ = 1.8, sd = 0.1
Kruskal-Wallis		H(2) = 1.2, $p > 0.05$	H(2) = 1.8, $p > 0.05$
Expected values			English L1 7–9 characters

**Due to the nature of the metrics jumping barkers are excluded from this analysis.*

Table 4.
Fixation count and saccadic amplitude over the whole text excluding jumping barkers.

Without a reference to the number of fixations per word it is difficult to determine whether the barkers have fixations similar to any other type of reading. However, it can clearly be seen that, on average, barkers have fewer fixations than the poor and moderate readers which once again could indicate the lack of cognitive processing that is occurring.

In summary, while none of the differences are significant it is noticeable that the behaviour of the barkers mimics that of very good readers (apart from the speed), even giving the impression that they are experiencing less difficulty with the text than the readers.

5.3 First pass reading of text and per word analysis

The mean first fixation duration for all words over the whole text was calculated for each participant as a measurement of a first pass at the text. Furthermore, the average fixation duration, the total fixation duration and fixation count was calculated as a function of the words—that is, each word was treated as a separate AOI and the mean values were calculated as such. This will give an indication of the behaviour on a per word level showing how long, on average, each word required and how many revisits or refixations each word required. The summary of the metrics is given in **Table 5**.

Similar to the fixation duration over the whole text, barkers have the shortest first fixation duration. This metric is indicative of the cognitive processing which is required to process the word on the first pass reading. In this instance, the poor readers required the longest initial processing time which confirms the fact they could be experiencing difficulty on the first pass which is not unexpected. The barkers are clearly not spending more time processing the words. When comparing the first fixation duration to the overall fixation duration, the values for the barkers is very similar, only differing by 4 ms. The poor readers have, on average, first fixations which are approximately 8 ms longer but the moderate readers have lower first fixations than overall fixations. However, when inspecting mean fixation durations per word in the **Table 5**, it is only the barkers who remain unchanged while both the poor and moderate readers have lower mean fixation durations, showing an increase in processing when first encountering the word. The difference between these and the values in the previous section could be attributed to the settings of the AOIs, hence there are some fixations which are outside the bounds of the individual words but within the body of the text.

The number of fixations and visits per word are very similar between the groups indicating that on this level the reading behaviour closely resembles one another (**Table 6**). This confirms that the minor difference in saccadic amplitude

	N	First fixation duration (ms)	Mean fixation duration (ms)	Total fixation duration (ms)	Mean visit duration (ms)
Barkers*	23	$\bar{x}$ = 300.4 sd = 64.7	$\bar{x}$ = 300.4 sd = 61.6	$\bar{x}$ = 495.2 sd = 93.3	$\bar{x}$ = 335.7 sd = 75.4
Poor readers	25	$\bar{x}$ = 318.8 sd = 46.8	$\bar{x}$ = 309.2 sd = 46.2	$\bar{x}$ = 485.2.4 sd = 96.4	$\bar{x}$ = 347.6 sd = 54.4
Moderate readers	19	$\bar{x}$ = 307.9 sd = 74.0	$\bar{x}$ = 306.3 sd = 66.3	$\bar{x}$ = 502.6 sd = 151.9	$\bar{x}$ = 345.3 sd = 77.7
Kruskal-Wallis		$H(2) = 2.8$, $p > 0.05$	$H(2) = 0.7$, $p > 0.05$	$H(2) = 0.3$, $p > 0.05$	$H(2) = 0.7$, $p > 0.05$

**Barkers includes jumping and regular barkers due to the nature of these metrics.*

Table 5.
A summary of the metrics for first pass reading of text.

	N	Fixation count (n)	Visit count (n)
Regular barkers*	13	$\bar{x}$ = 1.6 sd = 0.2	$\bar{x}$ = 1.5 sd = 0.2
Poor readers	25	$\bar{x}$ = 1.6 sd = 0.2	$\bar{x}$ = 1.4 sd = 0.2
Moderate readers	19	$\bar{x}$ = 1.6 sd = .2	$\bar{x}$ = 1.5 sd = 0.2
Kruskal-Wallis		$H(2) = 1.7, p > 0.05$	$H(2) = 1.7, p > 0.05$

**Due to the nature of the metrics jumping barkers are excluded from this analysis.*

Table 6.
The average number of fixations and visits per word excluding the jumping barkers.

is not of the order that barkers fixate on individual words less. The number of fixations is much higher than the average of 1.2, which is used as a measurement of age appropriate difficulty, suggesting that in all instances the participants were perhaps experiencing some difficulty. Of course, the fact that they were reading a scientific text as opposed to a piece of fiction could naturally change their reading behaviour.

5.4 Reading behaviour spread over text (uniformity)

In order to investigate whether the reading behaviour was uniform over the whole text, some metrics were calculated for each line. These metrics were average fixation duration per line, reading speed (milliseconds per character) and mean number of fixations per word.

The metrics were compared for barkers and non-barkers separately as a repeated measure to determine if their behaviour changed significantly as they read the text. A Friedman ANOVA was used for this purpose.

Additionally, some graphs are given in order to illustrate the distribution of behaviour over the text, in some instances the metrics are not analysed statistically.

5.5 Fixation duration

There was a significant difference in the line reading for barkers ($\chi^2 = 23.4$, $p < 0.05$, $p < 0.01$), poor readers ($\chi^2 = 24.8$, $p < 0.05$, $p < 0.01$) but not for moderate readers ($\chi^2 = 0.9$, $p > 0.05$) for the mean fixation duration. For barkers, the significant difference could be attributed to a difference between lines 1 and 2, 4, and 5. For poor readers, line 1 differed significantly from lines 2, 3, 4 and 5.

From the graph below, it can clearly be seen that the mean fixation durations for line 1 are lower than for the other lines from **Figure 4**.

The number of words per line in increasing order is lines 1, 3, 5, 4, 2. Interestingly the fixation duration of the barkers imitates this order in ascending order with the lowest average fixation duration on line 1 and the highest average fixation duration on line 2. This is not true for the poor and moderate readers who have, in ascending order of mean fixation duration, lines 1, 2, 4, 5, 3 and lines 1, 5, 2, 3, 4 respectively. In this respect, it appears the barkers adjust their behaviour according to the length of the line they are currently reading.

In terms of the difficulty, the two longest lines, namely lines 2 and 4 are also the lines which contain the most scientific content and concepts. Line 1 can be considered the easiest as it contains only everyday language and line 3 contains easier words and shorter sentences than lines 2 and 4. Hence in terms of length lines 1 and 3 are the shortest and in terms of difficulty also the easiest while lines

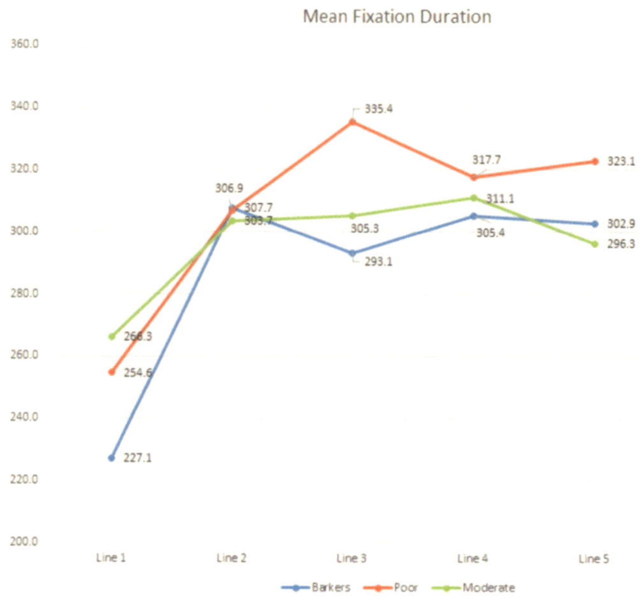

Figure 4.
Mean fixation durations per line for each participant group.

2 and 4 are both the longest and most difficult. Line 5 contains some words which may be unfamiliar to the participants but contains no scientific concepts and can thus be considered to be easier than lines 2 and 4. Therefore, the difficulty of the lines coincidentally mimics the length of the lines. Therefore, further investigation is required in order to determine whether the difficulty of the words in the line impacted the behaviour of the barkers or not.

Figure 5 gives an indication of mean time spent on words in the order the words appeared in the text. The vertical dashed lines indicate the lines of text. Clearly the first line has the lowest fixation durations for all groups but there are clear spikes and dips in the durations for each of the groups. An in-depth analysis of the length and difficulty of the word, together with the surrounding words, or concept, will possibly shed more light on the behaviour difference detected. However, that is beyond the scope of this chapter and will be analysed in a further study.

5.6 First fixation duration

Figure 6 shows the first fixation duration per word, in order of words over the text. From the graph it can be seen that for all groups the first fixation durations fluctuate across the text. The values do not appear to plateau based on the position of the word nor do they hold steady as one might expect for mindless reading. While the patterns are similar in some instances, i.e. all the groups decrease or increase for some words, it can be said that in some other instances there are different patterns where some groups increase and others decrease. Similar to the mean fixation durations, an individual word analysis which may provide more insight into the cause of the reading behaviour is beyond the scope of this chapter. For interest sake, some of the words and their associated behaviour will be discussed in an anecdotal manner, leaving in-depth analysis for a further study. For example, the word "potential" caused an increase in first fixation duration. The word potential preceded the word "difference" as the scientific concept of potential difference was under discussion. However, the word "difference" did not cause an increase in first fixation duration, nor did it have

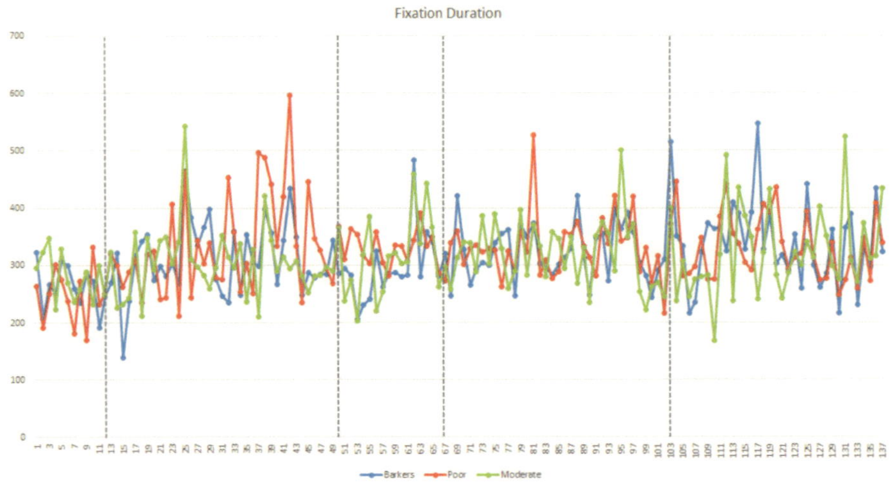

Figure 5.
Mean fixation duration per word, in word order for each participant group.

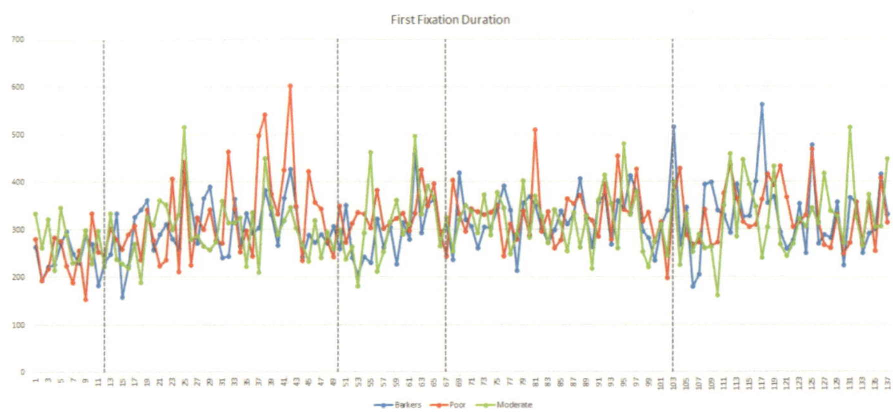

Figure 6.
First fixation duration per word for each participant group.

the same magnitude duration as "potential" suggesting that the participants were perhaps treating the text on a word-by-word basis and not processing concepts created by successive words. The poor readers had much higher instances of first fixation durations for many words in line 2, which was the most difficult line. Furthermore, for poor readers the words "collide" and "crystals" caused the highest and second highest first fixation duration on line 2. These could be considered to be more difficult words, hence the increase in first pass processing for this particular group.

5.7 Total fixation duration

Figure 7 shows the total fixation duration per word in the order the words appeared in the text. Similar to previous per word metrics, these also fluctuate. As one would expect there are some larger spikes on line 2 which was classified as the most difficult line. For example, looking at the larger duration on word number 25, the word is "enormous" and refers to an "enormous electrical field". The word "enormous" might have been a particularly difficult word for the participants. The first fixation duration on this word was also high for all groups. Barkers also had, on average, an increased duration on the word "potential" for the concept "potential difference", as with the first fixation duration. The increase for poor and moderate readers at word number 38 and 39 was caused by the words "ice crystals" at the start of the sentence "ice crystals inside the clouds...".

Comparing this graph to the graph of mean fixation durations for line 1, it appears that the participants spent a longer time in total at the start of the line, perhaps as they were getting into the reading pattern and settling down.

5.8 Reading speed

Reading speed was calculated for each line as milliseconds per character. There was no significant difference between the lines for the barkers (χ^2 = 9.3, p = 0.05) at an alpha-level of 0.05 but it can be considered significant at a level of 0.1. There was a significant difference for the poor readers (χ^2 = 45.9, $p < 0.05$) and moderate readers (χ^2 = 22.3, $p < 0.05$).

Significant differences are plotted in the **Table 7**, where B denotes barker, P denotes poor readers and M denotes moderate readers.

The table clearly shows that for the majority of the cases the same lines account for significant differences in each of the groups. Inspecting **Figure 8** shows that the

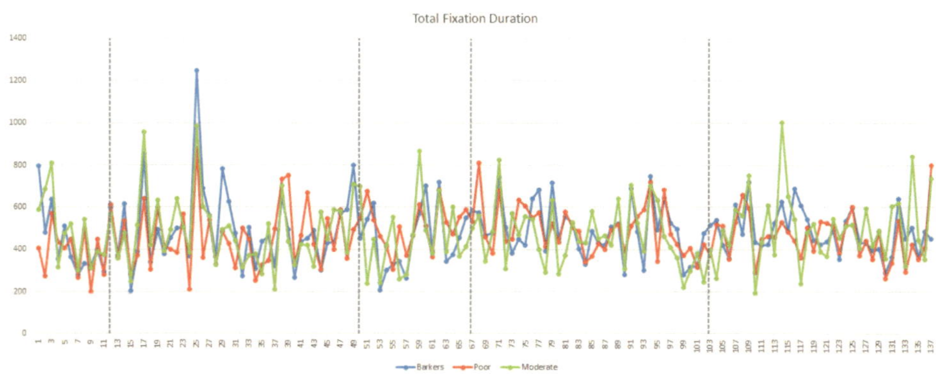

Figure 7.
Total fixation duration per word for each participant group.

	Line 2	Line 3	Line 4	Line 5
Line 1		B		
		P	P	P
		M	M	M
Line 2		B	B	B
		P	P	P
		M	M	M
Line 3			B	
			P	
Line 4				
				P

Table 7.
Summary of significant difference in reading speeds between lines.

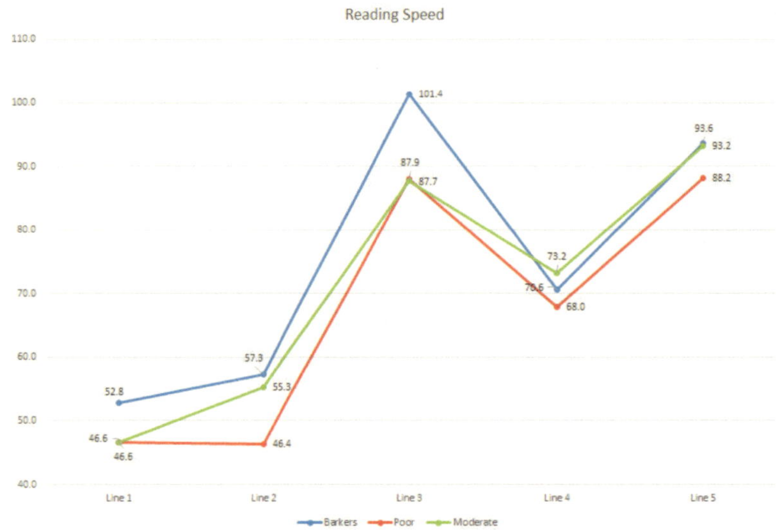

Figure 8.
Reading speed (milliseconds per character) for each line.

reading speed (in milliseconds per character) is significantly faster for lines 1 and 2. Line 3 is the shortest lines in terms of the number of words and it appears that participants slowed down when the line was shorter in this instance which is contrary to what one would expect given the mean fixation durations. Mean fixation durations for the barkers corresponded to the length of the line. Considering this, together with the reading speed, it can be posited that they had many short fixations on line 3.

5.9 Number of fixations

The number of fixations was calculated for each line and then spread over the number of words, hence the measurement is mean number of fixations per word for each line.

There was no significant difference between barkers ($\chi^2 = 3.04$, $p > 0.5$), but there was a significant difference between poor readers ($\chi^2 = 22.0$, $p < 0.05$) and moderate readers ($\chi^2 = 11.8$, $p < 0.05$).

For poor readers, line 1 differed significantly from lines 3, 4, and 5. Line 2 differed significantly from lines 3, 4, and 5 and line 3 differed from lines 4 and 5. For the moderate readers, lines 1 and 2 differed significantly from line 3.

Inspection of **Figure 9** shows that line 3 had the most fixations per word for all groups. This confirms the supposition that barkers on line 3 had many short fixations, accounting for the slower speed. To reiterate, line 3 was the shortest and did not contain any difficult words or concepts and, in particular, the barkers and the poor readers may have realised that the text in line 3 was understandable and hence they tried to read with more comprehension and cognitive processing, thus causing an increase in the number of fixations per word. An increase in cognitive processing also corresponds to the increase in fixation duration for poor readers. However, the same phenomenon is not seen with the barkers, who had lower fixation duration here, hence they seem to be processing the words by fixating on them more with short fixations, perhaps on a per syllable basis or with many refixations in order to understand the text. As mentioned previously, a word-by-word analysis will provide more details on this but is beyond the scope of this chapter.

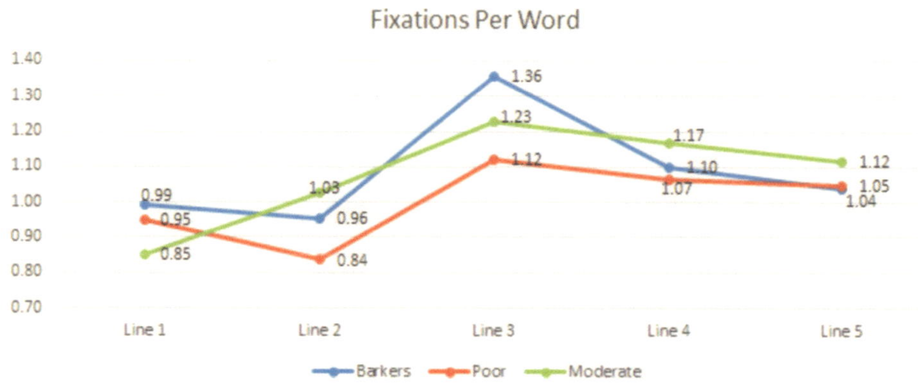

Figure 9.
Fixations per word for each line.

6. Discussion

The following research questions were posed at the start of this chapter.

1. How do the reading eye-movements of those participants who were barking at print compare to those of their peers of two levels of reading proficiency?

2. What are the eye movement characteristics of those participants who were barking at print?

3. How do the eye-movement characteristics of barking at print compare to those published for skimming, scanning and reading for meaning at various levels of proficiency?

The first two research questions will be answered together. There were no significant differences detected between barkers and non-barkers for any of the standard reading metrics. However, barkers do exhibit lower fixation durations, although durations are of a higher magnitude typical of second language reading, fewer regressions, coupled with a lower regression percentage. They also have fewer fixations and longer saccades although only marginally so. During first pass reading, barkers have shorter first fixation durations and shorter visits per word but the number of fixations and visits per word are similar to non-barkers. Barkers tend to adjust their mean fixation durations to the length and/or difficulty of the line currently being read as they read slower on easier and shorter sentences as a result of many short fixations, suggesting either more regressions or more fixations per word on the first pass reading.

In terms of fixation durations for skimming, scanning and thorough reading, barkers have shorter durations such as with skimming. Similarly, the longer saccades and fewer regressions [47] are similar to skimming. An in-depth comparison of these types of reading with our barkers will determine if there are significant differences or not but for now an anecdotal description can be provided. When mind wandering, first fixations and fixations are longer and number of regressions [42] and fixations are lower and the length of the saccades are shorter [43]. Hence, apart from the number of regressions, barking is not comparable to mind wandering on this level.

7. Significance, limitations, further investigation

Although this pioneering research into eye-movements during barking at print may have raised more questions than it has resolved, its significance particularly lies in pointing out that eye movements during barking at print are distinct from kinds of reading which exist in the eye-tracking literature. Findings from research into mindless reading and mind-wandering during reading, which are both associated with decoding with negligible comprehension, differ from the findings presented here in manners which show that comprehension, at least at the word level, for at least some of the words, does indeed affect eye-movement metrics. Except for the 'jumping barkers', eye movement was not found to be erratic in barking at print, whereas eye movement during mind-wandering is. Fixation durations of the barkers were shorter than those of the readers in this study and similar to second language reading, whereas mind-wandering and mindless reading are known to be associated with longer fixation durations than normal reading. Significant variation in eye-movement metrics between the lines of text, during barking at print, suggest changes in cognitive activity in response to textual features. In contrast, mind-wandering (cf. [5, 42, 43]) and mindless reading [15] are both associated with considerable uniformity in these metrics across lines. The low presence of regressions, however, is a point of similarity to both mind-wandering and mindless reading.

This chapter has provided a general description, with tentative metric ranges, for barking at print, at least by learners in this context. However, detection of these metrics does not necessarily diagnose barking, as evidenced by the lack of statistical significance between the barkers and the non-barkers in this sample. Therefore, detection of such metrics should be seen as indicating a high likelihood of barking, rather than as necessary detection of barking, with additional research required to enhance the validity of the diagnosis on the basis of eye-movements. Two limitations in this research are considered to have contributed to this lack of precision: (1) the assumption that regular eye-movement across text, at least for part of the text, indicates a high enough degree of decoding proficiency for a reader to potentially engage in barking at print (recall that in order to bark a reader must be able to decode); (2) the possibility that some of the learners classified as readers may also have been barking at print while reading screen 1, obscuring differences between the groups for the analysis performed here. Barking was deduced from the eye-movement behaviour and comprehension scores obtained as the learners answered questions on screen 2, which had screen 1's text repeated on one half of the screen, allowing the participants to re-read the text. It is possible that participants mitigated barking on screen 1 by undergoing reading with comprehension as they referred back to the text on screen 2, thus being able to answer the questions with reasonable comprehension, and therefore being categorised in one of the two non-barking groups despite their metrics actually displaying barking. This could explain the insignificant difference between the groups. If this is the case, it would mean that barking could be seen as an additional reading gear which at least some people can move into or out of depending on expectations, such as whether the reader realises that he/she is expected to answer questions about the text or not.

Future research could address these limitations by: (1) testing decoding accuracy explicitly using a fluency test while learners read text out loud (2) requiring the participants to answer questions immediately after reading, without being given the opportunity to refer back to the text. The limitation caused by the assumption that decoding proficiency is sufficient for barking to even be a possibility, is reduced by the fact that these were grade 8 and 9 learners reading in the language of learning and teaching (LoLT) which they had been schooled in for at least 5 years, and that the majority had been identified by their teachers as being academically strong.

Therefore, we can claim with considerable confidence that at least those learners who were classified as barking at print were indeed doing so. Our findings about the characteristics of these learners' eye movements during barking are therefore not negated by the possibility that some of the learners classified in other groups were actually also barking in the analysed data. We predict that the methodological changes suggested above would result in the same trends being found between the groups as we have reported here, but that these differences would then be statistically significant. Future research could also explore the variations in eye-movement metrics between the lines and, where appropriate, between the words, of the text, in an attempt to understand the cognitive processing the barkers are undergoing as they bark at print.

8. Conclusion

Given the pivotal role the ability to read with comprehension plays in cognitive development and academic achievement, it is vital that we enhance our understanding of reading difficulties, such as barking at print. This is done with the view of eventually being able to inform application of this knowledge to providing effective interventions. Eye-tracking technology is particularly powerful as a research method since it exposes the otherwise invisible and individual process which readers undergo. It is also a potentially powerful tool for intervention, once a phenomenon is understood sufficiently for valid application. This research has begun the investigation into understanding of a reading difficulty which is highly prevalent among the poor and marginalised, while also being in no way absent from more developed and affluent communities. Once a definitive classification can be proposed for readers in disadvantaged areas in South Africa, diagnostic and intervention programmes can be developed. Learners who are struggling can be evaluated using the diagnostic tools in order to determine whether their reading behaviour could be the reason for poor performance in an academic setting. Once each learner has been classified, the intervention programmes designed for their particular group can be applied. In this way, these learners can be identified and assisted and this could eventually lead to improved performance for these learners.

Author details

Tanya Beelders* and Angela Stott
University of the Free State, Bloemfontein, South Africa

*Address all correspondence to: beelderstr@ufs.ac.za

References

[1] Luckin R, Holmes W, Griffiths M, Forcier LB. Intelligence Unleashed: An Argument for AI in Education. London: Pearson; 2016

[2] Hutt S, Mills C, White S, Donnelly PJ, D'Mello SK. The eyes have it: Gaze-based detection of mind-wandering during learning with an intelligent tutoring system. In: Paper Presented at the 9th International Conference on Educational Data Mining; Raleigh, North Carolina, USA. 2016

[3] Brigham M, Levine E. Eye tracking and prompts for improved learning. In: Bachelor of Science. Worcester, Massachusetts: Worcester Polytechnic Institute; 2012

[4] Najar AS, Mitrovic A, Neshatian K. Utilizing eye tracking to improve learning from examples. In: Paper Presented at the International Conference on Universal Access in Human-Computer Interaction; Heraklion, Crete, Greece. 2014

[5] D'Mello SK, Mills C, Bixler R, Bosch N. Zone out no more: Mitigating mind-wandering during computerized reading. In: Paper Presented at the EDM. 2017

[6] Conati C, Merten C, Amershi S, Muldner K. Using eye-tracking data for high-level user modeling in adaptive interfaces. In: Paper Presented at the Proceedings of the National Conference on Artificial Intelligence. 2007

[7] Jaques N, Conati C, Harley JM, Azevedo R. Predicting affect from gaze data during interaction with an intelligent tutoring system. In: Paper Presented at the 12th International Conference on Intelligent Tutoring Systems; Honolulu, HI, USA. 2014

[8] Howie SJ, Combrinck C, Roux K, Tshele M, Mokoena GM, McLeod Palane N. PIRLS Literacy 2016 Progress in International Reading Literacy Study 2016: South African Children's Reading Literacy Achievement. Pretoria: Centre for Evaluation and Assessment; 2017

[9] Van der Berg S, Spaull N, Wills G, Gustafsson M, Kotzé J. Identifying Binding Constraints in Education. Stellenbosch: Department of Economics, University of Stellenbosch; 2016

[10] Pretorius EJ, Spaull N. Exploring relationships between oral reading fluency and reading comprehension amongst English second language readers in South Africa. Reading and Writing. 2016;**29**(7):1-23

[11] Samuels SJ, Farstrup AE. What Research Has to Say about Reading Instruction. Newark, DE: International Reading Assoc; 2011

[12] Dempster ER. Textual strategies for answering multiple choice questions among South African learners: What can we learn from TIMSS 2003? African Journal of Research in Mathematics, Science and Technology Education. 2007;**11**(1):47-60

[13] Samuels SJ. Reading fluency: Its development and assessment. In: Farstrup AE, Samuels SJ, editors. What Research Has to Say about Reading Instruction. Newark, DE: International Reading Association; 2002. pp. 166-183

[14] Applegate MD, Applegate AJ, Modla VB. "She's my best reader; she just can't comprehend": Studying the relationship between fluency and comprehension. The Reading Teacher. 2009;**62**(6):512-521

[15] Rayner K, Fischer MH. Mindless reading revisited: Eye movements during reading and scanning are

different. Perception & Psychophysics. 1996;**58**(5):734-747

[16] Carver RP. Reading rate: Theory, research, and practical implications. Journal of Reading. 1992;**36**(2):84-95

[17] Just MA, Carpenter PA. A theory of reading: From eye fixations to comprehension. Psychological Review. 1980;**87**(4):329-354

[18] Pikulski JT, Chard DJ. Fluency: Bridge between decoding and reading comprehension. The Reading Teacher. 2005;**58**(6):510-519

[19] Halladay JL. Revisiting key assumptions of the reading level framework. The Reading Teacher. 2012;**66**(1):53-62

[20] Rayner K. Eye movements in reading and information processing: 20 years of research. Psychological Bulletin. 1998;**124**(3):372

[21] Rayner K, Castelhano MS. Eye movements during reading, scene perception, visual search, and while looking at print advertisements. In: Wedel M, Pieters R, editors. Visual Marketing: From Attention to Action. New York: Erlbaum; 2007. pp. 9-42

[22] Morrison RE, Rayner K. Saccade size in reading depends upon character spaces and not visual angle. Perception & Psychophysics. 1981;**30**:395-396

[23] Murray WS, Liversedge SP. Referential context effects on syntactic processing. In: Clifton C, Frazier L, Rayner K, editors. Perspectives on Sentence Processing. Hillsdale, NJ: Erlbaum; 1994. pp. 359-388

[24] Hyrskykari A. Eyes in Attentive Interfaces: Experiences from Creating iDict, a Gaze-Aware Reading Aid. Academic Dissertation, Faculty of Information Sciences of the University of Tampere, Finland. Dissertations in Interactive Technology. 2006:4

[25] Biedert R, Hees J, Dengel A, Buscher G. A robust realtime reading-skimming classifier. In: Proceedings of the Symposium on Eye Tracking Research and Applications. 2012. pp. 123-130

[26] Rayner K. Eye guidance in reading: Fixation locations within words. Perception. 1979;**8**:21-30

[27] McConkie GW, Kerr PW, Reddix MD, Zola D. Eye movement control during reading: I. The location of initial eye fixations on words. In: Technical Report NO. 406, Center for the Study of Reading, University of Illinois. 1987

[28] Duggan GB, Payne SJ. Text skimming: The process and effectiveness of foraging through text under time pressure. Journal of Experimental Psychology: Applied. 2009;**15**(3):228-242. ISSN 1076-898X

[29] Carver RP. Silent reading rates in grade equivalents. Journal of Reading Behavior. 1989;**21**(2):155-166

[30] McConkie GW, Zola D, Grimes J, Kerr PW, Bryant NR, Wolff PM. Children's eye movements during reading. In: Vision and Visual Dyslexia. 1991. p. 13

[31] Rayner K. Understanding eye movements in reading. Scientific Studies of Reading. 1997;**1**(4):317-339. DOI: 10.1207/s1532799xssr0104_2

[32] Dolgunsöz E. Word familiarity effects in EFL reading: An eye tracking study. International Online Journal of Education and Teaching (IOJET). 2018;**5**(2):252-265

[33] Rayner K, McConkie GW. What guides a reader's eye movements? Vision Research. 1976;**16**:829-837

[34] Drieghe D, Brysbaert M, Desmet T, De Baecke C. Word skipping in reading: On the interplay of linguistic and visual factors. European Journal of Cognitive Psychology. 2004;**16**:79-103

[35] Williams R, Morris R. Eye movements, word familiarity, and vocabulary acquisition. European Journal of Cognitive Psychology. 2004;**16**(1-2):312-339. DOI: 10.1080/09541440340000196

[36] Balota DA, Pollatsek A, Rayner K. The interaction of contextual constraints and parafoveal visual information in reading. In: Cognitive Psychology. 1985;**17**(3):364-390

[37] Rayner K, Slattery TJ, Drieghe D, Liversedge SP. Eye movements and word skipping during reading: Effects of word length and predictability. Journal of Experimental Psychology, Human Perception and Performance. 2011;**37**(2):514-528

[38] Dolgunsöz E. Measuring attention in second language reading using eye-tracking: The case of the noticing hypothesis. Journal of Eye Movement Research. 2015;**8**(5):1-18

[39] Raney GE, Campbell SJ, Bovee JC. Using eye movements to evaluate the cognitive processes involved in text comprehension. Journal of Visualized Experiments. 2014;(83):e50780. DOI: 10.3791/50780

[40] Kuperman V, Van Dyke JA. Effects of individual difference in verbal skills on eye-movement patterns during sentence reading. Journal of Memory and Language. 2011;**65**:42-73

[41] Schad DJ, Nuthmann A, Engbert R. Your mind wanders weakly, your mind wanders deeply: Objective measures reveal mindless reading at different levels. Cognition. 2012;**125**(2):179-194

[42] Reichle ED, Reineberg AE, Schooler JW. Eye movements during mindless reading. Psychological Science. 2010;**21**(9):1300-1310

[43] Uzzaman S. The use of eye movements as an objective measure of mind wandering [masters thesis]. University of Toronto; 2010

[44] Cop U, Drieghe D, Duyck W. Eye movement patterns in natural reading: A comparison of monolingual and bilingual reading of a novel. PLoS One. 2015;**10**(8):e0134008

[45] Dednam E, Brown R, Wium D, Blignaut P. The effects of mother tongue and text difficulty on gaze behaviour while reading Afrikaans text. In: Proceedings of SAICSIT 2014. 2014. pp. 334-342

[46] Rayner K. Eye movements and attention in reading, scene perception, and visual search. The Quarterly Journal of Experimental Psychology. 2009;**62**(8):1457-1506

[47] Strukelj A, Niehorster D. One page of text: Eye movements during regular and thorough reading, skimming and spell checking. Journal of Eye Movement Research. 2018;**11**(1):1-22

[48] Sanders TJM, Gernsbacher MA. Accessibility in text and discourse processing. Discourse Processes. 2004;**37**(2):79-89

[49] Kaakinen JK, Hyönä J. Task effects on eye movements during reading. Journal of Experimental Psychology: Learning, Memory, and Cognition. 2010;**36**(6):1561-1566

[50] Flesch R. A new readability yardstick. Journal of Applied Psychology. 1948;**32**(3):221